ORAL HEALTH PROMOTION

Oral Health Promotion

•

LONE SCHOU
Department of Preventive Dentistry
University of Edinburgh

and

ANTHONY S. BLINKHORN
Department of Oral Health
University of Manchester

OXFORD UNIVERSITY PRESS

OXFORD
UNIVERSITY PRESS

Great Clarendon Street, Oxford OX2 6DP

Oxford University Press is a department of the University of Oxford.
It furthers the University's objective of excellence in research, scholarship,
and education by publishing world-wide in

Oxford New York

Auckland Bangkok Buenos Aires Cape Town Chennai
Dar es Salaam Delhi Hong Kong Istanbul Karachi Kolkata
Kuala Lumpur Madrid Melbourne Mexico City Mumbai Nairobi
São Paulo Shanghai Taipei Tokyo Toronto

Oxford is a registered trade mark of Oxford University Press
in the UK and in certain other countries

Published in the United States
by Oxford University Press Inc., New York

ISBN 0-19-262003-7

Printed in Great Britain by

Antony Rowe Ltd., Eastbourne

FOREWORD

Lois K. Cohen
Director, Extramural Program and Assistant Director for International Health, National Institute of Dental Research, Bethesda, MD, USA

Improvements in oral health depend, in large measure, on the appropriate application of preventive disease agents and strategies. These can be effected by the *individual*, by the health care *providers*, by *community* representatives who decide on the priority which should be given to competing preventive strategies, and by *political and other pressure groups* who determine legal and fiscal incentives for or against various parameters influencing health promotion.

Oral Health Promotion is a textbook which is intended to inform us about those methods and programmes required to bring to bear proven strategies for improving health. This is a volume whose time has come, for it places oral health in the context of health promotion; it covers a variety of theoretical constructs which may offer both the practitioner as well as the researcher, and all decision-makers in the field, options for intervening to effect positive personal behavioural change or societal changes which in turn can serve to reinforce and sustain optimal personal oral health behaviours.

One way to examine health outcomes is to systematically review the literature about all the determinants of health, illness, disease, and dysfunction. In reviewing the chapters in this book the reader will be able to understand the full range of these determinants. They encompass the biology of the human organism, lifestyle or individual self-care practices, the system of care delivery, and the more macro influences of the physical, social, and cultural environmental context in which the individual is located. These categories of variables interact and change their configurations as the individual develops and moves from the home, to school, into the workplace, and into old age. All of these variables reflect somewhat different practices and circumstances as they play out in industrialized nations or in the developing world. The challenge for all is to eventually understand how these determinants relate to roles and functions in a systematic plan for oral health promotion. By evaluating such plans and their implementation, feeding the results of effective and efficient strategies toward an even better and refined plan, it will then be possible to generate a variety of ways to achieve optimal oral health.

The practical value of attempting to enhance oral health through oral health promotion interventions, either through individual or large-scale programming, is the driving force of this effort. For oral health care professionals with training in clinical dentistry, in health education, in the behavioural and social sciences, or in public health, I heartily commend this valuable interdisciplinary material.

PREFACE

Dentistry has developed considerably since the beginning of this century, from being merely primarily concerned with pain relief to the development of highly sophisticated treatment for the whole range of oral health problems. A greater understanding of the aetiology and pathology of oral diseases has enabled the dental profession to not only offer a high standard of clinical care but also to diagnose both simple and advanced oral diseases. This improved scientific knowledge about the disease processes has prompted an increased interest in and understanding of the importance of preventing problems rather than placing all the emphasis on clinical intervention. Out of this interest in preventing rather than treating oral disease the discipline of oral health promotion has developed. The main impetus for concentrating on promoting health was the realization that dental diseases as diverse as oral cancer, periodontal disease, and caries are linked to human behaviour. If people adopt the appropriate oral health behaviour then their chances of developing oral health problems are greatly reduced.

Many dental health education programmes have been funded but it has become clear that education alone was not providing an effective solution; people do not change their behaviour just because they are informed about potential health risks. Health education is just one component of the overall process of *health promotion* which encompasses actions to protect or enhance health, including legal, fiscal, educational, and social measures. Health education is, however, a crucial component because individuals, politicians and health professionals need the basic information before other aspects of health can be discussed in a rational way. This book therefore includes advice and information on dental health education but offers a much broader range of options to the reader, in an attempt to introduce the concept of health promotion.

It seemed to the editors of this volume that a presentation on oral health promotion from diverse authors from different countries would be helpful to individuals charged with the task of improving oral health through education and health promotion. To that end 12 chapters on various aspects of health promotion are presented. Chapter 1 examines the historical background of oral health promotion, taking Britain as a role model. All too often we repeat the failures of our predecessors and may even forget the successes! Chapters 2 and 3 consider models and theories of health behaviour and the influence of social factors on oral health promotion. Changing human behaviour is a complex process, and all too often important influences on the way in which patterns of behaviour are shaped and altered are ignored or unidentified. Chapters 4 and 5 broaden the horizons of most professionals working in health promotion. Ignoring government health policy and the people who formulate it is a common mistake and may undermine the effectiveness of a health education campaign. Chapters 6A–6F and 7 review the literature and analyse specific settings and particular problems ranging in scope from establishing national campaigns to promoting oral health in the workplace. Chapter 6F is particularly important as it highlights ways of improving oral health in developing countries, at a time of increasing caries rates. The final chapter seeks to encourage an interest in planning and evaluation, which is essential if health promotion is to gain any academic credibility.

The book has been written primarily for the dental team, but clearly topics have been examined in greater depth than some readers will require. In order to help people to choose the sections they are interested in, the contents list is comprehensive, thereby providing a source of subject-specific references and information.

Other health professionals such as those interested in public health policy may find aspects of the oral health promotion model useful when considering strategies for general health promotion.

The major value of this book is that the authors come from a wide variety of backgrounds and give the reader the opportunity to gain a broad perspective on promoting oral health.

To the knowledge of the editors, no textbook has been published hitherto on this specific discipline of dentistry, and it is therefore possible that we have not included some important subjects and others may not have been covered to the extent that some readers may have wished. Comments would be welcome so that your suggestions could be incorporated into a second edition.

Edinburgh   L. S.
Manchester   A. S. B.
August 1992

CONTENTS

7 Evaluation and planning of oral health promotion programmes

ANTHONY S. BLINKHORN

CONTRIBUTORS

Anthony S. Blinkhorn
Department of Oral Health and Development, University Dental Hospital of Manchester, Higher Cambridge Street, Manchester M15 6FH
Telephone: +4461 275 6610 Fax: +4461 275 6776

Ray Croucher
Department of Dental Public Health, The London Hospital Medical College, Turner Street, London E1 2AD
Telephone: +4471 377 7632 Fax: +4471 377 7677

Murray Dickson
International Projects Unit, College of Dentistry, University of Saskatchewan, Saskatoon, Saskatchewan, Canada S7N 0W0
Telephone: +306 966 5108 Fax: +306 966 5126

Martin C. Downer
Department of Dental Health Policy, Institute of Dental Surgery, Eastman Dental Hospital, 256 Gray's Inn Road, London WC1X 8LD
Telephone: +4471 915 1192 Fax: +4471 915 1233

Helen C. Gift
Department of Health and Human Services, Public Health Service, National Institutes of Health, Bethesda, Maryland 20892
Telephone: +301 496 2883 Fax: +301 480 6648

Eino Honkala
Department of Preventive Dentistry and Cariology, Faculty of Dentistry, University of Kuopio, POB 6, 70211 Kuopio, Finland
Telephone: +358 71 162211 Fax: +358 71 162213

H. Asuman Kiyak
University of Washington, School of Dentistry and Department of Psychology, Seattle, Washington 98195
Telephone: +206 543 5197 Fax: +206 685 7222

Susan Reisine
The University of Connecticut Health Center, School of Dental Medicine, Farmington, Connecticut 06032
Telephone: +203 679 3823 Fax: 203 679 1342

Lone Schou
Department of Preventive Dentistry, 1 Surgeon's Square, High School Yards, Edinburgh EH1 1LZ
Telephone: +4431 650 2457 Fax: +4431 650 2502

Anne Johanne Søgaard
University of Tromsø, Institute of Community Medicine, Breivika, 9037 Tromsø, Norway
Telephone: +47 83 44 816 Fax: +47 83 44 831

Elizabeth M. L. Towner
Department of Child Health, Medical School, Framlington Place, Newcastle upon Tyne NE2 4HH
Telephone: +4491 222 7131 Fax: +4491 222 6222

Clive Wright
The University of Melbourne, Faculty of Medicine, Dentistry and Health Sciences, School of Dental Science, 711 Elizabeth Street, Melbourne 3000, Australia
Telephone: +61 3 341 0275 Fax: +61 3 341 0339

1

The history of dental health education: a case study of Britain

ELIZABETH M. L. TOWNER

Introduction

An understanding of the history of dental health education in any one country or area comes from an appreciation of the interplay of the particular social, political, economic, and technological forces over a period of time. Britain has been selected to illustrate this history because there is a particularly rich variety of primary and secondary source material which can be drawn upon in order to explore these various themes. Some of the primary sources include contemporary books, journals, and other literature, annual reports of local school medical officers and the Chief Medical Officer, government reports, and company records.

The evolution of dental health education can be seen from two main perspectives. The first is the professional, doctor/dentist version of history which illuminates 'the internal history of the profession' or describes 'the discovery or development of technical medical procedures' and which has a strongly biographical emphasis on 'the lives of the "great men" of medicine' (Berridge 1990). In contrast, the second perspective is that of the social historian where, 'developments can be most fully understood only when considered in relation to the network of social interaction' (Rosen 1951). Dental health education combines the scientific messages of the profession with the need to communicate those messages to the public. The social context is thus of considerable importance and the second approach, that of the social historian, is adopted for this review.

The review traces the history of dental health education in Britain in six main time periods: the period prior to professional responsibility for public dental health (before 1870), the period of growing responsibility (1870–1906), the early period of the School Medical Service (1906–1920), the period of mass dental health propaganda (1920–1939), the Second World War and early post-war period (1939–1956), and ending with the period of evaluation and accountability (1956 until the present day). Within each time period an attempt is made to set the scene of the social, economic, political, and technological conditions of the time. The contributions made by the state in the form of Health and Education Acts, by the dental profession, and by other agencies are examined to see how these can aid the understanding of the development of dental health education. Although this review is concerned specifically with Britain, it is hoped that the underlying themes identified will have relevance to developments elsewhere.

The period prior to professional responsibility for public dental health education (before 1870)

Health depends on a complex interaction between the environment, the genetic constitution of the individual, and individual and group behaviour. During the eighteenth century significant advances in recognizing the role of the environment in health emerged in Britain. The scientific revolution of the seventeenth century heralded the 'Age of Reason' and thirst for enquiry. During the eighteenth century there was a series of investigations into living conditions, stemming from the defence needs for a healthy army and navy (Acheson and Hagard 1984). The revelations of investigations of slum conditions and overcrowding for other groups of the population were not, however, considered appropriate areas for central government action and action was left to local initiatives (Berridge 1990).

In the nineteenth century a more interventionist role was adopted. Early in the century the effects of the interrelated agricultural and industrial revolutions created new social, physical, and economical conditions. The population grew rapidly from 9 million in 1781 to 20 million in 1851. Rapid and uncontrolled growth took place in towns and problems such as poor housing, overcrowded living conditions, and primitive methods of supplying water and disposing of sewage and waste became apparent. Conditions in rural areas were also bad (Walker 1979). The experience of infectious disease, such as cholera epidemics, brought the problems into public focus (Acheson and Hagard 1984). Reforms became both necessary and urgent and the Government was forced to take some responsibility for the nation's health.

In 1837 William Farr, a medical statistician, was appointed to estimate the extent of disease; his analysis of mortality figures established the close connection between living conditions and ill health (Davies 1983). Between 1839 and 1843 Edwin Chawick and Dr Southwood Smith instigated inquiries into the living conditions of the poor and in 1842 the *General report on the sanitary conditions of the labouring population of Great Britain* was published. This was followed by reports of Royal Commissions in 1844 and 1845. This evidence resulted in the setting up in 1848 of a General Board of Health which encouraged health districts to take up measures against insanitary conditions.

The development of public health in the nineteenth century was slow, with local bodies gradually assuming the responsibility for the health of local communities. This depended partly on political will but also on technology; the knowledge and experience of sanitary engineers and mass production methods of making drainage pipes were not available in the early nineteenth century (Walker 1979). Legislation and administration played an important role in the public's health; education and propaganda a relatively minor one. How does preventive dentistry and dental health education fit into the picture outlined above?

Until the end of the nineteenth century, there was no dental health education in the formal sense of planned or programmed efforts to bring about the promotion or continuation of health. Instead there was the scattered provision of informal dental health education by individual practitioners to their patients and in addition the written and oral traditions of transmitting information from an individual to a group or from person to person.

At times no specific objectives were apparent for dental health advice given, at other times the motives were more obvious: the prevention of bad breath, the promotion of the beauty of the teeth, and the prevention of tooth decay or gum disease (or a combination of these) can be traced in the dental health messages. The advice was most frequently connected with oral cleanliness; advice concerned with diet or dental visiting was less frequent.

The first book to be written in English on dental matters was Charles Allen's *The operator for the teeth*, published in 1685 and intended for the general public (Hillam 1990). In Menzies Campbell's *Dental bibliography*, Allen's was the only book on dental matters published in English in the seventeenth century but from then on books on dental advice grew in number and by the 1820s 34 books are listed, 15 of which were connected with practical advice on the prevention of dental disease (Menzies Campbell 1949). Examples of the books produced include Imrie's *Parents' dental guide* (Imrie 1834) and Saunders's *Advice on the care of the teeth*, which is reputed to have sold 11 000 copies in Britain (Saunders 1837). Although circulation of dental manuals was wide it was restricted to the middle and upper classes.

Much of the dental health advice in the oral tradition has been lost, but occasionally some evidence of it is available. The speeches delivered in market places by itinerant medical and dental practitioners were collected in the *Haranges, or speeches of several celebrated quack doctors* of 1745. This also included the songs of the accompanying jesters whose duty it was to attract a crowd and there were numerous references to the results of dental neglect (Menzies Campbell 1958). This would be one of the few instances where dental health advice was available for poorer members of society.

The nineteenth century was the time when the greatest increase in annual sugar consumption took place, rising from 20 pounds per person in 1830 to

60 pounds in 1880 (Hardwick 1960). Sugar was no longer a luxury item consumed by the wealthy and tooth decay was no longer an affliction solely of the wealthy. There would have been greater disease experience than in previous times but little preventive treatment and little or no advice on tooth-care for the vast majority of the population.

The period of growing professional responsibility for public dental health education (1870–1906)

In the years following the widening of the franchise (male urban workers obtained the vote in 1867 and male rural workers in 1884), public health, housing, and education all became issues of political importance. (Fraser 1984).

By the 1870s the great sanitary movement, initiated by Edwin Chadwick and others, was well under way. The State's responsibility for public health measures had been accepted and the 1875 Public Health Act set up a central government health department and established national minimum standards of hygiene (DHSS 1976; Davies 1983). Several Acts of Parliament sought to improve the housing of the working classes (Fraser 1984). The 1870 Education Act established in principle the right of every child to some form of schooling, and by 1891 education had become compulsory and free (Davies 1983; Walker 1979). At the same time as the State was beginning to extend its responsibility over some areas of health and welfare, there was still a firmly entrenched tradition of philanthropy (Fraser 1984).

The level of poverty which remained at the turn of the century was still very high. The social researches of Charles Booth in London and Seebohm Rowntree in York began to reveal and to quantify how deep was the deprivation and poverty which undermined the health of the people. Rowntree found that nearly 30 percent of York's population lived in poverty and were ill housed, ill clothed, and underfed (Rowntree 1901).

The reports of Booth and Rowntree caused some disquiet among those who worked among the poor and in public health departments. Greater public awareness of the poor health of the nation was stimulated by the evidence given by the Director-General of the Army Medical Services and the Inspectors-General of Recruiting which indicated that more than 40 percent of all recruits examined in the period 1901–2 were unfit for army service (Sutherland 1979). There was public alarm that the nation was undergoing a period of physical deterioration and debate on whether this was a biological phenomenon or the result of environmental factors which could be remedied (Pirrie and Dalzall-Ward 1962). Three highly critical authoritative reports (Royal Commission 1903; Interdepartmental Committee 1904; Interdepartmental Committee 1905) were published in the early years of the century. Following these, the government decided that a School Medical Service should be organized (DES 1975).

In the years between the 1870 Education Act and the 1907 Education Act when the School Medical Service was introduced, the concept of the school helping to promote health started to become apparent and arising from this the beginning of organized health education (Francis 1975). By 1905 school doctors had been appointed by 85 local education authorities and medical inspection of school children was being carried out in 48 areas (DES 1975). Some medical officers, like James Kerr, who was appointed medical officer of the London School Board in 1902, were particularly interested in the contribution that medicine might make to teaching (Francis 1975).

How did dental health education fit into this pattern of growing awareness of the health problems of the nation and increasing State responsibility for health and welfare? The Dentists' Act of 1878 set up a register of qualified and experienced practitioners and two years later the British Dental Association (BDA) was formed. The Dentists' Act helped to stimulate the growth in the profession's corporate responsibility to the dental health of the public as a whole, rather than solely to individual patients (Richards 1975; Fox and Maddick 1980).

One of the pioneers of the movement for a wider dissemination of dental health knowledge was William McPherson Fisher. In 1885, at the BDA Annual Conference, he urged: 'the necessity of compulsory attention to the teeth of school children' (Fisher 1885). He wanted dental health instruction to be given to children by dentists or teachers and in addition wanted the provision of cheap literature on teeth, 'to come within reach of the masses of the people, which at present does not exist' (Fisher 1885).

The extent of the problem of disease and the lack of public knowledge became apparent over the next few years. In 1886 the British Journal of Dental Science commented on the, 'ignorance concerning all dental matters among the public' (BJDS 1886). In 1890 the British Dental Association set up a committee to establish 'a system of instruction for the young of all classes'. Between 1891 and 1898 seven epidemiological reports conducted for the BDA painted a bleak picture of children's dental conditions (Interdepartmental Committee 1905). Once the problems had been highlighted in epidemiological reports, several Public and Poor Law schools appointed dental officers (Pickering 1900; BDA 1930).

The School Dentists' Society, inaugurated in 1898, emphasized hygiene and prevention and published the first available dental health education materials. These were a set of three wall charts on rollers, a set of lantern slides, and booklets on the care of teeth (Taylor 1977). The School Dentists' Society made pleas to lobby the National Union of Teachers at their annual conference to 'interest them in dental hygiene' and to get the subject included in the teachers' training (Rushton 1903). The Society also overcame the stumbling block of the lack of cheap toothbrushes by having toothbrushes made which could be offered to schools (Fox and Maddick 1980).

The recruiting statistics both before and during the Boer War highlighted not only the poor general health of potential recruits, but also their poor dental health. Newsholme (1903) had examined the rejections for the British Army over the previous 60–70 years and concluded that the figures indicated:

the importance of dental caries from a military standpoint, and the need for national action in the prevention of disease in the interest of an efficient Army as well as in the interest of public health.

He recommended three measures to combat the problem: compulsory teaching of hygiene in the senior classes of all elementary schools; the organization of daily cleaning of teeth in all residential schools; and the employment of a dentist by all school authorities.

Pedley was also concerned about the army recruiting figures in relation to dental disease, but he pointed out that in addition, dental disease could have economic and social consequences in other spheres of life. In 1899, 458 girls from parochial schools in the metropolis alone, entered domestic service in one year, and Pedley (1899?) observed:

The trouble of a domestic servant suffering from neglected teeth need little imagination to picture, but disordered digestion, irritability of temper and inability to perform the allotted duties are some of the most obvious results which may appeal to employees.

The call for a wider dissemination of knowledge relating to the prevention of dental disease came initially from a few committed individuals. Epidemiological data revealed the extent of the problem among school children to members of the dental profession but wider public awareness of the problem was heightened by Boer War recruiting statistics. Humanitarianism, coupled with military and economic necessity, all thus played a part in developing the dental profession's awareness of the need to educate the public in matters of dental health.

The early period of the School Medical Service (1906–1920)

The period from 1906 to the beginning of the 1920s was a time when the State became increasingly involved in the provision of health and welfare services. The period can be divided into two phases. The first is the period from 1906 to 1914 when the Liberal Government introduced a number of reforms. The second is the First World War, which had a profound impact on British society both during the war and its aftermath.

In 1906 a Liberal Government was elected with a large majority. With a group of 53 Labour members in the new Parliament, the Liberal Party needed to show that it was a party of concern and conscience which could legislate in the interests of the poor. The report of the Interdepartmental Committee on Physical Deterioration in 1904 urged that both medical inspection and feeding should be undertaken within the State educational system. In December 1906 the Education (Provision of Meals) Act was passed, which empowered Local

Authorities to feed necessitous school children. This was followed in 1907 by the Education (Administrative Provisions) Act, which established a medical department within the Board of Education to supervise a school medical service (Fraser 1984).

The First World War had an even greater impact on social policy. The pressures of war, with the need to mobilize the country's resources, led the Government to enact policies undreamt of before the war. The First World War, even more than the Boer War, exposed through deficient recruits the low physical condition of the British people. This strengthened the hand of the health reformers in their drive to create a Ministry of Health to unite the health services which were operating under different agencies (Fraser 1984). In 1919 a Ministry of Health was created, whose policy for the future included child health services, school medical services, sanitation in the community, industrial health, and the promotion of health education (Davies 1983). When the war ended there was a commitment to social reconstruction and a reaffirmation of the rights of a rising generation to health (Webster 1983).

The School Medical Service can be seen in the context of one of a number of social measures that were introduced before the First World War. The School Medical Service had initially been intended to be a preventive service, but disease was so prevalent in the early days of the school service that it was necessary to provide a treatment service (DES 1977). Similarly, the early pioneers of the school dental service were offering essentially unpleasant, even painful treatment to a population of children who were suffering from extensive dental disease but who had not received any dental care. John Knowles, the school dentist at Bradford, in his examination of 8657 children in 1910, found only six fillings (DES 1975).

Some of the early pioneers were interested not only in the establishment of school clinics but also in prevention and dental health education. George Cunningham was one of these pioneers. He established a school dental clinic in Cambridge before the 1907 Education Act was passed. It was subsequently taken over by the borough and became the first clinic of the new dental service (Davis 1969). As well as providing for treatment and inspection, oral hygiene instruction and dental health education played a large part in the clinic's programme. Cunningham saw two tasks for dental health education: firstly rousing the mass of the population to awareness of the need and desirability of good dental care, and secondly the instruction of the individual at the chairside. He founded the Children's Dental League : his methods were not to preach but to make dental health revelant and fun (Davis 1969).

In about 1909 toothbrush clubs began to be mentioned in reports (CMO 1910). Charles Wallis, for example, introduced the idea of toothbrush clubs to a number of day schools in London (Gelbier and Randall 1982). Teachers were involved in the scheme and in infant schools, the process of teeth cleaning in 'dumb show' was suggested as part of the children's daily drill. Lantern lectures on the care of the teeth given during school hours or immediately afterwards and compositions by children on the subject of the dental lectures all contributed to an incipient project approach (Wallis 1912?).

With the formation of toothbrush clubs, the idea of toothbrushing was being introduced to many children. At Shepparton Road LCC school a tooth-brush club had been introduced (Wallis 1912?) and 'through the personal exertions of the headmistress' positive results were noticed. When 290 girls were examined, 227 were found to have given the necessary attention to their teeth (BDA 1909). There are, however, no records of how many toothbrush clubs were formed in schools or how rapidly they spread.

In the early years of the twentieth century some workplaces also had prog-rammes of dental health education programmes for their employees. Messrs Cadbury Limited had a programme as part of its industrial dental clinic: 'Care of the teeth' charts were hung in lavatories, lectures given, and articles on dental subjects written for the works magazine. Workers under sixteen were supplied with free toothbrushes and powder and Cadbury's also supplied these to all local school children (Gelbier 1986).

The causes of tooth decay were beginning to be understood by the end of the nineteenth century with Miller's demonstration that bacteria in the mouth were responsible (Naylor 1980), but the work did not provide readily acces-sible dental health messages. Miller considered starches more harmful to teeth than sugar but Wallace later argued that sugars were more harmful (Wallace 1909).

By the end of the period there was still no widespread campaign although Watson in 1911 had called for an educational campaign with a central committee composed of 'the ablest of men' to direct it and targeted at teachers, the authorities, and the public (Watson 1911). Evidence collected from dental practitioners by the Committee of 1917–19 (whose recommendations were adopted in the Dentists' Act 1921), was unanimous 'as to the failure of the population to regard dental disease and its effect on health as in any way a serious matter'. Educational propaganda was required that could be distri-buted through agencies such as health visitors, school agencies, welfare super-visors, insurance societies, medical practitioners, the public health service, and the press (GMC 1944?).

The period of mass dental health propaganda (1920–1939)

Following a brief post-war boom, there was a sharp increase in unemploy-ment which came to dominate the inter-war years. From the end of 1920 to the summer of 1940 unemployment was never below one million and at times was over three million. Some areas such as south Wales, central Scotland, Lancashire, and north east England bore the brunt of the depres-sion while in London and the south east consumer and service industries were expanding.

In the years following the First World War the government was appre-
hensive about revolution and the spread of 'Bolshevism' and an ambitious
social policy was advocated by some, including Lloyd George, as a means of
creating social unity. In this strategy, housing occupied a critical position
(Fraser 1984). Despite the building of about a million homes for the working
classes during the inter-war period, the vast majority of the lower social
classes were still equipped with inadequate washing facilities. Shared lavatories and external water supplies were still common at the outbreak of the
Second World War (Webster 1983).

Conditions in some schools and houses meant that it was still not always
possible to practise toothbrushing. In some schools there were no supplies of
soap, water, or towels available (Kerr 1926). In the depressed homes of the
1920s and 1930s the toothbrush was still a luxury to the low paid or the
unemployed. Woolworths began, however, to retail brushes at 6 d, and many
more people were introduced to the habit of cleaning (Beaver 1980). The
availability of large quantities of toothbrushes at low prices and the fact that
they could be obtained at an outlet other than chemist shops, which were
mainly patronized by upper and middle classes, were both ways in which
commercial developments furthered the aims of dental health education (Fox
and Maddick 1980).

Concern over the health of children growing up between the wars was
prompted by an appreciation of their importance as the future labour force
and foundation of the national defence (Webster 1983).

In 1927 the Central Council for Health Education was set up by the Society
of Medical Officers of Health. It was funded by local authorities and voluntary
bodies and had the aims of promoting and encouraging education and
research in 'the science and art of healthy living' and assisting and coor-
dinating the work of all statutory bodies (Sutherland 1979). The first ten years
of the Council was the era of propaganda. 'Health education was realised
mainly in terms of mass publicity on all fronts' (HEJ 1953). Soon after the
Central Council had been set up, the Board of Education issued in 1928 a
Handbook of suggestions on health education for teachers in public elementary
schools. In content the book was little advanced since Chadwick's time with
the main effort being 'against filth' (Sutherland 1979).

Dental health education, in a similar way to health education, experienced
an era of mass propaganda in the inter-war period. Prior to 1923, no attempt
on a large scale had been made to educate the public in dental health, 'chiefly
because there was no body that was specially interested and had sufficient
funds at its disposal to carry out such education' (Rowlett 1930). During the
1920s and 1930s two bodies, the Dental Board of the United Kingdom and
the Ivory Castle League, funded by Messrs D. and W. Gibbs Limited provided
dental health propaganda materials on a nationwide scale.

The Dental Board of the United Kingdom had been established by the
Dentists' Act of 1921 to administer the affairs of the dental profession. In

1923 within the Board a Dental Health Propaganda Committee was formed; a year later its title was amended to the Dental Health Education Committee (Guy 1928). With an annual budget of £4000 the Board carried out an ambitious programme of propaganda, providing a great variety of leaflets, posters, exhibits, and films. A team of six lecturers was financed to tour the country speaking at Women's Institutes, miners' groups, factories, and so on. Full use was made of modern technology: wireless broadcasts were recorded and the Chairman of the Board, Sir Francis Dyke Acland, made a gramophone record entitled *The care of the teeth*. The Committee believed that advantage should be taken from time to time of 'any novel forms of advertisement likely to strike the public eyes'. To this end, a contract was made for the imprint on railway tickets issued by the London Midland and Scottish Railway of 'Maxims of dental health' (GMC 1944?). Posters were produced for use on the London Underground, on buses and trams, and displays of 'a series of large paintings conveying lessons on dental health' were provided for use on prominent sites in important railway stations (GMC 1944?).

The scale of the Board's propaganda activities can be demonstrated by two examples. In 1926 a book for teachers entitled *Hygiene of the mouth and teeth* was published (Dental Board of the United Kingdom 1926) and sent free of charge to all head teachers in public elementary and secondary schools in the British Isles; by 1928 31 000 copies had been distributed. In the second half of 1926 alone, over 1000 lectures on the care of teeth were given (GMC 1944?).

Records do not show whether there was any collaboration between the Dental Boards and Gibbs (Fox and Maddick 1978). Messrs D. and L. W. Gibbs & Co provided the other major source of dental health propaganda during this period, the Ivory Castle League. This represented the first major contribution by a commercial agency to dental health education. Before this Colgate had produced booklets for children and Beecham's promoted toothpaste, as well as pills, in the Beecham's Music Portfolio songbook of 1986 (Fox and Maddick 1980).

The Ivory Castle League was set up by Gibbs in 1923. The League gave 'material assistance to Teachers, Nurses, Superintendents of Clinics and Welfare Centres in their efforts to make mouth hygiene attractive to their proteges' (Ivory Castles 1927). Teachers were enrolled as members of the League and then encouraged their pupils to become 'Crusaders' to defend the 'Ivory Castles' of their teeth. Information was disseminated to teachers by means of a journal *Ivory castles* (Ivory Castles 1925–1932)and the materials available included readers, leaflets, posters, dental hygiene charts, and two films *A flight into fairyland* and *The ivory castle*. Toothbrush clubs were formed in schools throughout the country and photographs depicting them appeared in the magazine *Ivory castles* during the 1920s and 1930s. By 1932 the League had over 100 000 crusader members (Thornhill 1932).

There is a considerable amount of information from the inter-war period relating to the 'providers' of dental health education materials, namely the

Dental Board and the Ivory Castle League. What is more difficult to obtain is information relating to the 'users' of the materials. The widespread nature of the propaganda materials available may have been influential in modifying attitudes to dental cleanliness and the Gibbs scheme of supplying toothbrushes may have made the habit of toothbrushing more widespread, but there are no statistics available to support these contentions.

The most easily accessible sources of information relating to schools are the annual reports of the Chief Medical Officer of the Board of Education for Britain as a whole or for individual local education authorities. In some cases reports from individual schools are provided, such as this one from Miss Gertrude West, headmistress of an infant school in West Bromwich who described what was done in her school in connection with dental hygiene in 1932 (CMO 1933).

We began to equip the lowest (entrant) Nursery class for the exercise of Dental Hygiene in school ... and the exercise became in the lowest class a daily lesson.

Two years later, 'all eight classes were practising Dental Hygiene as a time-table lesson' (CMO 1933). This report suggests that a programme of oral hygiene had been in progress for about four years but there is no indication who initiated the scheme and whether any of the propaganda materials provided by the Dental Board or Gibbs were used. Further research into the records of other local education authorities would provide useful evidence of what occurred in schools in relation to dental health education.

Although much of the dental health education was directed at schools, some health departments were also concerned with other target groups (Connan and Smith 1925).

The health of the worker is an asset obvious both to himself and his employer ... in the Borough of Bermondsey employers take a very considerable interest in the health of their workers and our propaganda department has been approached with a view to giving 'dinner time' talks to the employees of various firms.

During the 1920s and 1930s the influential researches of Lady Mellanby began to distract attention from the oral environment. In particular she considered diet at the antenatal stage to be of primary importance (CMO 1934). Webster (1983) maintains that due to her influence:

The focus was therefore shifted from active care of the teeth of the child to the dietary supplementation of the mothers — itself beneficial to maternal health, but irrelevant to the dental condition of the progeny.

For the first time, during the inter-war period national campaigns of dental health education were launched in Britain. Vast quantities of materials were produced and circulated, many methods were tried, and a variety of target groups selected. Unfortunately no evaluation was conducted on the impact of the campaigns. The propaganda was directed primarily at improving dental hygiene and visiting the dentist, rather than at diet. Other developments during this period could simultaneously have assisted more widespread general and dental cleanliness, such as improvements in washing facilities in houses and wider availability of toothbrushes. It is not possible to isolate the impact of the mass propaganda on dental health attitudes and behaviour.

The Second World War and early post-war period (1939–1956)

The Second World War generated the political and social determination to overcome enormous difficulties and in its wake the spirit and practice of universalism affected the course of post-war social policy. The Second World War to an even greater extent than the First, was dependent on the efforts and support of the whole population, not just the military prowess of a professional army. The State was forced to adopt new and powerful policies; food shortages necessitated rationing, fears of inflation produced food subsidies, needs of production brought about direction of labour, and bombing of cities led to evacuation (Fraser 1984).

Two factors in particular transformed social attitudes towards health: these were evacuation and rationing. The 'official' picture of child health built up by the reports of the Board of Education and its ancillaries during the inter-war period was challenged by the evacuation, when the deprived children from the industrial cities came into contact with the better off (Webster 1983). Evacuation was part of the process by which 'British Society came to know itself' (Fraser 1984). The requirements of an overall food policy brought school meals and milk into greater prominence than before the war. In 1940 one child in 30 ate meals at school; by 1945 there had been a tenfold increase, and one child in three did so (Fraser 1984).

From a very early stage during the war, thoughts turned to post-war reconstruction. The Beveridge Report, published in December 1942, attacked the 'Five Giants of Want, Disease, Ignorance, Squalor and Idleness' (Fraser 1984). An essential part of the scheme was the introduction in 1945 of Family Allowances and in 1948 of a comprehensive National Health Service, in which a full medical service was made available to all the people in the country, without any payment at time of need, but financed by an insurance scheme (Davies 1983). The 1944 Education Act introduced by R. A. Butler created the office of Minister of Education and the duty of providing a national educational system.

In the field of general health education, the war created a tremendous sense of urgency, and the Central Council for Health Education stepped up its propaganda campaigns. The Council initiated the publication of a quarterly Health Education Journal in 1943 with the aim of increasing awareness of the part health could play in 'bettering the physical and mental health of the community' (CCHE 1946).

After the war the Central Council became more concerned with the training of professional health and education workers and less with direct programmes for the general public. Didactic methods of health education teaching were beginning to be questioned and methods less based on mass publicity and more on a personal basis were beginning to be introduced, as were some of the ideas developed during the war by the Army Bureau of Current Affairs (HEJ 1953).

During the war a high standard of dental care was available to members of all three services. This meant that for the first time dental treatment was available to a substantial section of the young adult population (Norman 1981). At the same time the school dental service was experiencing problems: the evacuation of large numbers of school children changed the pattern of demand, and the recruitment of school dental officers for service changed the provision of the service. Local education authorities were advised on how to make best use of their depleted staff. Rationing, however, produced a reduction in the incidence in dental caries (DES 1975).

During the war the propaganda activities of both the Dental Board of the United Kingdom and the Ivory Castle League were curtailed, so in contrast to general health education, dental health education was severely restricted. The Dental Board's income was reduced during the war years and allocation for dental health education was reduced from an average of £4000 per annum before the war to only £200 per annum in 1941 and the same in 1942 (GMC 1944?).

With the Government's increasing commitment to funding health and education, members of the Dental Board began to feel that it was inappropriate for an independent body to fund dental health education with fees paid by the dental profession. This function, it was felt, would be more properly carried out with Government funding on a national scale (GDC 1957). The Central Council of Health Education had a dental representative, but before the war appeared to have produced only one dental poster and was committed to other programmes of work (Fox and Maddick 1978). The Dental Board decided to continue producing some material in limited quantities to serve as an example. In particular, primary schoolchildren and their parents were selected as the group to target (GDC 1957).

In 1952 the Oral Hygiene Service was set up. In this year the first link between the dental profession and a commercial agency occurred when the profession approached Gibbs to make a film on dental health to open a FDI congress at the South Bank in London (OHS 1954). The Oral Hygiene Service was funded by Gibbs as an independent organization. It began to produce a range of non-branded materials including posters, leaflets, and films and to maintain good contact with the press (OHS 1955). The director of the service, Colin Davis, pioneered a number of imaginative approaches to dental health education, which did not rely on fear or didactic teaching methods (Fox and Maddick 1980).

In 1954 the British Dental Association investigated the position of dental health education in Britain and in conclusion urged the Ministry of Health to undertake 'a vigorous and continuous campaign of dental health education' (BDA 1954).

The period of evaluation and accountability in dental health education (1956–)

The general philosophy of social welfare flourished in the climate of growing affluence, full employment, and consensus politics of the 1950s and 1960s. Some challenge to the welfare consensus was apparent in the 1960s; by the 1970s the welfare ideal appeared to be in decline and this was further emphasized by the monetarist policies pursued by the governments of both the United Kingdom and the United States of America in the 1980s (Fraser 1984).

In the 1960s the challenges to the welfare consensus came from opposite ends of the political spectrum. On the left, the Welfare State was attacked for not achieving its goals on the abolition of poverty and the reduction of wealth. On the right, the monetarist view was that the Welfare State reduced freedom of choice and that services such as education or housing were more efficiently distributed by market forces than by welfare (Fraser 1984). The consensus of social democracy which had protected the Welfare State for a quarter of a century began to wither during the 1970s and 1980s and a policy of retrenchment persisted no matter which party was in power (Fraser 1984).

The first government report to stress the importance of health education was the Jameson Report of 1956 (Ministry of Health 1956). Sutherland (1979) considers that from this date a collective movement, no longer relying on the enthusiasm of individuals, can be traced. The Cohen Committee (Cohen 1964) examined health education and urged that

Health education must do more than provide information. It must also seek to influence people to act on the advice and information given.

It recommended a new profession of Health Educators and the establishment by the Government of a central board in England and Wales which would, 'promote a climate of opinion generally favourable to health education'.

In 1972 the Health Education Council commenced support for school education. The first curriculum development project set up by the Health Education Council was the 'Living Well' project. Between 1972 and 1976 teaching materials and teachers' guides to promote non-didactic methods in health education were produced (HEC 1977). This was followed by curriculum development projects for 5–8, 9–13, and 13–18 age ranges (SC/HEC 1977, 1982). The period from the mid-1970s has seen greater developments in health education in schools and in the community than in any corresponding period in the past (Campbell 1985). The greatest concentration of activity has been on school health education but increasingly other target groups are being catered for. The upward trend in health education in recent years stems from a declining belief in the high technology aspects of curative medicine and a strengthening belief in prevention.

In this review, 1956 is taken as the starting point in the modern phase of dental health education because it was the first time that a British study attempted to evaluate and quantify the effects of a programme (Davies *et al.* 1956). From this time onwards accountability became far more important. The study in question was conducted in St Albans where an experimental group of school children was provided with toothbrushes and given weekly lessons on dental health by their teachers over a period of a school term. Comparisons were made with a control group. The study concluded that fundamental oral hygiene habits were difficult to alter (Davis *et al.* 1956).

From 1956 onwards two main phases are apparent: an earlier phase when large scale campaigns were mounted in different parts of the country and then beginning in the early to mid-1960s, a phase of critically examining different themes in dental health education.

Among the large scale campaigns mounted in different parts of the country in the late 1950s and early 1960s was a continuous oral hygiene campaign carried out in Wellingborough from September 1958 to January 1960 (Goose 1960). Two problems were highlighted in the study's conclusion: the vested interests of school tuck shops and the poor variety of dental health education materials available (Goose 1960). In Dundee, the dental health education campaign, undertaken from November 1960 to March 1961, not only involved primary schoolchildren, but also attempted to involve the whole community (Finlayson and Wilson 1961). A substantial improvement in oral hygiene took place at the end of the survey but this was not sustained (Finlayson and Pearson 1967). In Guildford a dental health campaign was mounted throughout the community, with a priority being given to certain key groups (Davis and Land 1962). The large campaigns have been described as the 'blunderbuss approach' (Fox and Maddick 1980); many useful conclusions could be drawn from them but workers began to call for a more systematic approach.

Three main themes began to emerge in dental health education from the early to mid-1960s. The first of these was the need for more epidemiological data from which target groups could be delineated and attitudes to dental health determined. The second related to the value and effectiveness of the dental health messages and the third to the methods and materials employed in dental health education.

The need for more epidemiological data was highlighted by the Nuffield Provincial Hospital Trust report in 1962 (Moser *et al.* 1962). The type of information that was required to produce a picture of the dental health of the nation was provided initially in local studies, such as those conducted in the joint social–dental investigation in Britain which took place in Salisbury and

Darlington (Richards *et al.* 1965; Bulman *et al.* 1968*a*, 1968*b*) and those on the periodontal status of selected British populations (Sheiham 1969*a*, 1969*b*, 1970). National studies of adults and children began to provide more comprehensive data. Early studies included a survey of adult dental health in England and Wales in 1968 (Gray *et al.* 1970), in Scotland in 1972 (Todd and Whitworth 1974), and in Northern Ireland in 1979 (Rhodes and Haire 1981). For information relating to children's dental health, the first national survey took place in 1973 (Todd 1975). In addition to the national surveys, insights related to particular target groups came from the researches of a number of workers, including two unpublished doctoral theses from the University of Manchester: A. S. Blinkhorn's (1976) *Toothbrushing as part of primary socialization* and H. Hodges's (1979) *Factors associated with toothbrushing behaviour in adolescents*. In the 20 year period following Moser's report, the background picture of the nation's dental health has slowly been built up.

The value and effectiveness of popular dental health messages began increasingly to be questioned. For a long time the messages were based on the collective conventional wisdom of the dental profession, but not all of them were necessarily scientifically verified. In 1961, for example, a committee of the British Dental Association put forward five rules (BDA 1961). These were:

1. Eat nourishing meals, with nothing sweet or sticky in between.

2. Finish meals with raw fruit or vegetables and rinse the mouth with water.

3. Brush the teeth and gums after eating, and especially after breakfast and before going to bed.

4. Use a soft toothbrush, and an up-and-down motion.

5. Visit the dentist regularly for advice.

Variations on these messages appeared in dental health education materials and campaigns throughout the 1960s and early 1970s. In some cases conflicting advice appeared from different sources.

In 1971 the Health Education Council organized a seminar to determine the scientific evidence in support of the dental health educators' message and this was subsequently published (HEC 1972). In 1976 the Health Education Council and the British Association for the Study of Community Dentistry endeavoured to update the scientific basis of dental health education. Only scientifically proven and independently verified messages were accepted and all longstanding myths and new hypotheses eliminated (Craft and Holloway 1983). The resulting policy document was published by the Health Education Council (HEC 1979) and reprinted in the British Dental Journal (BDJ 1979) and by 1983 about 100 000 copies had been distributed (Craft and Holloway 1983).

Six years later the policy document was revised to take advantage of the more recent evidence on the cause and prevention of dental disease (Levine 1985) and further revisions took place in 1989 (Levine 1989).

The third theme to emerge was a more detailed investigation of the materials and methods employed in dental health education. At a symposium on dental health education in 1966 attended by the main bodies concerned, a call was made for the 'evaluation of the effectiveness of different methods and approaches to dental health education' (Cawson and Naylor 1966). An editorial in the British Dental Journal called for motivational research that could promote a desire for dental health by making it attractive to the public and voiced the need for inputs from outside the dental profession (BDJ 1965). Findings from the fields of sociology, psychology, anthropology, and education began to be incorporated into dental health education. Richards has summarized the contributions that applied studies in these fields could make (Richards 1975).

The interdisciplinary approach adopted in the United States slowly began to affect research opinion in Britain. From the field of education, an innovative approach to dental health education methods involving a programme of child-centred learning was developed with the cooperation of a dental officer and a classroom teacher (Maddick and Downton 1968). Curriculum development in the tradition of the Schools Council Health Education Project 5–13, was continued in dental health education by the 'Gleam Team' Programme (Towner 1984) and 'Teeth Time' (Maddick and Fox 1982; Wetton 1984). Both these were flexible programmes for use by infant teachers with their classes. Evaluation focused to a far greater extent on educational rather than dental objectives. The largest scale research study on dental health education has been the Cambridge Dental Health Study, led by Michael Craft. Funded by the Health Education Council from 1975 to 1986, the study developed two major programmes, the 'Good Teeth' Programme for preschool children and the 'Natural Nashers' Programme for adolescents. Both programmes have been extensively evaluated. For the preschool programme, the most substantive changes related to snacking behaviour (Croucher et al. 1985). The programme for adolescents brought about the largest recorded cognitive and affective gains of any dental health programme in the United Kingdom (Craft and Croucher 1979).

When the contributions made by the professional and commercial agencies to dental health education from 1956 to the present day are assessed, several changes are apparent. There has been a great increase in the number of agencies involved and in the type of agency involved. In 1956 the four professional agencies and one commercial agency were involved; this has grown to seven professional and four commercial agencies.

From 1956 onwards accountability has been a major influence on dental health education. Epidemiological studies and studies of dental attitudes have provided a sounder base on which to define target groups and a broad consensus on the dental messages has provided a more effective message.

Conclusion

The dental historian, Lillian Lindsay, writing in the 1920s observed (Lindsay 1925):

The study of the records of the health of a country reveals a likeness to those of its culture, and ... tends to disturb our complacency over what we have flattered ourselves were new ideas and reforms.

If the ideas and reforms of today's dental health education movement are examined, is it possible to find echoes of the past? In four areas this can perhaps be seen.

First, there has been a move away from propaganda and a reliance on didactic teaching methods, towards education which stresses involvement and participation in learning experiences. But it is worth recalling that this trend can be traced back to George Cunningham's 'Children's Dental League' in the early years of the century (Davis 1969) and the Oral Hygiene Service's 'Ivory Castle League' in the 1920s and 1930s. Second, over the last twenty years dental health education has increasingly sought inputs from outside the dental profession, from the fields of education, sociology, and psychology. Pedley and Harrison in 1908, for example, suggested that mothers should set an example of toothbrushing to their infant children (Pedley and Harrison 1908), while Kay in 1919 believed that parents should not be spoken to above their heads but should be addressed in their own language (Kay 1919). Thus concepts from other disciplines were applied but they were implicit rather than explicit. Third, dental health education has moved away from supplying information and towards seeking to modify attitudes and change behaviour. The tooth-brushing clubs of the early years of the century were pioneers of this approach. Fourth, dental health education has become less generalized and, in becoming more specific, has increased the number of target groups to which it is directed. Although most dental health education in the past was directed towards children, materials were produced for adults, such as those produced by the Dental Board of the United Kingdom in the inter-war period for use in the workplace.

In these four areas change over time has been one of degree. Instead of isolated examples of innovative good practice, many of the ideas are now incorporated into the main body of knowledge and general practice But there are two main areas which do not seem to have historical precedents and where there has been a break with the past.

The major change has been that of accountability, the need to evaluate what is done at every stage. Accountability has been facilitated by the emergence of the discipline of social science and appropriate techniques for research since the Second World War (Lussier 1984) and fuelled by the comtemporary political climate. A second area is that more confidence can now be placed on the messages of oral health education. They now have a much firmer scientific basis, for they represent a consensus, agreed on by members of the dental profession, of scientifically verified advice.

There are a number of areas where further research could contribute to an understanding of the history of dental health education in Britain. The role of oral history could be investigated to obtain information related to the 'audience' or 'users' of the dental health education over the years. Company records could be examined to estimate the extend of workplace campaigns in the past. Local studies using the reports of school medical officers, school log books, and local newspapers could also illuminate the national picture. A greater understanding of the history of dental health education helps an appreciation of the current practices in the field and furthermore can provide insights into society's attitudes to health generally.

References

Acheson, R. M. and Hagard, S. (1984). *Health, society and medicine. An introduction to community medicine.* Blackwell Scientific, Oxford.

Beaver, P. (1980). *Addis 1780–1980. All about the home.* Publications for Companies, Stevenage.

Berridge, V. (1990). Health and medicine. In *The Cambridge social history of Britain 1750–1950, Volume 3. Social agencies and institutions,* (ed. F. M. L. Thompson), pp. 171–242. Cambridge University Press, Cambridge.

BDA (British Dental Association) (1909). Majority report of representatives of the British Dental Association on the sub-committee of the Education Committee of the London County Council on the medical treatment of children. *Brit. Dent. J.,* **30**, 121–34.

BDA (British Dental Association) (1930). *The Jubilee book of the British Dental Association.* John Bale, Sons & Danielsson, London.

BDA (British Dental Association) (1954). Dental health of children. Child Dental Health Committee. *Brit. Dent. J.,* **96**, 199–220.

BDA (British Dental Association) (1961). BDA Dental Health Committee — oral hygiene basic rules. *Brit. Dent. J.,* **111**, 350.

BDA (British Dental Association) (1965). Editorial. *Brit. Dent. J.,* **119**, 51–2.

BDJ (British Dental Journal) (1979). The scientific basis of dental health education. *Brit. Dent. J.,* **146**, 51–4.

BJDS (British Journal of Dental Science) (1886). Editorial. Dental preventive medicine. *Brit. J. Dent. Sci.,* **30**, 19–21.

Bulman, J. S., Slack, G. L., Richards, N. D., and Willocks, A. J. (1986a). A survey of the dental health and attitudes towards dentistry in two communities. Part 2 - Dental data. *Brit. Dent. J.,* **124**, 549–54.

Bulman, J. S., Slack, G. L., Richards, N. D., and Willocks, A. J. (1986b). A survey of the dental health and attitudes towards dentistry in two communities. Part 3 — Comparison of dental and sociological data. *Brit. Dent. J.,* **125**, 102–6.

Campbell, G. (1985). Introduction. In *New directions in health education,* (ed. G. Campbell), pp. 1–3. Falmer Press, London.

Cawson, R. A. and Naylor, M. N. (1966). Symposium on dental health communication. *Brit. Dent. J.,* **120**, 141–4.

CCHE (Central Council for Health Education) (1946). *Annual Report 1945–1946*. CCHE, London.

CMO (Chief Medical Officer) (1910). *Annual report for 1909 of the Chief Medical Officer of the Board of Education*. HMSO, London.

CMO (Chief Medical Officer) (1933). *Annual report of the Chief Medical Officer of the Board of Education for the year 1932*. HMSO, London.

CMO (Chief Medical Officer) (1934). *Annual report of the Chief Medical Officer of the Board of Education for the year 1933*. HMSO, London.

Cohen, Lord (1964). *Report of a joint committee on the Central and Scottish Health Services Councils on Health Education*. HMSO, London.

Connan, D. M. and Smith, G. (1925). Education of the public in hygiene. *Brit. Dent.J.*, **46**, 986–9.

Craft, M. H. and Croucher, R. E. (1979). Preventive dental health in adolescents. Results of a controlled field trial. *R. Soc. Hlth J.*, **2**, 48–56.

Craft, M. and Holloway, P. J. (1983). A programme of dental health education. *Hlth Educ. J.*, **42**, 16–19.

Croucher, R. E., Rodgers, A. I., Franklin, A. J., and Craft, M. H. (1985). Results and issues arising from an evaluation of community dental health education: the case of the 'Good Teeth programme'. *Community Dent. Hlth*, **2**, 89–97.

Davies, J. B. M. (1983). *Community health, preventive medicine and social services*, (5th edn). Balliere Tindall, London.

Davis, H.C. (1969). George Cunningham: the man and his message. *Brit. Dent. J.*, **127**, 527–37.

Davis, H. C. and Land, D. (1962). Good teeth for Guildford. A case study in civic enterprise. *Brit. Dent. J.*, **122**, 430–4.

Davis, H. C., Parfitt, G. J., and James, P. M. C. (1956). A controlled study into the effect of dental health education of 1939 school children in St Albans. *Brit. Dent. J.*, **100**, 354–6.

Dental Board of the United Kingdom (1926). *Hygiene of the mouth and teeth*. Dental Board, London.

DES (Department of Education and Science) (1975). *The school health services 1908–1974*. HMSO, London.

DES (Department of Education and Science) (1977). *Health education in schools*. HMSO, London.

Finlayson, D. A. and Wilson, W. A. (1961). Results of Dundee's campaign. *Brit. Dent. J.*, **111**, 103–6.

Finlayson, D. A. and Pearson, J. C. G. (1967). Dundee dental campaign. A study of its value six years later. *Brit. Dent. J.*, **1213**, 535–6.

Fisher, W. M. (1985). *Compulsory attention to the teeth of school children. Brit. Dent. Ass. J.*, **6**, 585–93.

Fox, B. and Maddick, I. (1978). Development of dental health education. The contribution of the Dental Board. *Brit. Dent.J.*, **145**, 339–44.

Fox, B. and Maddick, I. (1980). *A hundred years of dental health education. Brit. Dent. J.*, **149**, 28–32.

Francis, H. W. S. (1975). Education and health: the English tradition (1) Hesitant beginnings (2) The rise and fall of routine medical inspections (3) The community medicine of education. *Publ. Hlth Lond.*, **89**, 129–35, 181–90, 273–7.

Fraser, D. (1984). *The evolution of the British Welfare State*, (2nd edn). Macmillan, Basingstoke.

GDC (General Dental Council) (1957). *Dental health education. A review of the work of educating the public in dental care carried on by the Dental Board of the United Kingdom and the General Dental Council. 1924–1957.* General Dental Council, London.

Gelbier, S. (1986). Dental health and the chocolate factory. *Dental Historian*, **12**, 17–25.

Gelbier, S. and Randall, S. B. (1982). Charles Edward Wallis and London's toothbrush clubs: 1909 style. *Dent. Hlth*, **21**, 12–15.

GMC (General Medical Council and Dental Board of the United Kingdom) (1944?). *Memoranda of evidence submitted on behalf of the Council and of the Board to the interdepartmental committee on dentistry 1943–1944.* General Medical Council, London.

Goose, D. H. (1960). An oral hygiene campaign in Wellingborough. *Dent. Practit.*, **10**, 258–62.

Gray, P. G., Todd, J. E., Slack, G. L., and Bulman, J. S. (1970). *Adult dental health in England and Wales in 1968.* HMSO, London.

Guy, W. (1928). The work and policy of the Dental Board. *Brit. Dent. J.*, **49**, 419–25.

Hardwick, J. L. (1960). The incidence and distribution of dental caries through the ages in relation to the Englishman's diet. *Brit. Dent. J.*, **108**, 9–17.

HEC (Health Education Council) (1972). Report of a conference on dental health education. *Brit. Dent. J.*, **133**, 353–8.

HEC (Health Education Council) (1977). *'Living Well' project.* Cambridge University Press, Cambridge.

HEC (Health Education Council) (1979). *The scientific basis of dental health education. A policy document.* Health Education Council, London.

HEJ (Health Educational Journal) (1953). Editorial. *Hlth Educ. J.*, **11**, 1–6.

Hillam, C. (ed.) (1990). *The roots of dentistry.* British Dental Journal, London.

Imrie, W. (1834). *The parents' dental guide.* John Churchill, London.

Interdepartmental Committee (1904). *Report of the interdepartmental committee on physical deterioration.* HMSO, London.

Interdepartmental Committee (1905). *Report of the interdepartmental committee on medical inspection and feeding of children.* Vols 1 and 2. HMSO. London.

Ivory Castles (1925–1932). Vol. 1, No. 1–Vol. 8, No. 3. Published quarterly by the Ivory Castle League & Crusade, funded by D. & W. Gibbs Ltd.

Kay, V. (1919). A dental address to mothers at school clinics. *Brit. Dent. J.*, **40**, 693–7.

Kerr, J. (1926). *The fundamentals of school health.* George Allen & Unwin, London.

Levine, R. S. (ed.) (1985). *The scientific basis of dental health education. A policy document.* Health Education Council, London.

Levine, R. S. (ed.). (1989). *The scientific basis of dental health education. A policy document,* (3rd edn). Health Education Authority, London.

Lindsay, L. (1925). The historical side of a burning question. *Brit. Dent. J.*, **46**, 1147–51.

Lussier, R. (1984). *History of health education.* In *Health education. Foundations for the future,* (ed. L. Rubinson and W.F. Alles), pp. 1–33. Timer Mirror/Mosby College, St Louis.

Maddick, I. H. and Downton, D. (1968). Teach yourself dental health. *Dent. News*, **5**, 1–3.

Maddick, I. and Fox, B. (1982). *The assessment of a teacher-based programme of dental health education for 5–7 year olds.* J. Dent. Res., **61**, 540 (37).

Menzies Campbell, J. (1949). *A dental bibliography.* David Low, London.

Menzies Campbell, J. (1958). *From a trade to a profession. Byways in dental history.* Collected and reprinted for private circulation.

Ministry of Health (1956). *An enquiry into health visiting,* (Jameson report). HMSO London.

Moser, C. A., Gales, K., and Morpurgo, P. W. R. (1962). *Dental health and the dental service.* Oxford University Press, London.

Naylor, M. N. (1980). The prevention of dental caries. *Brit. Dent. J.,* **149,** 17–20.

Newsholme, M. N. (1903). The relation of the dental profession to public health. *Brit. Dent. J.,* **24,** 533–45.

Norman, D. H. (1981). Public health dentistry before 1948. In *Dental public health. An introduction to community dental health,* (2nd edn), (ed. G.L. Slack and B.A. Burt,), (pp. 325–31). John Wright, Bristol.

OHS (Oral Hygiene Service) (1954). *Annual report.* Oral Hygiene Service. London.

OHS (Oral Hygiene Service) (1955). *Annual report.* Oral Hygiene Service, London.

Pedley, R. D. (1899?). *The hygiene of the mouth: a guide to the prevention and control of dental diseases.* Segg and Co., London.

Pedley, R. D. and Harrison, F. (1908). *Our teeth. How built up. How destroyed. How preserved.* Blackie & Son, London.

Pickering, H. J. (1900). The condition of school children's teeth — its results and suggested remedies. *J. Brit. Dent. Ass.,* **21,** 619–31.

Pirrie, D. and Dalzall-Ward, A. (1962). *A textbook of health education.* Tavistock Publications, London.

Rhodes, J. R. and Haire, T. H. (1981). *Adult dental health survey. Northern Ireland 1979.* HMSO, Belfast.

Richards, N. D. (1975). *Towards a policy in dental health education.* Health Education Council, London.

Richards, N. D., Willocks, A. J., Bulman, J. S., and Slack, G. L. (1965). A survey of the dental health and attitudes towards dentistry in two communities. Part 1. Sociological data. *Brit. Dent. J.,* **118,** 199–205.

Rosen, G. (1951). The new history of medicine: a review. *J. Hist. Med. Allied Sciences,* **6,** 516–22.

Rowlett, A. E. (1930). The Association, the Dental Board and dental health education. *Brit. Dent. J.,* **51,** 157–9.

Rowntree, B. S. (1901). *Poverty: a study of town life.* Macmillan, London.

Royal Commission (1903). *Royal Commission on Physical Training (Scotland). Report.* HMSO, London.

Rushton, W. (1903). Education of the public in the care of their teeth. *Brit.Dent. J.,* **24,** 545–51.

Saunders, E. (1837). *Advice on care of the teeth.* Thomas Ward, London.

SC/HEC (Schools Council/Health Education Project) (1977). *Health education 5–13.* Thomas Nelson & Sons, London.

SC/HEC (Schools Council/Health Education Project) (1982). *Health education 13–18.* Forbes Publications, London.

Sheiham, A. (1969a). The prevalence and severity of periodontal disease in Surrey schoolchildren. *Dent. Practit.,* **19,** 232–8.

Sheiham, A. (1969b). The prevalence and severity of periodontal disease in British populations. *Brit. Dent. J.,* **126,** 115–22.

Sheiham, A. (1970). Dental cleanliness and chronic peridontal disease studies on populations in Britain. *Brit. Dent. J.,* **129,** 413–18.

Sutherland, I. (1979). History and background. In *Health education. Perspectives and choices*, (ed. I. Sutherland), (pp. 1–19). George Allen & Unwin, London.

Taylor, A. G. (1977): The school dentist's society. *Brit. Dent. J.*, **142**, 133–5.

Thornhill, M. B. (1932). *100 000 Crusaders*. Ivory Castles 8, (2), 10, 11, 14.

Todd, J. E. (1975). *Children's dental health in England and Wales 1973*. HMSO, London.

Todd, J. E. and Whitworth, A. (1974). *Adult dental health in Scotland 1972*. HMSO, London.

Towner, E. M. L. (1984). The 'Gleam team' programme: development and evaluation of a dental health education package fo r infant schools. *Community Dent. Hlth*, **1**, 181–91.

Walker, J. (1979). *British economic and social history. 1700–1971*, (2nd edn), revised by C. W. Munn. Macdonald & Evans, Plymouth.

Wallace, J. S. (1909). Remarks on the hygienic and the artificial methods of preventing dental caries. *Brit. Dent. J.*, **31**, 241–58.

Wallis, C. E. (1912?). *School dental clinics. Their foundation and management*. Claudius Ash, Sons, London.

Watson, A. M. (1911). A plea for an educational campaign. *Brit. Dent. J.*, **32**, 452–6.

Webster, C. (1983). The health of the school child during the depression. In The fitness of the nation — physical and health education in the nineteenth and twentieth centuries, (ed. N. Parry and D. McNair), (pp. 70–85). Procs of 1982 annual conference of the History of Education Society of Great Britain. History of Education Society, Leicester.

Wetton, N. M. (1984). *Teeth time. A dental health education programme for 5–7 year olds. The research findings and some conclusions*. Unpublished report. University of Southampton.

2

Theories and models of health behaviour

ANNE JOHANNE SØGAARD

Theory can serve many purposes. According to McQueen (1991), theories for health education should fulfil some basic aims:

(1) to help organize research questions about health education;

(2) to be empirically verifiable;

(3) to be falsifiable;

(4) to lead to a better understanding of the phenomena under study;

(5) to lead to practical research;

(6) to build on existing knowledge in the field;

(7) to help health education address questions which are of importance for public health;

(8) to lead to research which is utilized.

The terms 'theory', 'model', and 'paradigm' are frequently used interchangeably in the health behaviour and promotion literature. This adds to the difficulty of research in this field. Although this chapter is divided into one part with basic theories and one with health behaviour models, the general 'names' and labels of the different theories and models make a consistent use of the terms impossible.

According to Bandura (1986) **theories** specify the determinants and mechanisms governing the phenomena of interest. Theories consist of one or more general and logically interrelated propositions offered to explain a class of phenomena (Bauman 1980). Theories are usually concerned with very general and global classes of behaviour and do not deal directly, as conceptual models do, with specific types of behaviour in specific contexts. Also, theories generally represent reality from a discipline-specific perspective, whether sociological, economic, or biological. Because they are discipline-specific, theories often specify level-specific causes.

Earp and Ennett (1991) define a conceptual **model** as a set of concepts believed to be related to a particular public health problem. A conceptual model can be formed by more than one theory and conceptualized at multilevels — from micro to macro. As importantly in an applied field, it allows the inclusion of processes or characteristics not grounded in formal theory, but which represent empirical findings or the experience of practising professionals.

A sound theoretical framework will provide a substantial basis for practice. It should explain how individuals make health-related decisions. It will attempt to define the ways in which social and environmental factors influence these decisions and will provide insight into the nature of both inter- and intrapersonal dynamics governing behaviours. If we have some under- standing of the constellation of factors influencing human behaviour in health and illness, we will be in a better position to devise strategies and formulate methods which will achieve our health education goals — no matter what our philosophy or what model we choose to follow (Tones *et al.* 1990). Again, if we understand the existing relationships between, for example, knowledge, beliefs, skills, attitudes, social pressures, and environmental constraints, we should have some insight into the likely effects of a given educational programme and might, thus, select out indicators of success in a more rational and meaningful way.

It could be fruitful, as stated by Rise (1986), to distinguish between theories explaining behaviour and theories of changing behaviour i.e. issues for explanatory vs. intervention research. Because the process of behavioural influence is complex, and all behaviour can be seen as a product of ongoing process rather than a reflection of fixed internal entities, this distinction is not made in this chapter. Life is a continuing process of opening and resolving problems, a process of interactions between situational demands and historical factors and between learned and innate factors. Therefore, it is difficult to clearly distinguish between theories explaining health behaviour and theories of health behaviour change.

To make a broad overview of theories and models in health behaviour science is an enormous task, which goes far beyond the scope of this chapter. I take the liberty for those particularly interested in this topic, to recommend McGuire's (1991) distinguished paper published in a special 'theory' - issue of *Health Education Research* (Vol. 6 (2), 1991) where he systematizes 16 cate- gories of theories of human behaviour.

This chapter will firstly describe some basic theories highly relevant for health promotion. Secondly, models particularly constructed for and tested in health education and health promotion will be reported. Some of these will be well known for most readers, while others are referring to specific fields, such as nursing, or practical problems, such as compliance, and are just commented on briefly. Thirdly, some comprehensive systems models or metamodels are referred, before a short conclusion closes the chapter.

Basic Theories

The Yale model

The Yale approach (Hovland *et al.* 1953) provides a structured list of variables or factors that have a direct bearing on the impact which persuasive messages have on attitudes — for example the credibility of the source, the use of one-sided vs. two-sided messages, interpersonal communication vs. mass media, and the level of involvement of the receiver. This model concentrates on 'Who said what to whom with what effect?' The Yale model has been elaborated upon and extensively advocated by McGuire (1978, 1984) as the classic **information processing model**. McGuire has suggested the 'persuasion matrix' as a way of conceptualizing the change process and understanding the complexities of the relationships between outcomes (changes in knowledge, attitudes, and behaviour) and inputs (the persuasive communication and its properties).

The columns of McGuire's persuasion matrix are shown in Fig. 2.1. According to this approach the fundamental processes in behaviour change are

Independent Variables: The Communication Components / Dependent Variables: Steps in Being Persuaded	Source	Message	Channel	Receiver	Destination
Message presentation → exposure					
Attention → awareness					
Comprehension → knowledge					
Yielding → beliefs/attitudes					
Retention → persistence/ maintenance					
Action → behaviour					

Fig. 2.1   A matrix of persuasion for assembling and evaluating advertising (from McGuire 1978).

attention, comprehension, yielding, and retention. These processes are affected by source, message, recipient, and channel factors. The model assumes that information (if provided by a credible and familiar source, in an appropriate form, and via appropriate channels; and if attended to, comprehended, and accepted) leads to changes in knowledge and beliefs. These cognitive changes are then assumed to lead to changes in attitudes (affective changes) and behaviour (conative changes). These assumptions have, however, been questioned by many researchers (for review see Flay 1981; Søgaard 1986, 1989). 'It sounds like a logical framework — new knowledge produces a change in attitude which produces a change in behaviour. The only problem is it doesn't work.' (Silversin 1979).

Flay suggests that the information processing model is best restricted to explaining changes in the cognitive structure (knowledge and beliefs), whereas changes in the affective and behavioural structure require consideration of additional models.

McGuire's information processing model does not tell us anything about those conditions that might increase the likelihood of changes in belief leading to attitude change, or changes in attitude leading to changes in behaviour. Flay (1981) has extended the model — integrating other theories which better describe the affective and behavioural structures, such as the theory of reasoned action (Ajzen and Fishbein 1977) and the Health Belief Model (Becker 1974). In combination with the model of 'two-step flow of communication' (Katz 1957), the information processing model with Flay's additions has been used to explain the effect of mass media health education campaigns in Norway (Søgaard 1988; Fønnebø and Søgaard 1990). The information processing model was also incorporated in Hølund's recently published dental health (dietary) behaviour study (Hølund 1991).

The possible orders or hierarchies of effects among cognitive, affective, and conative elements has been studied by Ray (1973). He suggests that the three most probable processes are the **learning hierarchy** (cognition → affection → conation), the **dissonance attribution hierarchy** (conation → affection → cognition) and the **low involvement hierarchy** (cognition → conation → affection). The learning hierarchy occurs when there is high involvement and clear differences between behavioural alternatives; the dissonance–attribution hierarchy generally occurs when there is high attitudinal involvement and almost indistinguishable or equal alternatives, and the low involvement hierarchy occurs when involvement is low and the differences between alternatives are minimal. The model most often underlying health education programmes is the learning hierarchy.

Regarding dental health behaviour, we do not know which one of these hierarchies will be the most likely to work. People are not highly involved in dental health issues (Kegeles 1974), at least not those we want to reach. This should point at the low involvement hierarchy. However, the differences between alternatives (e.g. daily use or no use of dental floss) might be perceived as distinctive. Based on this assumption none of the hierarchies mentioned will be the typical one elicited in the context of dental health education. Thus, more research is needed to test out which model — or combination of models (Flay 1981) — is applicable to dental health issues. As Heløe and König (1978) stated: 'The mechanisms of adopting dental health habits and the diffusion of dental knowledge are seemingly manifold and confusing'.

Group-dynamic model

In contrast to the methodology of Yale tradition (Hovland *et al.* 1953), the approach developed by Kurt Lewin is based on a field-theory orientation (Lewin 1947, 1951). It assumes that the individual is more than an isolated, passive processor of information. Instead the person is viewed as a social being, with an intimate dependence on others for knowledge about the world and even about him/herself. This theory takes social interactions into account. A major factor that causes people to change their attitudes, beliefs, and perceptions of the world, is the discrepancy that exists between an individual's attitude or behaviour and the group norm. A dissonance between one's own knowledge, attitudes, and practice on the one hand, and one's perception of these factors in the group on the other, will be experienced as group pressure.

One of the more interesting aspects of the group dynamics approach is its emphasis on the effects of active participation during group interaction. Lewin's experiment on housewives' attitudes to and use of organ meats instead of more common cuts (Lewin 1943) has become classical. One group was asked to discuss openly the positive aspects of using organ meats while another group was told about the benefits of organ meats by means of a formal, informational lecture. The active discussions left housewives more favourable toward the ideas and more likely to indicate that they would try organ meats at home than did the lecture. Actively taking a position in the presence of other uncritical, and sometimes supportive, people may be sufficient to exert a powerful impact on one's self-image.

Many encounter groups also employ this technique. Some call it role-playing, others call it sharing, and still others refer to it as 'interpersonal trusting'. The **role-playing approach** is based upon a study by Janis and King (1954), in which the effects of actively presenting arguments on an issue were compared with the effects of passively listening to arguments presented by another person. Each subject had to role-play an attitude position on one topic and listen to the two subjects role-playing the attitude position on two other topics. The results of this experiment was that the role-playing subjects changed their opinion more in the direction of the communication than did the passive listeners. Added to this there is evidence to conclude that role-playing produces more persisting attitude change than passive exposure because people remember better the arguments that they generate than arguments generated by others. Later research has shown role-playing to be an effective technique for changing attitudes on a wide variety of issues as long as people have enough background information on the issue to permit improvization of arguments (Janis and Mann 1977).

Jensen (1981a, 1981b) has employed many of the ideas from Lewin's 'field-theory' in his dental health education project among schoolchildren, their teachers, and their parents.

Social learning theory

The basic idea in this theory (Rotter 1954; Bandura 1969, 1977a) is that the likelihood of a specific behaviour is determined by the consequences the person expects will follow the performance of that behaviour, but only as those consequences are interpreted and understood by the individual. Major elements are identification, reinforcement, feedback, and reward.

The social learning theory (SLT), which recently has been relabelled social cognitive theory (Bandura 1986), holds that behaviour is learned observationally through modelling, by visualizing, by self-monitoring, and by skill-training.

From observing others, one forms ideas of how new behaviours are performed, and on later occasions this coded information serves as a guide for actions. Bandura maintains that behaviour is determined by expectancies and incentives. The **expectancies** are divided into:

(1) expectancies about environmental cues (beliefs about how events are connected — about what leads to what);

(2) outcome expectancies (opinions about how individual behaviour is likely to influence outcomes);

(3) efficacy expectancies (self-efficacy — expectancies about one's own competence to perform the behaviour needed to influence outcomes).

Incentive is defined as the value of a particular object or outcome. The outcome may be health status, approval of others, or economic gain.

Thus, for example, individuals who value the perceived effects of changed lifestyles (incentives) will attempt to change if they believe: that their current lifestyle poses threats to any personally valued outcome, such as health or appearance (environmental cues); that particular behavioural changes will reduce the threats (outcome expectations); and that they are personally capable of adopting the new behaviours (efficacy expectations). The distinction between outcome expectations and efficacy expectations is important because both are required for behaviour change (Fig. 2.2).

Self-efficacy (Bandura 1977b) is increasingly utilized in health promotion programming and research (Sherer et al. 1982; Schunk and Carbonari 1984; Davis et al. 1984; Strecher et al. 1986; Clark 1987; Yalow and Collins 1987; Rosenstock et al. 1988). This part of Bandura's theory states that psycho-

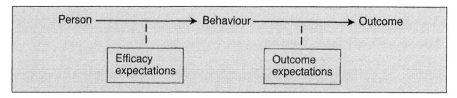

Fig. 2.2 Constructs from social learning theory — illustrating the difference between efficacy expectations and outcome expectations (Bandura 1977b)

logical procedures, whatever their form, alter the level and strength of self-efficacy. It hypothesizes that expectations of personal efficacy determine whether coping behaviour will be sustained in the face of obstacles and aversive experiences and physiological states. In the proposed model, expectations of personal efficacy are derived from four principal sources of information: performance accomplishments, vicarious experience, verbal persuasion, and physiological states.

Social learning theory has been tested in several studies, for example in school-based dental health education and in smoking reduction programmes in Norway, with positive short-term effects on dental health knowledge, attitude, behaviour, and gingival health (Søgaard *et al.* 1987; Søgaard and Holst 1988) and reduction in consumption of cigarettes (Aarø *et al.* 1983). SLT has also been the basic theory in large-scale community action programmes in the North Karelia project (Puska *et al.* 1985), in the Stanford Three Community Study (Maccoby *et al.* 1977), and in the Minnesota Heart Health Program (Mittelmark *et al.* 1986).

Health locus of control, derived from the locus of control concept of Rotter's social-learning theory (Rotter *et al.* 1972), measures to what extent people believe that their health is influenced either by their own behaviour or by external causes. Central to the concept of 'locus of control' is the understanding of one's behaviour as a function of one's expectancy of the reinforcement value (positive or negative) that one's actions will bring. These expectancies are developed through prior experience. Health-specific locus of control beliefs are measured by a multidimensional scale with three dimensions (Wallston *et al.* 1978). These dimensions are labelled 'internal control', 'external control' or 'powerful others control', and 'chance control'. Locus of control thus contains ideas similar to the concept of self-efficacy. But while efficacy is situation specific, focused on beliefs about one's personal abilities in specific settings, locus of control is a generalized perception of who or what is in control of one's health. In this view locus of control relates more to outcome expectations than to efficacy expectations (Fig. 2.2). Studies comparing the predictive power of these two constructs have shown self-efficacy to be more strongly related to health behaviour than locus of control, and so self-efficacy has recently become more prominent in health promotion research (Hølund 1991).

Theory of reasoned action

This model (Fig. 2.3) concentrates on explaining the attitude–behaviour relations, and argues that a person's attitude toward an object influences the overall pattern of his or her responses to the object, but that it need not predict any action (Ajzen and Fishbein 1977, 1980). This model posits that volitional behaviour, e.g. consumption of sweets, is predicted by one's intention to perform the behaviour ('How likely is it that you will cut down on the amount of sweets during the next month?'). Behavioural intention is a function of attitude toward performance of an impending behaviour ('How pleasant or unpleasant is eating sweets?') and subjective norms ('Do most people, who are important to you, think you should cut down on the amount of sweets you eat?'). Attitude is a function of beliefs about the consequences of the behaviour ('How strongly would you agree or disagree that sweets damage your teeth?') weighted by an evaluation of the importance of that attribute ('How important to you is preventing dental decay'). Subjective norms are a function of expectation by significant others ('Do your parents think you should cut down on the amount of sweets you eat?') weighted by motivation to conform ('How important is it for you to please your parents?').

This model has been tested in several studies (for review see Norman 1985) — for instance to predict sugar consumption (Freeman 1984), toothbrushing behaviour (Bateman 1985), and demand for dental care (Hoogstraten *et al.* 1985). Bentler and Speckart (1979) included 'past behaviour' as an additional predictor of behaviour in study of drug consumption, and found that attitudes and past behaviour accounted for a significant degree of drug consumption behaviour not accounted for by intentions.

The original model has been criticized for assuming a simple causal structure. A much more complex model is needed because research suggests that intention to act is not a necessary and sufficient cause of behaviour. A further criticism is that attitudes do not mediate completely the effect of cognitions on intentions. Liska (1984) has proposed a revision of the model, which specifies contingency conditions as explicit conditions of the model and includes additional causal pathways between the variables.

Ajzen (1985) observed that the original theory of reasoned action was particularly valuable when describing behaviours that were totally under volitional control. However, most behaviours are located at some point along a continuum that extends from total control to a complete lack of control. To take account of such barriers, real and perceived, Ajzen (1985) has added a third concept of perceived behavioural control to the original Fishbein and Ajzen's model.

Testing this expanded version of the model, labelled **theory of planned behaviour**, Schifter and Ajzen (1985) found that the best predictor of weight loss was the perceived control over one's own weight. Intentions had only a low correlation with the actual weight loss.

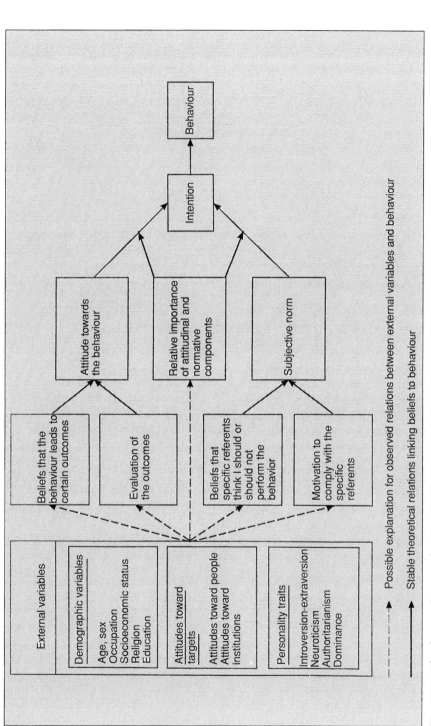

Fig. 2.3 The theory of reasoned action (Fishbein's model) (from Ajzen and Fishbein 1980).

The notion of perceived behavioural control is closely similar to Bandura's concept of self-efficacy (Ajzen and Madden 1986) and to Triandis's concept of facilitating conditions in his model of social behaviour (Triandis 1980) and Antonovsky's (1984) 'manageability' (see descriptions later in this chapter). It reflects personal beliefs as to how easy or difficult adoption of the behaviour is likely to be, and beliefs about resources and opportunities may thus be viewed as underlying perceived behavioural control.

Attribution theory

Attribution theory (Bem 1972; Kelly 1973, 1978; den Boer *et al.* 1991) is one in a range of cognitive theories that attempt to explain human behaviour. Several concepts in this theory show great similarity with concepts in Bandura's (1982) self-efficacy theory. These theories have in common the assumption that behaviour is determined by the cognitions people have about their behaviour. Attribution theory addresses two issues:

(1) how people derive attributions from previous behavioural outcomes;

(2) the consequences of these attributions on future behaviour.
    Kelly (1978) termed these latter analyses attributional theories.

Attribution theory attempts to describe the way in which we generate reasons for our own and other people's actions. The aim of the theory is to explain the way in which people try to account for human actions. There are no motivational constructs in the theory, such as a need to reduce dissonance or pressures toward uniformity. Instead, it attempts to understand how we perceive the motives, intentions, and causes of people's actions. The theory does not tell us whether the motives we infer others to have are the true ones. It simply provides an explanation for the way in which we reach our conclusions about motives and other causes for a person's actions. Recently there has been an enormous increase in the use of attributional techniques to change people's behaviour. Den Boer *et al.* (1991) present results from different studies and discuss how attribution theory is related to self-efficacy theory and **relapse prevention theory** (Marlatt and Gordon 1985), and how insights from attribution theory can be applied in health behavioural inter-ventions.

Cognitive–dissonance theory

Festinger advanced the notion that discrepancies or inconsistencies between people's own and other similar people's attitudes cause an uncomfortable tension that people try to reduce or eliminate (Festinger 1957, 1962; Aronsen 1969). He assumed the discrepancy itself to exist entirely within the indi-vidual's own cognitive system.

According to this theory, two cognitive elements can be either consistent, inconsistent, or irrelevant to one another. Two elements are consistent (consonant) when one follows from the other, and inconsistent (dissonant) when knowledge of one suggests the opposite of the other. Finally two elements can be irrelevant when knowledge of one tells you nothing about what you might expect regarding the other. The magnitude of dissonance experienced by an individual is a function of three variables: the **importance** of each of the cognitive elements, the **ratio** of dissonant to consonant cognitions that exist at that time, and the **functional equivalence** of the objects or activities represented by each cognition.

The crucial issue of the theory is the importance of dissonance reduction. Festinger suggests three models:

1. The person can change one of the elements to make two elements more consonant.

2. He/she can add consonant cognitions.

3. He/she can reduce the dissonance by changing the importance of the cognitions.

To change attitudes according to the cognitive dissonance theory, behaviour change should be induced under manipulated conditions of high choice and minimally adequate justification. When providing an opportunity for the new attitude to be expressed, the result will be a changed attitude.

As mentioned previously, role-playing can be a powerful technique in producing attitude change. One explanation of this attitude change could be cognitive dissonance, assuming that when a person engages in a behaviour that is inconsistent with a prior attitude, dissonance is aroused. One means of reducing the dissonance is to change one's attitude to bring it into line with the discrepant behaviour.

The consistency theories, which were popular during the 1960s, are extensively reviewed by Abelson *et al.* (1968).

Diffusion of innovation model

The basic concept of this theory (Rogers and Shoemaker 1971; E. M. Rogers 1983) is how different people pass through the five stages: awareness, interest, trial, decision, and adoption (Fig. 2.4). Rogers and Shoemaker have established that the communication process follows a pattern of prevalence diffusion, and they describe five groups of adopters: innovators, early adopters, early majority, late majority, and laggards.

Those who adopt an innovation earliest, the **innovators**, tend to be middle-class people who are more adventurous and actively seek information about new ideas. Media are a source of new ideas for innovators (E. M. Rogers 1983). **Early adopters** are respected members of the established social system. The **early majority**, the third category, adopt a new idea deliberately, just before the average member of the social system. In all the first three groups the people adopt a change primarily on the basis of their reasoning about the

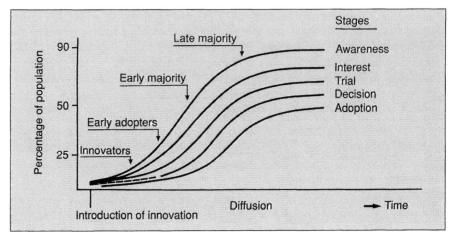

Fig. 2.4 Diffusion of innovation — five stages of adoption for four groups of adopters. The model shows how a message spreads to different groups of the population and have different effects over time (after Green *et al.* 1980).

costs and benefits of an innovation. The next group, the **late majority**, is lower in social influence and social status, and learns of new ideas primarily from peers through social influence, rather than from media channels. **Laggards**, the last adopter category (not shown in Fig. 2.4), are more socially isolated from traditional networks and their behaviour is less responsive to new ideas, peer influence, or other social pressures.

The diffusion of innovation model is the only model which consciously uses the dimension of *time* as its major explanatory variable. The model concentrates on the 'process' of change through time, independent of what 'message' is being adopted in the target population.

The model tries to integrate mass communication with interpersonal communication. It has been adapted to health behaviour and lifestyle changes (Green *et al.* 1980; Green and McAlister 1984) — and used to explain the adoption and implementation of fluoride rinse programmes in schools (Coombs *et al.* 1981).

The described model for the spread of innovations in a population is closely related to other models and concepts applied in mass media communication research. In Katz and Lazarsfeld's (1955) early theoretical contributions, the well-known **two-step flow hypothesis** was proposed. Mass media does not influence the audience as efficiently and directly as assumed in the childhood of radio and television. The lack of such direct effects was attributed to processes in the environment of the receivers, and it was assumed that some individuals in the audience served a special function as opinion leaders.

The opinion leaders interpret, emphasize, and modify the message they receive. The two-step hypothesis has been modified many times. It is possible that the diffusion process is more complex, and that the communication flows in more than two steps. All people are probably receivers of the message, but only the most influential and well informed have the special qualifications on how the message should be understood and assessed. It is also asserted that the opinion leaders themselves, although more exposed to mass media than are those they influence (Katz 1957), are influenced first of all through other people.

Social marketing model

Marketing is a systematic approach to planning and achieving desired exchange relations with other groups (Kotler 1975). Even though there are many differences between marketing and strategies for changing health behaviour, some of their basic ideas and approaches can be used to understand human behaviour. The adoption of an idea, like the adoption of any product, requires a deep understanding of people's needs and perceptions, preferences of the reference groups, and behavioural patterns of the target audience. Also needed are knowledge about the tailoring of messages, the effect of media, 'costs', and facilities to maximize the case of adopting the idea.

In the field of marketing many of the theories of behaviour previously referred have been used to influence consumer behaviour (Engel and Blackwell 1982).

Models of Health Behaviour

Over the past three decades a number of theoretical frameworks have appeared which attempt to account for individuals' health behaviour. The models differ considerably in their theoretical perspectives, in the type of health behaviour they attempt to explain, and in the terms employed to label their respective dimensions and variables.

Most models are derived from psychological and behavioural theory. A single theory is usually insufficient to incorporate all variables of interest to conceptual models in health promotion. Therefore, alternative models have been suggested based on a variety of theoretical frameworks (e.g. economic, sociodemographic, sociocultural, and organizational approaches).

Health belief model

The health belief model (HBM) (Rosenstock 1966, 1974; Becker 1974; Becker and Maiman 1975; Janz and Becker 1984) is a decision-making theory based on *the field theory* of Kurt Lewin (Lewin 1951). The HBM hypothesizes that a decision to undertake a health action will not be made unless the individual is psychologically ready to take action relative to a particular health threat or condition (Fig. 2.5). Readiness to act is defined by the extent to which:

(1) the individual feels susceptible to the condition in question and the extent to which its possible occurrence is viewed as having serious consequences;

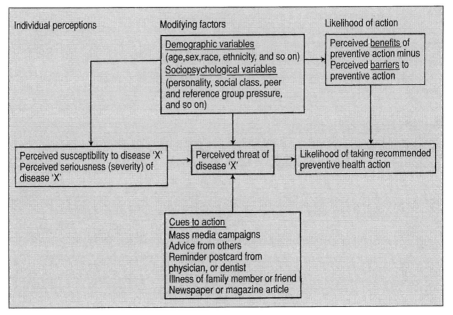

Fig. 2.5   The health belief model (from Becker and Maiman 1975).

(2) the individual believes that there are actions which would be beneficial in reducing his/her susceptibility to and/or severity of the condition/disease;

(3) the individual believes that the psychological costs associated with taking the health action are outweighed by the benefits to be derived.

The HBM has not proved useful in predicting children's dental health behaviour in terms of dental visits (Kegeles 1963), participation in a preventive programme (Weisenberg *et al.* 1980), or adherence to at-home mouth rinsing (Kegeles and Lund 1982, 1984). Given the negative effects from study to study, the authors conclude that health beliefs have helped in neither the prediction, nor the explanation, of children's preventive dental health behaviour (Kegeles and Lund 1984).

Thus, the findings of empirical studies of the HBM have not uniformly supported the model. However, most of the studies have been retrospective rather than prospective, with greater support for the model coming from retrospective studies, which may imply that it is, in reality, **past behaviour** which predicts actual behaviour (Kegeles and Lund 1984).

In addition to the 'theory of reasoned action', the HBM is probably the model most frequently employed in health education research. Norman (1985) has made a highly deserving and recommendable review and comparison of these two — and other health behaviour models. It has been noted by a number of authors that the health belief model is closely related to the social cognitive theory (Bandura 1986), as both theories build upon Lewin's field theory (Lewin 1951). Recently the HBM has been revised, incorporating self-efficacy as a separate individual variable along with the traditional health belief variables (Rosenstock *et al.* 1988). The 'model-builders' point out that social learning theory has made at least two contributions to explanations of health-related behaviour that should be included in the HBM: 'The first is the emphasis on the several sources of information for acquiring expectations, particularly on the informative and motivational role of reinforcement — and on the role of observational learning through modelling the behaviours of others. The second major contribution is the introduction of the concept of self-efficacy (efficacy expectation) as distinct from outcome expectation' (Rosenstock *et al.* 1988).

With this new addition the overlap between the two models is even more obvious. However, Bandura does not explicitly include the important traditional health belief variables of perceived susceptibility, severity, benefits, and barriers, as emphasized by Rosentock *et al.* (1988).

Antonovsky and Kats (1970) have tested an integrated model related to the traditional HBM. They hypothesize that it is the combination of effective motivation and blockage variables which predict preventive dental health behaviour. These variables, in turn, are explicable by reference to the conditioning variables, i.e. the variables which presumably condition the motivating and blockage variables (such as education, previous experience, or passive orientation).

Health action model

This model (Tones 1987; Tones *et al.* 1990) serves as a theoretical basis for researching the various factors governing health decisions.

The health action model (HAM) provides an overview of these influences (Fig. 2.6); it describes the interaction of knowledge, beliefs, values, attitudes, drives, and normative pressures and seeks to show how these relate to individual intentions to act. It also indicates how environmental circumstances, information, and personal skills may facilitate the translation of intentions into health actions.

HAM is concerned with deliberate discrete single-time choices. It attempts to define the factors leading to an individual deciding to perform a specific act such as visiting a dentist for a yearly check-up or writing to a local Public Health Office to complain about sports sponsorship by tobacco manufacturers.

As indicated above, the choice may also be the first step towards changing a lifelong habit — for instance, not adding sugar to tea. It may similarly be the first step in establishing a completely new practice such as regular physical activity.

Whatever the nature of the choice three major systems influence it. These are the belief system, the motivation system, and the normative system (Fig. 2.6).

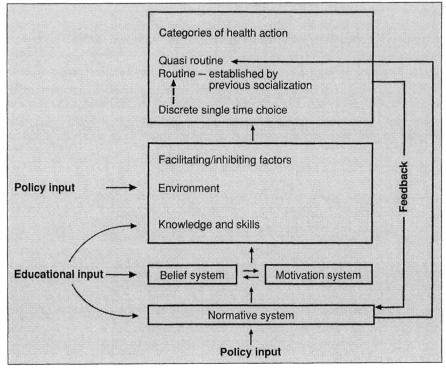

Fig. 2.6   The health action model (from Tones 1987).

The health action model incorporates the main elements of the health belief model. It also draws on Ajzen and Fishbein's theory of reasoned action (Ajzen and Fishbein 1977, 1980) and takes account of those approaches which adopt a sociological perspective such as Baric's (1979) **social intervention model**.

Medically orientated analyses such as Freidson's **lay referral system** (1960) may also be accommodated. HAM does, however, differ from these approaches in certain important ways. For instance, in addition to emphasizing the import-ance of those inhibiting and facilitating factors discussed earlier, it also acknowledges ways in which powerful 'drive factors' may overwhelm socially acquired competing values and attitudes in determining behavioral outcomes.

Protection motivation theory

Another composite model is the **protection motivation theory** (PMT) (R. W. Rogers 1975, 1983; Prentice-Dunn and Rogers 1986). Originally the theory was proposed to provide conceptual clarity to understanding fear appeals (R. W. Rogers 1975), but the theory was later expanded to incorporate information about health-threatening behaviour (R. W. Rogers 1983). As the health belief model and the theory of reasoned action, the PMT can also be labelled a value-expectancy theory (Fig. 2.7).

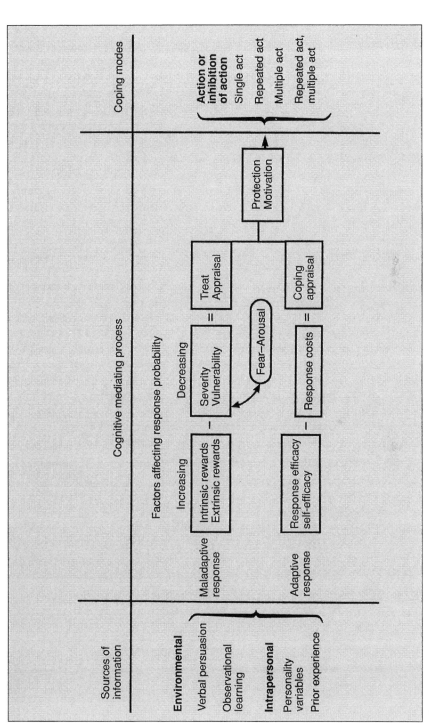

Fig. 2.7 The protection motivation model (from R.W. Rogers 1983).

When a person receives a message about a health threat, two cognitive processes are initiated: **threat appraisal** and **coping appraisal**. The **threat appraisal** process evaluates the factors that increase or decrease the probability of making the maladaptive response. The maladaptive action can be a behaviour that could be enacted, such as beginning to smoke, or it could be a current behaviour, such as not wearing a seat-belt. Variables that increase the likelihood of the maladaptive response are intrinsic rewards (e.g. bodily pleasure) and extrinsic rewards (e.g. social approval). Factors reducing the probability of the maladaptive response are the assessed severity of the threat and the perceived vulnerability to the threat. Fear arousal influences perceived severity, but has only an indirect effect on the eventual behaviour enacted. The total threat appraisal is an algebraic sum of the variables that increase and decrease the maladaptive behaviour likelihood.

In addition to evaluating threat, the individual also makes a **coping appraisal**. This consists partially of judgements about the efficacy of a preventive response that will avert the perceived threat (response efficacy) plus the assessment of one's ability to successfully initiate and complete the adaptive response (self-efficacy). The self-efficacy component is crucial to the successful avoidance of the threatening situation (Bandura 1977b, Bandura 1986). An important feature of PMT, the explicit role of personal mastery, has been neglected in virtually all expectancy-value theories. Thus, the implication is that the existence of an effective alternative to the maladaptive health beha-viour is not sufficient; one must also believe himself of herself capable of carrying out the preventive regimen. It should be noted that an individual's sense of self-efficacy is conceptually independent of the 'barriers' referred to in the HBM. Self-efficacy influences not only the initiation of the coping response, but also the amount of energy expended and the person's persistence in the face of obstacles (Bandura 1982).

Theory of social behaviour

Triandis has provided a relatively comprehensive set of predictors and equations in the **theory of social behaviour** (Triandis 1980). Like Ajzen and Fishbein, Triandis regards intention as a major predictor of behaviour. Intention is not the only important one, however, especially not in the case of behaviours termed habitual. In the case of behaviour sequences which have become automatic, habit is of importance, and may receive more weight than intention.

In this model **behavioural intention** is determined by:

(1) a cognitive component identical to Fishbein's beliefs about the consequences of performing the act and the evaluation of those consequences;

(2) an affective component expressed as the individual's emotional response to the thoughts of performing a given behaviour;

(3) a social component, which is relative to the behaviour studied;

(4) personal normative beliefs, which measure the individual's belief concerning the felt obligation to perform the behaviour in question.

The variables most often used are **normative beliefs**, that is, the appropriateness of performing the behaviour for a member of the reference group, and **role beliefs**, that is, the appropriateness of performing the behaviour for a person occupying a specific position in the social structure.

In predicting the probability of an act, Triandis has introduced the terms 'physiological arousal' of the individual and 'facilitating conditions'. These two factors should be multiplied by the weighted sum of intention and habit to predict behaviour. Physiological arousal exists when the individual is in a high drive state, or in a situation that is relevant to the individual's values. Facilitating conditions are defined as objective environmental factors that several judges or observers agree make an act easy to do.

Compared with some of the other models presented, the Triandis theory of social behaviour is more detailed as far as social factors are concerned. The distinction between normative beliefs and role beliefs is important. The normative beliefs tend to be uniform within one subculture. The role beliefs may be unique for a class of persons occupying one particular kind of position within a culture, a community, or a social system. A set of role beliefs may be common only to all persons belonging to one category of roles.

The Triandis model does not include any feedback from behaviour to beliefs. It does not allow for the perspective of Bem's (1972) **self perception theory**. Bem regards behavioural attitudes and opinions as a product of how we perceive own behaviour. He maintains that we perceive our own behaviour in the same way as we perceive others' behaviour.

Wallston and Wallston (1984) compared the use of the social learning theory, the health belief model, the theory of reasoned action, and Triandis's theory of social behaviour — and concluded by suggesting an integrated model composed of the three latter theories (or models). The fundamental equation of this model is that behaviour is predicted by behavioural intention, habit, and facilitating conditions. This integrated model is similar to Triandis's equation, but differs in some respect. The facilitating conditions in Wallston and Wallston's proposal consist of knowledge of the action, the ability to perform the behaviour, and arousal. This model has been tested empirically by Feldman and Mayhew (1984) in a prospective study of nutrition behaviour. The authors underline that nutrition behaviour encompasses varying types of behaviour, and that social–psychological factors play a differential role depending upon the type of behaviour.

Problem-behaviour theory

Jessor (1984) emphasizes the unsatisfactory state of theory in the field of adolescent health, regarding the understanding of the nature of adolescent risk behaviour. Jessor bases the **problem-behaviour theory** on the theoretical perspectives of Kurt Lewin. The theory, initially formulated in 1977 (Jessor and Jessor 1977), rests on the social–psychological relationships that obtain within and between each of three major systems: the personality system, the perceived environment system, and the behaviour system. Within each of the systems, the structure of the variables they encompass is inter-related and organized so as to generate a theoretical dynamic state called **proneness**, that summarizes the likelihood of occurrence of problem behaviour or health-risk behaviour. Thus, it is theoretically possible to speak of personality proneness, environmental proneness, and behavioural proneness, and of their combination as psychosocial proneness towards problem behaviour. Psychosocial proneness is the key theoretical basis for predicting and explaining variations in youthful behaviour.

Several studies have confirmed that the problem-behaviour theory provides a theoretical framework useful to identify aetiological factors predictive of drinking and driving among adolescents (Klepp 1987), alcohol use among adolescents (Hay et al. 1987; Jessor 1987), use of seat-belts (Maron et al. 1986), and dental health behaviours in schoolchildren (Rise et al. 1991).

PRECEDE framework

Proposed by Green et al. (1980), the **PRECEDE framework** (PRECEDE being an acronym for **p**redisposing, **r**einforcing and **e**nabling **c**auses in **e**ducational **d**iagnosis and **e**valuation), is a model for health education planning, rather than a theory of health behaviour. However, one part of the model especially relevant in explaining health behaviours is the 'educational diagnosis', which is concerned with assessing causes of health behaviour (Fig. 2.8).

The factors influencing health behaviours are seen to be of three distinct kinds: predisposing, enabling, and reinforcing. Green et al. (1980) point out that the configuration of these factors is not thought to form an all-inclusive causal model of health behaviour change. Rather, these factors have been selected because of their convenience for sorting the determinants of behavioural change most responsive to health education.

Predisposing factors include knowledge, attitudes, beliefs, values, and perceptions, as well as demographic factors such as socioeconomic status, age, and gender. These predisposing factors are antecedent to the behaviour and provide the rationale or motivation for the behaviour. In this connection Green et al. (1980) mention the utility of the health belief model.

Enabling factors are factors antecedent to behaviour that allow a motivation or aspiration to be realized. Resources and skills necessary to facilitate health behaviours (for example health care facilities, personnel, and schools) are vital in this context. Examples of skills can range from the appropriate use of relaxation techniques and physical exercise, to the use of the variety of medical instruments and diagnostic procedures frequently required in self-care programmes. The concept of modelling, as employed by Bandura (1969), clearly plays an important role in enabling persons to adopt

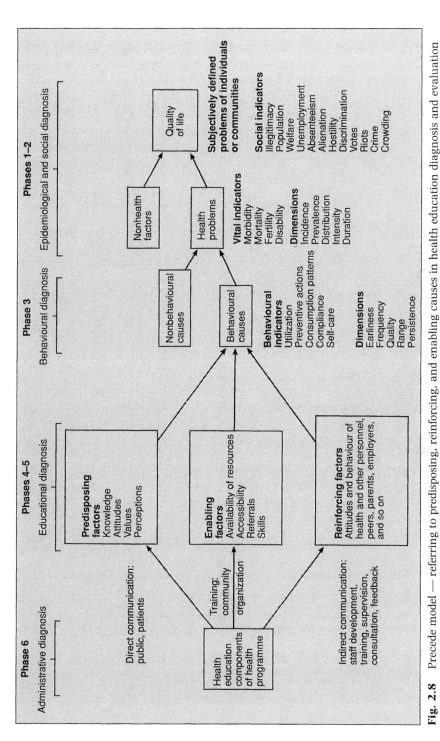

Fig. 2.8 Precede model — referring to predisposing, reinforcing, and enabling causes in health education diagnosis and evaluation (after Green *et al.* 1980).

behaviours conducive to health, and also in predisposing them toward such behaviours.

Reinforcing factors are those factors subsequent to behaviour which provide the continuing reward, incentive, or punishment for a behaviour and contribute to its persistence or disappearance.

Mullen *et al.* (1987) compare the health belief model, theory of reasoned action, and PRECEDE model to predict changes in smoking, exercise, and consumption of sweet and fried foods over an eight-month interval. The PRECEDE model accounted for more variance in behaviour (except for smoking) than both the other models, but it required far more questions. When intention, self-efficacy, and social network were added to the HBM, this 'new' model predicted about as much or more behaviour change as PRECEDE, except in the case of the number of cigarettes smoked.

Sense of coherence theory

Although Antonovsky's (1979) **sense of coherence** is a theoretical construct in understanding and dealing with health issues, the contribution of his construct to the field of behavioural health is obvious. Antonovsky has launched what he calls the salutogenic paradigm, which suggests that the normal state of affairs of the human organism is one of entropy, of disorder, and of disruption of homeostasis. The very core of the salutogenic paradigm is the focus on successful coping, on what may well be called behavioural immunology. The question is no longer 'What keeps one from getting sicker?' but 'What facilitates one's becoming healthier?' wherever one is at any given time on the health–disease continuum.

The sense of coherence (SOC) is defined as 'a global orientation that expresses the extent to which one has a pervasive, enduring though dynamic feeling of confidence that one's internal and external environments are predictable and that there is a high probability that things will work out as well as can reasonably be expected' (Antonovsky 1979). The construct includes three components (Antonovsky 1984), and is measured by means of a 29-item scale:

1. **comprehensibility** refers to the extent to which individuals perceive the stimuli that confront them as making cognitive sense; whether they have confidence that sense and order can be made of a situation.

2. **manageability** is the extent to which people perceive that resources at their disposal are adequate to meet the demands posed by stimuli. There is some similarity to Bandura's (1977*b*) concept of self-efficacy described previously. When people are high on manageability, they have the sense that, aided by their own resources *or by those of legitimate others*, they will be able to cope.

3. **meaningfulness** is the emotional counterpart to comprehensibility. People who are high on meaningfulness feel that life makes sense emotionally.

The stronger their SOC, the more people can avoid threat or danger. They are more likely to engage in activities that are health-promoting and to avoid those that are health-endangering. People's belief that life is meaningful, that they have resources to manage, and that life is ordered and predictable provides sound basis for such behaviours.

Spiral of silence theory

A number of theories can guide the development of programmes to change community environments in order to influence people's subjective norms and intentions. One guideline is Noelle-Neumann's **spiral of silence theory** (Noelle-Neumann 1974, 1977). This theory stresses the importance of dominating communication channels so the public perceives that the position being advocated is held by a majority in the community. According to Noelle-Neumann, and the evidence she gathered from repeated public opinion surveys, when a particular position is perceived as the majority position, those who oppose it will be less likely to voice their opposition because they fear social isolation. On the other hand, those who favour the position will be more likely to speak up, resulting in an upward spiralling of the amount of communication favouring the position which finally establishes the opinion as a community norm.

Health promotion model

Pender (1987) has presented the **health promotion model** as an organizing framework to guide research on health-promotion behaviour. Drawing from Bandura's social learning theory, this model proposes that the likelihood of engaging in health-promoting behaviours is associated with certain cognitive–perceptual factors, such as perceived importance of health and perceived control over health; demographic, biological, interpersonal, situational, and behavioural factors which may affect the predisposition to health-promoting behaviours; and internal or external cues to action. Many of the factors included in this model are based upon previous research. A number of studies have established a positive relationship between perceived personal control, perceived self-efficacy, and health behaviours such as success in weight loss, wearing seat-belts, and maintenance of smoking cessation.

Thus, Pender's model does not add any new concepts or dimensions regarding health behaviour prediction. It is suggested, however, that this model is particularly relevant to persons with disabilities, because Pender's contention is that health and illness are qualitatively different concepts: 'Health is the actualization of inherent and acquired human potential through goal-directed behaviour, competent self-care, and satisfying relationships with others while adjustments are made as needed to maintain structural integrity and harmony with the environment' (Pender 1987). In this definition, absence of illness or impairment is not a prerequisite for health.

Utility model of preventive behaviour

Within the framework of the economic theory of demand, Cohen (1984) has presented a **utility model of preventive behaviour**. The utility model assumes that all preventive behaviour can be expressed as the consumption of those 'goods' that affect the risk of illness or injury. Total utility yielded by risk-affecting goods is the sum of that derived from the use value of the goods, if any, and that from reduced anxiety which results from reduced risk.

The utility model retains the three elements from the HBM:

(1) the size of the threat, incorporating perceptions of likelihood and severity;

(2) the efficacy of the preventive action in reducing the size of the threat;

(3) the barriers to preventive actions.

But Cohen postulates that the primary motivating factor in preventive behaviour is the **anxiety associated with the threat**, rather than the threat itself. Anxiety results from an awareness of being at risk and, generally, any perceived reduction in risk will result in a reduction in anxiety.

The initial level of anxiety is dependent on:

(1) the perceived level of risk, which, in common with the 'threat' in the HBM, contains both a probability and a severity dimension;

(2) *when* the outcome is expected;

(3) the individual's attitude to present vs. future time;

(4) the degree to which the individual is averse to risk.

The benefits of consumption — that is, the reduction in anxiety — depend on the perceived efficacy of the good, service, or activity in reducing the perceived risk.

A major advantage of this approach is that it explains the consumption of all goods, whether preventive, hazardous, or neutral.

Some other less known models will be presented briefly.

Self-care deficit theory

Orem (1985) argues in this theory that although people may have the basic knowledge and skill to practise a health behaviour, they may lack motivation toward practising it consistently, representing a self-care deficit.

Self-regulation theory

The **self-regulation theory** is an information-processing theory that addresses how people cope with a stressor. It consists of three components: a schema (generalized, cognitive representation), a set of coping techniques, and a feedback process (Lauver 1987).

Model of positive health

A new **model of positive health** proposed by Seeman (1989) is based on a human-system framework — which is comprehensive in that

1. It encompasses all of the human system's behavioural subsystems (bio-chemical, physiological, perceptual, cognitive, and interpersonal).

2. It permits a higher asymptote of health conceptualization and measurement than that afforded by Western biomedical theory.

Model of adherence

Gritz *et al.* (1989) tested a six-factor **model of adherence** (DiMatteo and DiNicola 1982), including:

(1) effective provider communication;

(2) rapport with provider;

(3) client's beliefs and attitudes;

(4) client's social climate and norms;

(5) behavioural intentions;

(6) supports for and barriers to adherence.

Compliance studies have also used HBM — for example, regarding the compliance of periodontal patients given oral hygiene instructions (Kühner and Raetzke 1989). The HBM has proved to be a rather reliable predictor of patient compliance in medicine (for review see Haynes 1976; Becker 1979). Studies applying the HBM to dental compliance problems have not yielded unequivocal results (for review see Kühner and Raetzke, 1989). This is largely due to inadequate study designs and the problem that health beliefs are only a part of the social matrix in which behaviour occurs. However, significant correlations between health beliefs and compliance prevail as far as health behaviour of adults is concerned.

Social competence theory

Meichenbaum *et al.* (1981) use the term competence, similar to the concept of coping in that it also may be considered as a foundation or underlying factor related to the promotion of all identified health-related behaviours.

Categories of models of dental health behaviour

Kirkegaard and Borgnakke (1985) and Petersen (1985) have reviewed models employed to explain dental health behaviour. They distinguish between economic models, social–psychological models, interaction models, and models built on a conflict–sociological perspective.

Economic models

The **economic models** are developed mainly to explain how price and income influence the demand for health services. Holst (1982) has described how third-party payment systems can be assumed to influence the output, and examined the relationship between three major groups of structural determinants: objectives, organization, and financing.

Cohen's (1984) **utility model of preventive behaviour** should also be listed in this category. Cohen presents this alternative model of preventive behaviour in the belief that the insights provided from the perspective of another discipline can help in understanding those aspects of behaviour not fully explained by psycho-sociological analysis. Both this and another 'economic model', the social marketing model, are previously described.

Social–psychological models

The **social–psychological models** focus on perception of the disease, assessment of need, attitudes, and motives. Many of these models, which are among the most employed models in health behaviour research (such as the health belief model and the theory of reasoned action), are presented previously.

Interaction models

While many social–psychological models hold that attitudes are prerequisites for behaviour, those involved in the development of **interaction models** believe that behaviour causes attitude (Bem 1972). These are more complex models and incorporate a sociological perspective. Craft *et al.*'s (1981) trials of an integrated curriculum package in preventive dental health among English adolescents could be categorized under the label 'interaction model'.

Conflict theory

Petersen (1981) has constructed a model, built on **conflict theory**, to explain dental health behaviour of employees in a Danish manufacturing firm. The model is based on a holistic view. People's health-related behaviour is explained as a result of the social systems of which they are a part.

Comprehensive systems models — metamodels

Researchers have recently tried to bring the different models and theories together. Cummings *et al.* (1980) presented an excellent analysis of 14 empirical models, all of which had one common objective: to define and test a predictive model of health action from a psychosocial perspective. Their analysis suggests that while these models included a wide range of variables (109 variables), there are six sets of factors common to all models (judgements were obtained from the original authors of these models). These are:

(1) accessibility to health care;

(2) evaluation of/attitude to health care;

(3) perception of symptoms and threat of disease;

(4) social network characteristics;

(5) knowledge about disease; and

(6) demographic characteristics.

These six common factors are probably most relevant for health-care seeking, and not traditional health-promoting behaviour, in that the important dimensions of self-efficacy/HLC/manageability/perceived control are not incorporated.

A 'systems model' has been constructed by Kersell and Milsum (1985). Their model integrates social, environmental, psychological, and physiological factors, and takes into account social structure, cultural factors, situational factors, and intrapsychic factors. Kersell and Milsum have defined four levels within the model:

(1) external antecedent condition — parental and hereditary/genetic process and sociocultural environmental milieu;

(2) personal antecedent condition — personal demographic dynamics, personal socialization process, and personal health dynamics;

(3) social–psychological condition — perception of the self, perception of social influences, perception of health status, and perception of environmental factors;

(4) behavioural condition — intention formation process, skills, and behavioural repertoire.

Hunt and Martin's (1988) model of behavioural change draws together empirical findings and theoretical speculations from several disciplines, and is based on the proposal that the most used models (such as the value expectancy models) involve the questionable assumption that action is based upon a reasoned process. Its major drawback is its failure to deal with the fact that although behaviours may be health-related, they are not necessarily carried out *because of* their health implications.

Drawing together fragments of evidence from the wide variety of studies reported, it would seem that self-initiated behavioural change often occurs when some formerly routine activity is brought into awareness for a prolonged period of time, such that it becomes salient or problematic. This often takes place in conjunction with a change in the context in which the particular behaviour is being carried out, for example, a smoker going to live with a non-smoker.

Hayes and Ross (1987) as well as Ben-Sira (1991) support this conclusion. Ben-Sira's theoretically justified and empirically supported framework of health-protective behaviour suggests a distinction between types of behaviour according to the type and effort needed to engage in each (that is, the type of stimulus and enabling factors). His study highlights that health is not necessarily *the* incentive for health-protective behaviour. Other factors, such as external appearance, may have a greater weight than concern with health in motivating health-protective behaviour. Taking this line of reasoning a step further, Ben-Sira postulates that the data from his study (Ben-Sira 1991) as well as those of Hayes and Ross (1987) and Mullen *et al.* (1987) may explain the limitations of those models that conceive of 'susceptibility' (Rosenstock 1974) as the stimulus for inducing healthy persons to engage in health-protective behaviour.

Levy (1991) proposes a metaparadigm which is basically an analogical representation of a set of phenomena (Levy 1974). It is less than a full-blown theory and is not meant to result in immediate explanatory links between variables. It is a beginning or a crude approximation of the salient concepts to be refined with more precise and definitive functional relationships between variables.

Combining Endler's (1983) **interaction model of personality** with Levy's (1974) **conceptual paradigm for the study of play behaviour**, Levy suggests the following formula for the 'dynamic model of interaction':

$$B = f(P \times E),$$

where B = behaviour, f = function, P = person, and E = environment.

Foshee (1989) combines social learning theory (Bandura 1977*a*) with **social control theory** (Hirschi 1969) in an attempt to understand the parental influence on adolescent smoking.

Based upon field theory and attitude theories, Kar's (1983–84) **health promotion model** holds that in populations with comparable sociodemographic and biological status (exogenous variables) a health behaviour is a function of direct and interaction effects of *five* key intrapsychic and external variables.

(1) behavioural intentions;

(2) social support;

(3) accessibility of means for action;

(4) personal autonomy;

(5) action situation.

Thus the model is based upon a systems approach which integrates elements of Lewin's field theory (Lewin 1951), Fishbein's behavioural intention model (Ajzen and Fishbein 1977, 1980), psychosocial models of preventive health actions (Parsons 1951; Mechanic 1968; Leventhal and Gleary 1980; Rosenstock 1974), models of individual health behaviours (Cummings *et al.*

1980), and a cross-cultural validation of Kar's own model with large data sets from Venezuela, Kenya, and the Philippines (See Kar 1983–4). Findings from these studies suggest that while health promotion strategies deal with intrapsychic determinants of behaviour, key extrapsychic factors (such as social support, quality and accessibility of health-care measures, and situational factors) all have direct and independent effects on health behaviour as well. Health promotion research and interventions which aim exclusively at intrapsychic determinants would thus have rather limited overall value.

In the field of dental health Hølund (1991) and Faresjö *et al.* (1981) have constructed and tested **comprehensive models for dental health action**. Hølund's (1991) model is a combination of social learning theory, the information processing model, the group dynamic approach, and role-playing and used to test adolescents' sugar behaviour. She found the most important predictor of sugar consumption to be previous consumption, which in turn was mainly determined by peer group norms. Cognitive factors in terms of knowledge and beliefs, affective factors in terms of attitudes, and environmental factors in terms of socioeconomic status and gender did not add to the explanation of sugar consumption.

The intervention programme, based on group dynamics and role-playing, had no impact on knowledge and beliefs, while attitudes and behaviour changed. The intervention also included a special 'learning by teaching' approach. The 14-year-old target group gave lectures for 10-year-old schoolchildren.

Hølund concludes that the processes behind sweet-consumption among adolescents seem to be too complex to be explained by simple cognitive models. She asks for more interactionistic models of explanation (Hølund 1991).

Faresjö's model included:

(1) a general frame — including physical structure (e.g. fluoride) and societal structure (e.g. organization of dental services);

(2) individual components — including material (e.g. economy, education), social/political (e.g. dental care utilization), mental (e.g. knowledge, attitudes), and physical (e.g. sex, age).

All the factors were connected to the dental health action of the individual, and ultimately dental health. However, Faresjö *et al.* (1981) used only dental health, not behaviour, as the dependent variable when testing the model.

The elements of a comprehensive model (Aarø 1986) have to be borrowed from several academic disciplines:

(1) personality and individual psychology;

(2) social psychology;

(3) sociology;

(4) mass communication research and marketing research;

(5) political science and political economy.

Aarø and Nylenna (1987 have launched such a macro model built on many of the theories described previously, as well as empirical results from health education studies. They do not take a stand on the relationship between knowledge, attitude, and beliefs, but incorporate these three elements as a 'block' which is influenced through health education and which in turn influences the next 'block' of elements, namely: climate of opinions, social norms, and behavioural norms (Fig. 2.9). These elements then influence health behaviour, which ultimately influences health. In this model feedback processes between the 'blocks' are incorporated.

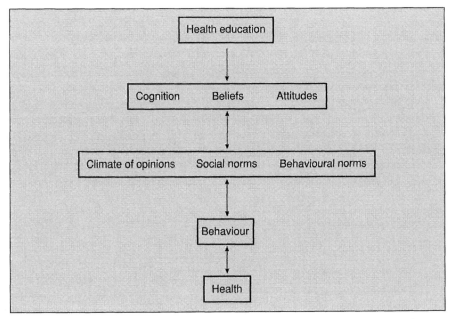

Fig. 2.9   The macro model of health behaviour (after Aarø and Nylenna 1987).

Concluding remarks

Different types of preventive health behaviour may be products of specific contexts, which may well include specific beliefs about the behaviour and specific circumstances associated with the decisions to adopt a particular preventive health behaviour (Calnan 1985).

Health behaviours may be considered as a dependent set of variables which are predicted by personal factors and environmental factors. Behaviour itself should also be considered as a predictor in a more dynamic and open system.

Furthermore, the economic and political structure of a society should be considered as an important predictor of the process leading to differences in health behaviour and health. The whole process of changes in health behaviour may be described at a macro level, emphasizing the time dimension and describing how innovations spread in a population.

The models of health behaviour reviewed here differ in some aspects in their theoretical perspectives. Many of them include variables and interrelationships which have not been empirically validated. Some of the models may be relevant to specific settings and specific types of preventive health behaviour.

Regardless of which theory, model, or combination of these we prefer, it is important to consider that each individual is surrounded by multiple sets of intercorrelating factors which influence his or her behaviour. Some factors are within the individual, some are in the formal and informal social network, and some are in the structure of the community as a whole. 'No individual is an island.'

Most of the models mentioned so far are based on the assumption that the ultimate success of preventive regimens is dependent upon people's willingness to undertake or maintain the required health behaviours. Such a perspective has serious limitations (Sheiham 1986): it places the responsibility for health mainly on the individual and does not take into account that the major determinants of health are the socioeconomic and environmental conditions under which people live. It is these conditions which to a large extent lead to unhealthy lifestyles.

Therefore, any discussion of health behaviour should be analysed against the more important background of environmental forces which predispose individuals towards unhealthy behaviours. For example, it is logical to assume that the sugary food a person eats was chosen by him. Yet, behind that choice lies a complex set of factors relating to the political, economic, cultural, and industrial reasons why sugar is so widely available and heavily promoted in industrialized societies (Sheiham 1986). Only a few of the models and theories reviewed have taken these dimensions into account. These are the PRECEDE, Kar's, and Levy's models.

Indeed, it may be unrealistic to expect a model to explain such complex behaviours as health behaviours. Without any ambition to find the 'final solution' Gadgil and Søgaard (unpublished) have, nevertheless, tried to synthesize the different models of knowledge, attitude, and behaviour change currently found in the literature. The interrelationship between these models is shown in Fig. 2.10 which highlights all possible sequences of the relationship between cognition, affect, and behaviour. All these linear hierarchies are models of processes going on continuously in the individual, depending on what kind of internal and external context the individual finds himself or herself in. It becomes a matter of punctuation of events in time, and the statement of observer preference, as to which hierarchical model(s) we prefer to use in order to explain changes within the individual. If this 'context model' is

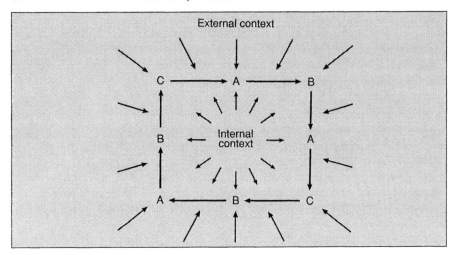

Fig. 2.10   The six possible linear hierarchies of the elements cognition (C), affect (A), and behaviour (B) — influenced by the internal and external contexts of the individual.

combined with the theory of diffusion of innovation, we may explain why different models of behaviour change may work or not work at different times, for different target groups (Fig. 2.11).

According to McQueen (1991) there is still no solid emergent theory of behavioural change, no grand synthesis of disciplinary perspectives leading to a new and better theoretical basis for research. Although no grand theory or model explaining health behaviour has been developed, several of the theore-

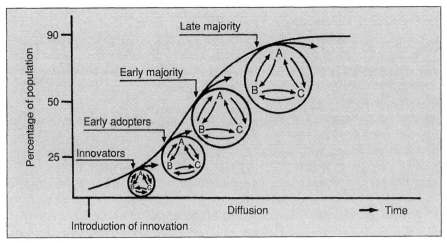

Fig. 2.11   The hierarchies of the elements cognition (C), affect (A), and behaviour (B) incorporated in the diffusion of innovation model.

tical perspectives referred to in this chapter contribute to a better understanding of the limitations of the present models and the specific needs for new theoretical perspectives.

It is important to remember that social science explanations are, at best, partial theories which can capture only some of the important influencing forces of behaviour. Each theory is an approximation of a different slice of reality or a different perspective on the same slice. Modelling will always be an oversimplification of the problem (Rise 1986). This means that the different social science disciplines should be regarded as complementary rather than competing strategies. The reader should seek to assimilate all the theories presented rather than to select a favourite.

References

Aarø, L. E. (1986). *Health behaviour and socioeconomic status. A survey among the adult population in Norway*. Thesis. University of Bergen, Bergen.

Aarø, L. E. and Nylenna, M. (1987), Helseopplysning. In *Kunnskap er makt — og bør deles med andre*, festskrift til Ole K. Harlems 70-års dag, (ed. P. Fugelli and M. Nylenna), pp. 70–81. Universitetsforlaget A/S, Oslo.

Aarø, L. E., Bruland, E., Hauknes, A., and Løchsen, M. P. (1983). Smoking among Norwegian school children 1975–1980. III. *Scandinavian Journal of Psychology*, **24**, 277–83.

Abelson, R. P., Aronsen, E., and McGuire, W., *et al.* (1968) *Theories of cognitive consistency*. Rand McNally, Chicago.

Ajzen, I. (1985). From intention to actions: a theory of planned behaviour. In *Action-control: from cognition to behavior*, (ed. J. Kuhl and J. Beckmann), pp. 11–39. Springer, Heidelberg.

Ajzen, I. and Fishbein, M. (1977). Attitude – behavior relations: a theoretical analysis and review of empirical research. *Psychological Bulletin*, **84**, 888–918.

Ajzen, I. and Fishbein, M. (1980). *Understanding attitudes and predicting social behavior*. Prentice-Hall, New Jersey.

Ajzen, I. and Madden, T. J. (1986). Prediction of goal-directed behavior: attitudes, intentions, and perceived behavioral control. *Journal of Experimental Social Psychology*, **22**, 453–74.

Antonovsky, A. (1979). *Health, stress and coping*. Jossey-Bass, San Francisco.

Antonovsky, A. (1984). The sense of coherence as a determinant of health. In *Behavioral health. A handbook of health enhancement and disease prevention*, (ed. J. D. Matarazzo, S. M. Weiss, J. A. Herd, *et al.*), pp. 114–29. Johan Wiley and Sons, New York.

Antonovsky, A. and Kats, R. (1970). The model dental patient: an empirical study of preventive health behavior. *Social Science and Medicine*, **4**, 367–80.

Aronsen, E. (1969). The theory of cognitive dissonance. In *Advances in experimental social psychology*, **4**, (ed. L. Berkowitz), pp. 2–35. Academic Press, New York.

Bandura, A. (1969). *Principles of behaviour modification*. Holt, Rinehart and Winston, New York.

Bandura, A. (1977a). *Social learning theory*. Prentice Hall, London.

Bandura, A. (1977b). Self-efficacy: towards a unifying theory of behavioral change. *Psychological Review*, **84**, 191–215.

Bandura, A. (1982). Self-efficacy mechanism in human agency. *American Psychologist*, **37**, 122–47.

Bandura, A. (1986). *Social foundations of thought and action: a social cognitive theory.* Prentice-Hall, New Jersey.

Baric, L. (1979). Non-smokers, smokers, ex-smokers: three separate problems for health education. *International Journal of Health Education*, **22** (no 1), supplement.

Bateman, P. M. (1985). *Understanding and predicting toothbrushing behaviour in adolescents.* MSc Report. London Hospital Medical College, London.

Bauman, K. E. (1980). *Research methods for community health and welfare.* Oxford University Press, New York.

Becker, M. (ed.) (1974). The health belief model and personal health behavior. *Health Education Monographs* **2**, 1–146.

Becker, M. H. (1979). Understanding patient compliance: the contributions of attitudes and other psychological factors. In *New directions in patient compliance*, (ed. S. Cohen), pp. 1–31. Health, Lexington, MA.

Becker, M. H. and Maiman, L. A. (1975). Sociobehavioral determinants of compliance with health and medical care recommendations. *Medical Care*, **13**, 10–24.

Ben-Sira, Z. (1991). Eclectic incentives for health protective behavior: an additional perspective on health oriented behavior change. *Health Education Research*, **6**, 211–29.

Bem, D. J. (1972). Self perception theory. An alternative interpretation of cognitive dissonance phenomena. In *Advances in experimental social psychology*, 6, (ed. L. Berkowitz), pp. 1–62. Academic Press, New York.

Bentler, L. F. and Speckart, G. (1979). Models of attitude – behavior relationship. *Psychological Review*, **86**, 451–64.

Calnan, M. (1985). Patterns in preventive behaviour: a study of women in middle age. *Social Sciences and Medicine*, **20**, 263–8.

Clark N. M. (1987). Social learning theory in current health education practice. In *Advances in health education and promotion*, (ed. W. B. Ward), vol 2, pp. 251–75. JAI Press, Greenwich, Conn.

Cohen, D. (1984). Utility model of preventive behaviour. *Journal of Epidemiology and Community Health*, **38**, 61–5

Coombs, J. A., Silversin, J. B., Rogers, E. M., and Drolette, M. E. (1981) The transfer of preventive health technologies to schools: A focus on implementation. *Social Science and Medicine*, **15**, 789–99.

Craft, M., Croucher, R., and Dickinson, J. (1981). Preventive dental health in adolescents: short and long term pupil response to trials of integrated curriculum package. *Community Dentistry and Oral Epidemiology*, **9**, 199–206.

Cummings, K. M., Becker M. H., and Maile, M. C. (1980). Bringing the models together: an empirical approach to combining variables used to explain health actions. *Journal of Behavioral Medicine*, **3**, 123–45.

Davis, K. E., Jackson, K. L., Kronenfeld, J. J., *et al.* (1984). Intent to participate in worksite health promotion activities: a model of risk factors and psychosocial variables. *Health Education Quarterly*, **11**, 361–77.

den Boer, D. -J., Kok, G., Hospers, H. J., *et al.* (1991). Health education strategies for attributional retraining and self-efficacy improvement. *Health Education Research*, **6**, 239–48.

DiMatteo, M. R. and DiNicola, D. D. (1982). *Achieving patient compliance: the psychology of the medical practitioner's role*. Pergamon Press, Elmsford, NY.

Earp, J. A. and Ennett, S. T. (1991). Conceptual models for health education research and practice. *Health Education Research*, **6**, 163–71.

Endler, N. S. (1983). Interactionism: a personality model, but not yet a theory. In *Nebraska symposium on motivation 1982*: Personality — current theory and research, (ed. M. M. Page), pp. 155–200. University of Nebraska Press, Lincoln, Nebraska.

Engel, J. F. and Blackwell, R. D. (1982). *Consumer behavior* (4th edn). The Dryden Press, New York.

Faresjö, T., Gamsäter, G., Hamp, S. -E., *et al.* (1981). Influence of social factors on the effect of different prophylactic regimens. *Swedish Dental Journal* Supplement 7.

Feldman, R. H. L. and Mayhew, P. C. (1984). Predicting nutrition behavior: the utilization of a social psychological model of health behavior. *Basic and Applied Social Psychology*, **5**, 183–95.

Festinger, L. (1957). *A theory of cognitive dissonance*. Row Peterson, Evanston, Illinois.

Festinger, L. (1962). Cognitive dissonance. *Scientific American*, **107**, 99–113.

Flay, B. R. (1981). On improving the chances of mass media health promotion programs causing meaningful changes in behavior. In *Health education by television and radio*, (ed. M. Meyer), pp. 57–91. K. G. Saur, München.

Fønnebø, V. and Søgaard, A. J. (1990). The penetrating educational effect of a mass media-based fund-raising campaign 'Heart for life'. *Scandinavian Journal of Social Medicine*, **18**, 185–93.

Foshee, V. (1989). *The role of parents in the initiation of adolescent cigarette smoking: an empirical investigation of control theory*. PhD dissertation. University of North Carolina, Chapel Hill, North Carolina.

Freeman, R. (1984). *Understanding and predicting sugar consumption in adolescents: factors affecting choice intention*. Thesis. London Hospital Medical College, London.

Freidson, E. (1960). Client control and medical behavior. *American Journal of Sociology*, **65**, 377–82.

Green, L. W. and McAlister, A. L. (1984). Macro-intervention to support health behaviour: some theoretical perspectives and practical reflections. *Health Education Quarterly*, **11**, 322–39.

Green, L., Kreuter, M. W., Deeds, S. G., and Partridge, K. B. (1980). *Health education planning. A diagnostic approach*. Mayfield Publishing Company, California.

Gritz, E. R., DiMatteo, M. R., and Hays, R. D. (1989). Methodological issues in adherence to cancer control regimens. *Preventive Medicine*, **18**, 711–20.

Hay, R. D., Stacy, A. W., and DiMatteo, M. R. (1987). Problem behaviour theory and adolescent alcohol use. *Addictive Behaviours*, **12**, 189–93.

Hayes, D. and Ross, C. (1987). Concern with appearance, health beliefs and eating habits. *Journal of Health and Social Behavior*, **28**, 120–30.

Haynes, R. B. (1976). A critical review of the 'determinants' of patient compliance with therapeutic regimens. In *Compliance with therapeutic regimens*, (ed. D. L. Sackett and R. B. Haynes), pp. 26–39. Johns Hopkins Press, Baltimore.

Heløe, L. A. and König, K. G. (1978). Oral hygiene and educational programs for caries prevention. *Caries Research*, **12**, Supplement 1, 83–93.

Hirschi, T. (1969). *Causes of delinquency*. University of California Press, Berkeley, CA.

Holst, D. (1982). *Third party payment in dentistry. An analysis of the effect of a third party system and of system determinants*. Thesis. University of Oslo, Oslo.

Hølund, U. (1991). *Explanation and change of adolescents' dietary behavior.* Thesis. The Royal Dental College, Aarhus.

Hoogstraten, J., De Haan, W., and Ter Horst, G. (1985). Stimulating the demand for dental care: an application of Azjen and Fishbein's theory of reasoned action. *European Journal of Social Psychology,* **15**, 401–14.

Hovland, C. I., Janis, I. L., and Kelley, H. H. (1953). *Communication and persuasion.* Yale University Press, New Haven.

Hunt, S. M. and Martin, C. J. (1988). Health-related behavioural change — a test of a new model. *Psychology and Health,* **2**, 209–30.

Janis, J. L. and King, B. T. (1954). The influence of role-playing on opinion change. *Journal of Abnormal and Social Psychology,* **49**, 211–18.

Janis, J. L. and Mann, L. (1977). *Decision making: a psychological analysis of conflict, choice and commitment.* The Free Press, New York.

Janz, N. K. and Becker, M. H. (1984). The health belief model: a decade later. *Health Education Quarterly,* **11**, 1–47.

Jensen, K. (1981a). Involvement of gatekeepers in school health education. *International Journal of Health Education,* **14**, Supplement, 1–23.

Jensen, K. (1981b). *Sundhedspædagogisk udviklingsarbejde.* Et demonstrastions — forskningsprosjekt om forebyggende tandpleje i skolen. Aarhus Odontologiske Boghandel, Århus.

Jessor, R. (1984). Adolescent development and behavioral health. In *Behavioral health: a handbook of health enhancement and disease prevention,* (ed. J. D. Matarazzo, S. M. Weiss, J. A. Herd, *et al.*), pp. 69–90. Wiley, New York.

Jessor, R. (1987). Problem-behaviour theory, psychosocial development, and adolescent problem drinking. *British Journal of Addiction,* **82**, 331–42.

Jessor, R. and Jessor, S. L. (1977). *Problem behavior and psychosocial development: a longitudinal study of youth.* Academic Press, New York.

Kar, S. B. (1983–4). Psychosocial environment: a health promotion model. *International Quarterly of Community Health Education,* **4**, 311–41.

Katz, E. (1957). The two-step flow of communication: an up-to-date report on an hypothesis. *Public Opinion Quarterly,* **21**, 61–78.

Katz, E. and Lazarsfeld, P. (1955). *Personal influence.* Glencoe, Illinois.

Kegeles, S. S. (1963). Why people seek dental care: a test of conceptual formulation. *Journal of Health and Social Behavior,* **4**, 166–73.

Kegeles, S. S. (1974). Current status of preventive dental health behavior in the population. *Health Education Monographs,* **2**, 197–200.

Kegeles, S. S. and Lund, A. K. (1982). Adolescent's health beliefs and acceptance of a novel preventive dental activity: replication and extension. *Health Education Quarterly,* **9**, 192–208.

Kegeles, S. S. and Lund, A. K. (1984). Adolescents' health beliefs and acceptance of a novel preventive dental activity: a further note. *Social Science and Medicine,* **19**, 979–82.

Kelly, H. H. (1973). The processes of causal attribution. *American Psychologist,* **28**, 107–28.

Kelly, H. H. (1978). A conversation with Edward E. Jones and Harold H. Kelley. In *Directions in attribution research* (ed. J. H. Harvey, W. J. Ickes, and R. F. Kidd), vol 2, pp. 371–88. Erlbaum, Hillsdale, NJ.

Kersell, M. W. and Milsum, J. H. (1985). A systems model of health behavior change. *Behavioral Science*, **30**, 119–26.

Kirkegaard, E. and Borgnakke, W. S. (1985). *Tandsykdomme, behandlings-behov og tandplejevaner hos et repræsentativt udsnit af den voksne danske befolkning.* (Voksenundersøgelsen). Licentiatafhandling. Institutt for Børnetandpleje og Samfundsodontologi. Århus Tandlægehøjskole, Århus.

Klepp, K. I. (1987). *Onset and development of drinking and driving among adolescents.* Thesis. University of Minnesota, Minneapolis.

Kotler, P. (1975). *Marketing for nonprofit organizations.* Prentice Hall, New Jersey.

Kühner, M. K. and Raetzke, P. B. (1989). The effect of health belief on the compliance of periodontal patients with oral hygiene instructions. *Journal of Periodontology*, **60**, 51–6.

Kühner, M. K. and Raetzke, P. B. (1989). Die Bedeutung des Health Belief Models, der Zahnheilkunde. In *Bedeutung der Patientenmitarbeit in der Zahnheilkunde*, (ed. T. Schneller and M. Kühner), pp. 22–38. Deutscher Aertze-Verlag, Køln.

Lauver, D. (1987). Theoretical perspectives relevant to breast self examination. *Advances in Nursing Science*, **9**, 16–24.

Leventhal, H. and Gleary, P. D. (1980). The smoking problem: a review of research and theory in behavioral risk. *Psychological Bulletin*, **88**, 370–405.

Levy, J. (1974). An applied intersystem congruence model of play, recreation, and leisure. *Human Factors*, **16**, 545–57.

Levy, J. (1991). A conceptual meta-paradigm for study of health behaviour and health promotion. *Health Education Research*, **6**, 195–202.

Lewin, K. (1943). Forces behind food habits and methods of change. *Bulletin of the National Research Council*, **108**, 35–65.

Lewin, K. (1947). Group decision and social change. In *Readings in social psychology*, (ed. T. Newcomb and E. Hartley), pp. 197–211. Holt, New York.

Lewin, K. (1951). *Field theory in social science.* Harper, New York.

Liska, A. E. (1984). A critical examination of the causal structure of the Fishbein/Azjen attitude – behavior model. *Social Psychology Quarterly*, **47**, 61–74.

Maccoby, N., Farquhar, J. W., Wood, P. D., *et al.* (1977). Reducing the risk of cardiovascular disease: effects of a community-based campaign on knowledge and behavior. *Community Health*, **3**, 100–14.

McGuire, W. (1978). An information-processing model of advertising effectiveness. In *Behavioral and management science in marketing*, (ed. H. L. Davis and A. J. Silk), pp. 156–80. Wiley, New York.

McGuire, W. J. (1984). Public communication as a strategy for inducing health-promoting behavioral change. *Preventive medicine*, **13**, 299–319.

McGuire, W.J. (1991). Using guiding idea theories of the person to develop educational campaigns against drug abuse and other health-threatening behavior. *Health Education Research*, **6**, 173–84.

McQueen, D. V. (1991). Editorial. *Health Education Research*, **6**, 137–9.

Marlatt, G. A. and Gordon, J. R. (1985). *Relapse prevention. Maintenance strategies in the treatment of addictive behaviors.* The Guilford Press, New York.

Maron, D. J., Telch, M. J., Killen, J. D., *et al.* (1986). Correlates of seat-belt use by adolescents: implications for health promotion. *Preventive Medicine*, **15**, 614–23.

Mechanic, D. (1968). *Medical sociology: a selected view.* The Free Press, New York.

Meichenbaum, D., Butler, L., and Gruson, L. (1981). Towards a conceptual model of social competence. In *Social competence*, (ed. J. Wine and M. Smye), pp. 32–89. Guilford Press, New York.

Mittelmark, M. B., Luepker, R. V., Jacobs, D. R., *et al.* (1986). Community-wide prevention of cardiovascular disease: education strategies of the Minnesota Heart Health Program. *Preventive Medicine*, **15**, 1–17.

Mullen, P. D., Hersey, J. C., and Iverson, D. C. (1987). Health behavior models compared. *Social Science and Medicine*, **24**, 973–81.

Noelle-Neumann, E. (1974) The spiral of silence: a theory of public opinion. *Journal of Communication*, **24**, 43–51.

Noelle-Neumann, E. (1977). Turbulence in the climate of opinion: methodological applications of the spiral of silence theory. *Public Opinion Quarterly*, **41**, 143–58.

Norman, R. M. G. (1985). *The nature and correlates of health behaviour*. Health Promotion Studies Series no. 2. Health Promotion Directorate, Health and Welfare, Ottawa.

Orem, D. E. (1985). *Nursing concept of practice* (3rd edn) McGraw-Hill, New York.

Parsons, T. (1951). *The social system*. Free Press of Glencoe, New York.

Pender, N. S. (1987), *Health promotion in nursing practice* (2nd edn). Appelton and Lange, East Norwalk, Connecticut.

Petersen, P. E. (1981). *Tandplejeadfærd, tandstatus og odontologisk behandlingsbehov blant arbejdere og funktionærer på en stor dansk industrivirksomhed. En socialodontologisk bedriftsundersøgelse*. Thesis. Odense Universitetsforlag, Odense.

Petersen, P. E. (1985). Sundheds — og sygdomsadfærd; begreber og teorier i sundhedssosiologien. *Tandlægebladet*, **89**, 451–8.

Prentice-Dunn, S. and Rogers, R. W. (1986). Protection motivation theory and preventive health: beyond the health belief model. *Health Education Research*, **1**, 153–61.

Puska, P., Nissinen, A., Tuomilehto, J., *et al.* (1985). The community-based strategy to prevent coronary heart disease: conclusions from the ten years of the North Karelia Project. *Annual Review of Public Health*, **6**, 147–93.

Ray, M. (1973). Marketing communication and the hierarchy-of-effects. In *New models for mass communication research*, (ed. P. Clark), pp. 147–76. Sage, Beverly Hill, CA.

Rise, J. (1986). Explaining health behavior. Response to Sheiham. In *Promotion of self care in oral health*, (ed. P. Gjermo), pp. 116–24. Scandinavian Group for Preventive Dentistry, Dental Faculty, Oslo.

Rise, J., Wold, B., and Aarø, L. E. (1991). Determinants of dental health behaviors in Nordic schoolchildren. *Community Dentistry and Oral Epidemiology*, **19**, 14–9.

Rogers, E. M. (1983). *Diffusion of innovations* (3rd edn). The Free Press, New York.

Rogers, E. M. and Shoemaker, F. F. (1971). *Communication of innovations. A cross-cultural approach* (2nd edn). The Free Press, New York.

Rogers, R. W. (1975). A protection motivation theory of fear appeals and attitude change. *Journal of Psychology*, **91**, 93–114.

Rogers, R. W. (1983), Cognitive and physiological processes in fear appeals and attitude change: a revised theory of protection motivation. In *Social psychology: a sourcebook*, (ed. J. R. Cacioppo and R. E. Petty), pp. 153–76. Guilford Press, New York.

Rosenstock, I. M. (1966). Why people use health services. *Milbank Memorial Fund Quarterly*, **44**, 94–127.

Rosenstock, I. M. (1974). The health belief model and preventive health behavior. *Health Education Monographs*, **2**, 354–86.

Rosenstock, I. M. Strecher, V. J., and Becker, M. H. (1988). Social learning theory and the health belief model. *Health Education Quarterly*, **15**, 175–83.

Rotter, J. B. (1954). *Social learning and clinical psychology*. Prentice Hall, New York.

Rotter, J. B., Chance, J., and Phares, E. J. (1972). *Applications of a social-learning theory*. Holt, Rinehart and Winston, New York.

Schifter, D. E. and Ajzen, D. E. (1985). Intention, perceived control and weight loss: an application of the theory of planned behavior. *Journal of Personality and Social Psychology*, **49**, 843–51.

Schunk, D. H. and Carbonari, J. P. (1984). Self-efficacy models. In *Behavioral health. A handbook of health enhancement and disease prevention*, (ed. J. D. Matarazzo, S. M. Weiss, J. A. Herd, *et al.*), pp. 230–47. John Wiley and Sons, New York.

Seeman, J. (1989). Towards a model of positive health. *American Psychology*, **8**, 1099–109.

Sheiham, A. (1986). Theories explaining health behavior. Position paper. In *Promotion of self care in oral health*, (ed. P. Gjermo), pp. 105–16. Scandinavian Working Group of Preventive Dentistry, Dental Faculty, Oslo.

Sherer, M., Maddux, J. E., Mercandante, B., *et al.* (1982). The self-efficacy scale: construction and validation. *Psychological Report*, **51**, 663–71.

Silversin, J. B. (1979). Strategies for improving your community's oral health. In *The handbook of health education*, (ed. P. M. Lazes), pp. 77–91. Aspen Systems Corporation, Germatown, Maryland.

Søgaard, A. J. (1986). Present state of dental health knowledge, attitudes and behavior and developmental trend in Scandinavia. In *Promotion of self care in oral health*, (ed. P. Gjermo), pp. 53–70. Scandinavian Working Group for Preventive Dentistry, Dental Faculty, University of Oslo, Oslo.

Søgaard, A. J. (1988). The effect of a mass media dental health education campaign. *Health Education Research*, **3**, 243–55.

Søgaard, A. J. (1989). *Health education and self-care in dentistry — surveys and inter-ventions*. Thesis. Institute of Community Medicine, University of Tromsø, Tromsø.

Søgaard, A. J. and Holst, D. (1988). The effect of different schoolbased dental health education programmes in Norway. *Community Dental Health*, **5**, 169–84.

Søgaard, A. J., Tuominen, R., Holst, D., and Gjermo, P. (1987). The effect of 2 teaching programs on the gingival health of 15-year-old schoolchildren. *Journal of Clinical Periodontology*, **14**, 165–70.

Strecher V. J., DeVellis B. M., Becker M. H., and Rosenstock, I. M. (1986). The role of self-efficacy in achieving health behavior change. *Health Education Quarterly*, **13**, 73–91.

Tones, K. (1987). Devising strategies for preventing drug misuse: the role of the Health Action Model. *Health Education Research*, **2**, 305–17.

Tones, K., Tilford, S., and Robinson Y. K. (1990). *Health education: effectiveness and efficiency*. Chapman and Hall, London.

Triandis, H. C. (1980). Values, attitudes and interpersonal behavior. In *Nebraska symposium on motivation, 1979; beliefs, attitudes and values*, (ed. M. M. Page), pp. 195–259. University of Nebraska Press, Lincoln, Nebraska.

Wallston, B. S. and Wallston, K. A. (1984). Social psychological models of health behavior: an examination and integration. In *Handbook of psychology and health*, (ed.

A. Baum, S. E. Taylor, and J. E. Singer), pp. 22–53. Lawrence Erlbaum, Hillsdale, New Jersey.

Wallston, K. A., Wallston, B. S., and DeVellis, R. (1978). Development of the multi-dimensional health locus of control (MHLC) scales. *Health Education Monographs*, **6**, 160–70.

Weisenberg, M., Kegeles, S. S., and Lund, A. K. (1980). Children's health beliefs and acceptance of dental preventive activity. *Journal of Health and Social Behavior*, **21**, 59–74.

Yalow, E. S. and Collins, J. L. (1987). Self-efficacy in health behavior change: Issues in measurement and research design. In *Advances in health education and promotion*, (ed. W. B. Ward), vol 2, pp. 181–99. JAI Press, Greenwich, Conn.

3

Social factors in oral health promotion

HELEN C. GIFT

Introduction

The purpose of this chapter is to consider the range of social factors which are either correlates or determinants of oral health, oral disease prevention, or health promotion strategies. Social factors represent customs, values, and behaviours of cultures, societies, and social networks, and arise, directly or indirectly, from the associations of individuals with each other, social groups, and society.[1] Social factors are associated with many of the major processes that lead to oral diseases or dysfunction, including: exposure of individuals to conditions that lead to illness; susceptibility of people to disease; socially determined habits, customs, and values; as well as general social changes such as economic cycles and technological development which alter resources and ultimately health.

To effect the most positive changes in oral health through oral health promotion strategies, social factors must be acknowledged, understood, and addressed through individual, social group and network, organizational, institutional, community, political, societal, and cultural mechanisms. Thus, oral health promotion goes beyond the biological emphasis on disease in the medical model, and recognizes the complex of physical, biological, cultural, and societal,

---

[1] For the purposes of this chapter, *culture* is defined as the sum total of the attainments and activities of any specific race or people including their beliefs, customs, institutions, attitudes, and technology. An *institution* is the established order of organized society as seen, for example, in the family. *Social organizations* are arrangements and relations of individuals to one another to assist in subsistence and protection, as exemplified by the food industry. The *community* is the basic unit of organized culture. It is a system encompassing social norms or values and cultural behaviours in interdependent institutions within a specific geographic space. The term *oral health promotion*, as used in this Chapter, encompasses primary disease prevention as well as strategies which help maintain good oral health through improved knowledge, lifestyle, and environment.

While a global approach is taken in this chapter, it is written from the perspective of the social sciences and health literature published in the English language, which may result in a bias toward Western, industrialized countries.

economic, health-delivery system, and patterned lifestyle factors with positive or negative effects on health and/or health-related behaviours (Fig. 3.1).

While most of the aggregate burden of oral dysfunctions in any population can be reduced through known preventive and early intervention approaches, many people manifest oral diseases and disorders and do not exhibit appropriate oral health promoting behaviours. Beyond employing known preventive and therapeutic approaches, success of oral health promotion also requires:

(1) a supportive social and physical environment which provides the health services and education, as well as community and work environments, which are safe and healthy;

(2) knowledgeable and positively orientated health services practitioners who are accessible to individuals and groups requiring dental care;

(3) knowledgeable and positively orientated individuals and groups who believe oral health is important.

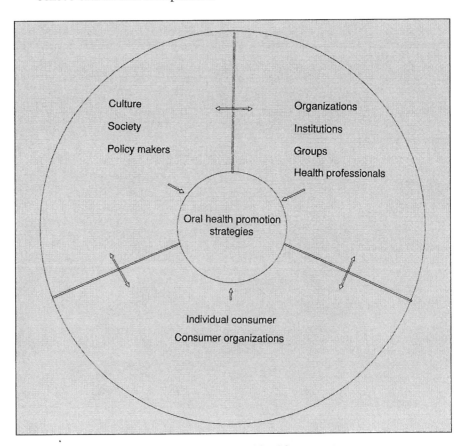

Fig. 3.1   Interaction of social factors with oral health promotion.

Effective oral health promotion strategies must focus on the structure and process of assuring the availability of, and access to, appropriate oral health education and services, particularly preventive technology. Oral health promotion is the mechanism unifying primary preventive regimens with their adoption and consistent use by communities, professional organizations, or other institutional groups, and individuals. Social and environmental factors have the greatest impact on this translation into practice.

To fully understand the interrelation of social factors with oral health promotion, the concept of risk factors is important. Risk factors occur at the biological, environmental, and behavioural levels and result in an increased probability of an unwanted outcome. The ideal outcome of oral health promotion is to modify risk factors, through environmental channels, professional behaviours, and individual actions, in order to prevent oral conditions before they occur. To do this, it is important to know the risk factors and what is available to ameliorate them. The next section in this chapter provides a brief overview of oral diseases and disorders, as well as their associated biological and other known risk factors, and available preventive approaches. This material provides the basis for the discussion of social determinants on oral health outcomes which follows later in the chapter.

Oral function and dysfunction, established risk factors, and known preventive interventions

Oral function can affect quality of life by permitting optimal chewing, eating, speaking, and other primary human needs. Oral dysfunction can affect quality of life by interacting with systemic functional status and self-perception of general and oral well-being. The most notable conditions or diseases that may lead to oral dysfunction are untreated caries and periodontal diseases; tooth loss; oral mucosal alterations related to soft tissue lesions, precancers, and cancer; acquired defects such as those associated with trauma; and congenital conditions as exemplified by cleft lip or palate anomalies and malocclusion.

Dental caries

The dental caries process is a result of the interaction of several risk factors accompanied by plaque formation: a susceptible tooth surface; the presence of sufficient numbers of cariogenic micro-organisms; and ingestion of a caries-conducive diet. Other contributing factors are inadequate fluoride exposure and sealant coverage; a history of high caries experience; reduced or altered salivary flow; and poor oral hygiene. In the case of severe caries, pain can be a major dysfunction.

The most effective and practical means of reducing caries demonstrated to date is the provision of optimal exposure to systemic and topical fluorides.

Fluorides act primarily by facilitating the remineralization of enamel, may strengthen the enamel, and serve as an antibacterial agent against cariogenic micro-organisms. In the presence of optimal fluoride, the impact of diet on caries is not as clear-cut. Therapeutic fluorides are available in a variety of modalities, which have been shown to be effective against caries in varying degrees when used either singly or in combination. Community water fluoridation has been a major effort for a generation, particularly in the United States. In localities without central water systems the fluoridation of the water supplies serving individual schools has been useful; for example, in rural areas where schools are in consolidated buildings that have a separate water supply (Horowitz 1983, 1984). Also, other school-based approaches have been demonstrated to be effective, including daily use of fluoride tablets and weekly mouthrinsing with fluoride solutions.

Those surfaces of the tooth that benefit the least from fluorides are those that contain pits and fissures, e.g. the chewing surfaces of posterior teeth. A key method for reducing the susceptibility of these tooth surfaces is through the provision of dental sealants. Thus, a combination of fluorides and dental sealants can result in teeth with low resistance to dental caries. Lack of access to a professional who applies sealants is a key contributing factor to caries incidence in children and adolescents with erupting permanent teeth at risk to caries.

Self-administered oral hygiene procedures can help in the removal of plaque. However, toothbrushing as performed by most individuals has been shown to reduce caries only if it is employed with a fluoride-containing dentifrice.

The incidence of dental caries can be affected by reducing consumption of cariogenic food or by adequate oral hygiene immediately following the ingestion of cariogenic foods (Newburn 1982; Schou 1991). The impact which dietary practices have on the development of caries is most evident in 'baby bottle tooth decay' — the major dental problem among children under three years of age (Ripa 1988). This has been attributed to nursing at will or allowing a child to feed for an extended period or sleep with a bottle containing liquid conducive to the formation of caries.

Controlling dental caries through diet modification is complex and has met with only limited success. The precise cariogenicity of any food is not easily predicted, people eat a mixed diet, and the sequence of eating various foods and the form of the foods may affect the cariogenic potential (Newburn 1982). Also, it appears that the association between sugar consumption and caries experience weakens when caries decline in general, possibly when the level of sugar intake is high in a population, and in the presence of optimal fluoride (Schou 1991). Children appear to know the association of sugars with dental decay, but their behaviours are not health-promoting in this regard (Horowitz and Larach 1991). Community-based or school programmes directed at dietary changes have indicated short-term successes (Schou *et al.* 1990*b*), and attempts have been made at the population level to replace sugar with substitutes in snack foods, beverages, and chewing-gums (Corbin 1991). The complexity of these individual behaviour modifications or social changes suggests that population-wide oral health promotion based on diet modification is less practical than other caries prevention strategies (Corbin 1991; Horowitz and Larach 1991; Schou et al. 1990b).

Periodontal diseases

Periodontal diseases are infections of the gingival and supporting-bone tissues of teeth thought to be caused by bacteria contained in plaque. The most widely accepted methods for controlling periodontal conditions are personally and professionally applied mechanical oral hygiene measures.

Oral mucosal alterations

Oral mucosal alterations are often a result of local conditions such as poorly fitting dentures; saliva secretion; long-term use of antibiotics; medications with xerostomic side effects; and systemic conditions. Close monitoring and treatment of these conditions, through collaboration among health care providers, could lead to reductions in soft tissue lesions for medically high-risk individuals among whom the chronic diseases themselves, or associated medications or treatments, result in oral lesions.

Immunodeficiencies may result in oral soft-tissue manifestations. For example, being HIV-positive is a factor contributing to oral soft tissue lesions. HIV-infected individuals (those with AIDS, AIDS-related complex (ARC), and healthy individuals who are seropositive) may exhibit oral manifestations, such as candidiasis and hairy leukoplakia.

Oral precancers and cancer

Oral precancers and cancer are potentially the most damaging of oral diseases. Many precancers and cancer are the result of excessive use of tobacco (smoking and smokeless) and alcohol. These can be prevented through elimination of tobacco use and reduction in alcohol consumption. Due to the serious nature of these lesions, their early identification is critical. Surgical interventions to remove cancers of the head and neck are invasive and, in fact, result in a common disease-related source of acquired craniofacial defects.

Oral and facial trauma

The primary causes of oral and facial trauma are falls, accidents, sporting events where the face is unprotected, and physical abuse or interpersonal violence. Protective mouth and head gear for sports and occupant restraints in automobiles are the primary ways of reducing oral and facial trauma from some of these sources. Dental personnel can work closely with social services workers to decrease the impacts of such trauma.

Cleft lip and palate

Cleft lip and palate, and most instances of malocclusion, are notable among oral conditions as traits which have their origins in inherited genetic materials. While direct genetic factors associated with cleft and malocclusion are difficult to address, rehabilitation potential is great. The dysfunctional aspects of cleft conditions can be reduced through early intervention and linkages among professionals working in health care and social work fields. Even though prevention is not presently an option, malocclusions can generally be corrected by professional interventions.

Tooth loss

Tooth loss is the ultimate sequel of untreated caries, untreated advanced periodontal diseases, oral cancer, trauma, and extractions as part of orthodontic treatment, and is an expression of the kinds of preventive or treatment services received or not received. Reductions in tooth loss in the population could be achieved by preventing the diseases or conditions that cause tooth loss and by receipt of appropriate interceptive and restorative care.

Other oral structures and functions

Other oral structures and functions, including salivary gland function, oral chemosensory performance (taste and smell), and oral motor function are less well understood. Risk factors include iatrogenic causes such as medications (including chemotherapy) and inadequate or inappropriate dental care.

The impact of any intervention or preventive measure is dependent on several factors operating together: its availability, its actual clinical efficacy, its cost and degree of access, and the presence of combined efforts of the community, profession, and individual in ensuring that the measure is used appropriately. At the community level, prevention of oral diseases can be provided to target populations as a public health measure. Community-based measures have the advantage of reaching a large number of individuals but do not maximize individual variations and needs. Health professionals (dentists, dental hygienists, nurses, health visitors, teachers, physicians, and so on) can provide preventive procedures either in the dental/medical office or in school-based and community-based settings. The provision of disease-prevention services within a clinical-care setting has the advantage of being individualized to specific needs, yet has the burdens of time and cost. Only those individuals who become patients, however, have the benefit of these professionally provided measures. Individually based measures are intended for use at home, work, or school. The long-term benefits of self-administered or professionally-provided preventive regimens, such as diet control, can be excellent, but are dependent on compliance of the professional, patient, or parent in applying these regimens appropriately. Maximizing oral health promotion requires an interdisciplinary team as well as an appropriate mix of these community-based and professionally and/or individually administered preventive interventions.

The social process and context of oral function and dysfunction

Illness is not solely a biological and physical phenomenon, but occurs within a social context. Social factors may initiate or promote a disease process. These factors may also affect the definition or recognition of, or response to, a disease as a problem. When it is so defined, it becomes an illness. For example, the necessary biological conditions must be present for oral cancer to occur, yet the social behaviour of excessive tobacco use is a known cofactor, as is excessive alcohol consumption. In this case, these behaviours actually interact with biological factors to produce the illness. Herpes labialis results from the effects of herpes simplex virus, yet the condition is exhibited most often when environmental or social conditions such as emotional stress or overexposure to ultraviolet light exist. Additionally, social factors may create stress which alters physiological balance and symptoms of disease, thus aggravating or facilitating the biological or physical disease-causing agents. Also, stress may affect the acceptance or completion of an episode of professionally provided dental care.

While the consequences specific to oral diseases are considerable, all evidence suggests that oral diseases and disorders and lack of treatment for these conditions may compound not only existing systemic medical conditions but also socially based dysfunctions associated with low income, minority status, or disadvantaged housing; functions which on the surface seem remote from health care or prevention services. As an extreme illustration, a poor, depressed, edentulous person with oral lesions, may have arthritis and severe cardiovascular disease, and live in a third-floor apartment with access only by stairs. This individual has economic, emotional, dental, and systemic health problems in addition to housing problems (Brody 1990). It is all too easy for a dentist to suggest that coming to the office for dental services is necessary. Health promotion strategies, however, require that the solutions for oral problems be considered within the context of the individual's general health care strategies and be achievable within the social environmental constraints operating for that individual.

Social factors operate in many ways to affect the efficacy of oral health promotion (Gift 1991). Social factors are often *indicative of inequities or barriers* to care (e.g. language as an inability to communicate or understand meaning). An individual's involvement in oral health promotion is not a random event but rather is structured by a variety of demographic, social status, organizational, and environmental resources, such that individuals in lower socioeconomic groups are exposed to a more unhealthy environment (lifestyle), and deprivation may result in health inequality. Alternatively, it is possible that persons in poor health tend to move down the socioeconomic and occupational scale because they are unable to act on opportunities. Others contend that individuals choose behaviours and harm their health through poor choices (King 1972; Petersen 1990).

Social inequalities may occur at the community and society level. For example, communal water fluoridation, healthy work environments, relevant social policies, and availability of health care services can affect oral health promotion. The interaction of community and organizational characteristics with the individual's background (as measured by factors such as having a usual source of care, the utilization of that care, and past oral health state) can affect the individual's current state of oral health, knowledge, beliefs, expectations, and actual exposure to any oral health promoting event.

Social and cultural factors are often *'proxies' for attitudes and beliefs.* Many obstacles or incentives have their roots in sociocultural norms of the society in which individuals live, while others can be traced to family practices independent of societal practices or norms. Individual attitudes, knowledge, and behaviours determine what a person knows about oral diseases and their prevention and control; how information is interpreted and decided upon; and what action is ultimately taken. For example, attitudes appear to be more highly correlated with dental visits among those who have to pay for their own care (Davies *et al.* 1987; Kiyak 1989). Some attitude measures, such as perceived need, appreciation of action for delayed benefit, and value ascribed to health, are salient in predicting both utilization of services and oral hygiene behaviours, and represent the linkage between values and actions occurring within a social system. Individual attitudes, knowledge, and behaviours may be mediated by psychological barriers (such as fear, anxiety, or suspicion). Similarly they can be mediated by incentives, such as concerns for personal appearance; priority toward oral health and dental care; access to knowledge regarding oral health or prevention and treatment techniques; access to knowledge regarding financial assistance programmes and dental care programmes; regular self-care activities; and regular use of dental services.

Many social characteristics may be *indirect measures of other undetected factors.* For example, ethnic status may indicate a particular dietary pattern as well as other genetic or social risk factors. Measures of social factors may overlap or be related to other risks (Alvarez *et al.* 1988). For example, Hispanic ethnicity in the United States is highly correlated with language barriers, low income and education, as well as lack of insurance and a regular source of health care (Andersen *et al.* 1986).

A social factor, or a combination of social factors, may result in *differing responses to oral health and behaviours:* how individuals feel about themselves, or how they interact with their environments. One factor, such as ethnicity, may change those responses even if other social conditions, such as poverty and discrimination, are shared commonly with other groups. An individual's assessment of physical well-being appears to be influenced by social factors, such as position in the socioeconomic structure, being male or female, black or white, high or low income, educated or uneducated, rural or urban (Kiyak 1989).

Social factors represent and create a *lifestyle*. This lifestyle represents patterns of behaviours and social support networks and is strongly associated with dental visits, oral hygiene self-care practices, and oral health status.

The lifestyle concept is well illustrated by tobacco use in relation to oral hygiene, periodontal diseases, and oral cancers. Behaviours deeply seated in cultural norms, such as use of tobacco, betel nuts, pan chulta, and bid cigarettes in south-east Asia, result in exceptionally high rates of oral precancers and cancers (Binnie *et al.* 1983). Factors influencing smoking and chewing in Western societies include the cultural association of smoking with relaxation, attractiveness, and emancipation; the social structure of tobacco production, processing, distribution, and legislation; and explicit advertising based on influential personalities and peers who favour smoking. The social environment, which implicitly encourages people to start and continue smoking, and individual behaviours, are key social factors which have been addressed with some success in oral health promotion among selected groups in the United States (Smoking and Tobacco Control Taskforce 1991).

Another example of the lifestyle interpretation is the intercorrelation of social factors with dental utilization. Women and school-age children traditionally attend the dental office more often than males and other age groups. Non-white, poor, uninsured, less educated, and rural portions of the population have lower rates of utilization of oral health services than do whites and those with economic advantages and access. In the Rand Health Experiment in the United States, younger persons, those with lower incomes, and those with less generous dental insurance were less likely to see the dentist than were other, more advantaged individuals, regardless of underlying differences in oral health, perceptions, attitudes, and regular source of care (Davies *et al.* 1987).

In the past decade, the influence of social factors on individual attitudes, knowledge, and behaviours, as well as the importance of perceptions of self and others, has become better understood. Also, additional information is now available on the influence of social factors on oral health promotion at the institutional and organizational levels (as represented by provider characteristics and dental services delivery mechanisms), and at societal and cultural levels.

Social factors associated with oral health promotion

Social factors can determine the nature or character of oral health promotion, its processes and outcomes. These factors can operate at the individual (micro) level, at the institutional, organizational, and social network (meso) level, and at the cultural, societal, and political (macro) levels (Petersen 1990). The individual factors are typically described in sociodemographic or economic terms to depict those segments of the population in which oral diseases and disabilities are concentrated. Social factors at the meso level are often descriptive of interactions among individuals in the context of social groups and organizations which, in turn, affect individual values and behaviours. The macro-level factors represent the influence of general societal conditions or cultural norms on the nature of social institutions and their associated technologies. Also, macro-level political and economic challenges may place limitations on individuals and social groups. These levels interact with each other; but for the purposes of this presentation will be considered sequentially, and social factors will be grouped under only one level.

Individual characteristics at the micro level

Often oral diseases and disabilities are concentrated in selected segments of the population. Micro-level social factors are direct measures of the individual's ability to garner resources from or achieve status in a particular cultural, societal, community, or family group described later in this chapter. For example, individual characteristics such as age, gender, race, and ethnicity may designate an individual's position in the social structure. They also may serve as proxy measures to reflect the impact of social policies on oral health promotion for specific groups. An individual's ability to pay, as measured by income or insurance, for example, can reflect the availability of jobs in the community, the availability of insurance or access to public assistance associated with employment, or eligibility for state programmes. Individual factors can be thought of as enabling an action to occur in that education, type of employment, experience with the dental delivery system, social isolation, or availability and quality of child-care either singly, or in combination, can serve to encourage or inhibit an appropriate oral health behaviour.

Age

Age is correlated with the occurrence of oral diseases and conditions, as well as with the use of dental services. Yet, there is little evidence that ageing itself, representing changes in host resistance, is a cause of oral diseases and disorders. Rather, exposures to general systemic diseases, trauma, and adverse environmental and social conditions are more common in certain age groups and, overall, result in a cumulative impact represented by chronological age.

Age becomes a proxy for societal and cultural influences evidenced in cohort effects and becomes an example of managing social political change. Within any age group other social factors interact to affect outcomes of oral health promotion. For example, some older adults can face critical barriers related to limitations of fixed income, lack of transportation, restricted housing, physical or social isolation, or other constraints.

Additionally, age appears to reflect congruent attitudes. For example, older adults who perceive barriers to seeking oral health care are often those who stereotype themselves; believe that poor oral health is a product of ageing; do not see oral health as part of general health; think that nothing can be done to maintain acceptable oral health levels; perceive themselves as frail; and perceive that income will not meet expenses (Antczak and Branch 1985; Schou and Eadie 1991).

The environmental conditions and cultural norms existing at the time an individual is young may create an imprint which affects not only actual levels of oral health in later years but also basic attitudes. Since most of today's older individuals were raised in a time and circumstance when fluoride vehicles for caries prevention and oral hygiene aids were less widespread, and restorative techniques were less refined, it is not surprising that older adults have more oral diseases and lower expectations of the delivery system. As the next century approaches, however, a more knowledgeable older age cohort will, no doubt, exhibit greater expectations for continuous and regular preventive as well as restorative services.

Gender

Men and women often occupy different positions in a society's social structure. Traditional role values may be expressed by women who are the caretakers and who arrange health care appointments for all family members. When both parents work, however, the father may bring the child for dental care, receive advice, yet not transmit that information to the mother who is the primary care-giver in the home. Differences in roles of genders for specific age cohorts, occupational groups, or family structures should be recognized by planners of health promotion programmes in order to target given oral health promotion activities more appropriately.

Historical gender differences in utilization of oral health services appear to be decreasing. Recent evidence in the United States suggests that men visit the dentist more for symptomatic needs while women tend to be more routine attenders. Women appear to both engage in self-care and to visit dental offices more regularly than do men (Davies *et al.* 1987). Other gender differences are based on behaviour patterns, for example, men are more likely than women to experience orofacial trauma and oral cancers.

Race and ethnicity

Racial, ethnic, and immigrant minority populations in most countries are at a health disadvantage. The unmet needs are greater and the use of services less frequent among minorities in all types of delivery systems (Blaxter 1983), A disproportionate concentration of racial and ethnic minorities living in industrialized countries is at the lower end of the socioeconomic scale, particularly as measured by education and income (Andersen *et al.* 1986). Thus, in addition to culture, language, shared norms, values, and practices, which differ from the predominant population and may create barriers, ability to pay becomes a critical problem. In the United States, for example, 20 per cent of all children under the age of 18 are being raised in families with incomes below poverty standards, and of these children 45 per cent are black and 39 per cent are Hispanic. In addition, minority groups often live in areas with ineffective schools, high rates of dependence on public assistance, severe problems of crime and drug use, fewer sources of routine care, and low and declining employment (Jaynes and Williams 1989).

There are some specific sociocultural factors which are significant in considering the economic and health status of ethnic and racial minorities. Social isolation, as reflected by language or culture, usually restricts availability of information. Yet, information about oral health promotion opportunities, including availability of services, costs and eligibility for programme enrolment, are critical to obtain access. This is a particular concern for newly arrived immigrant populations. While preserving their cultural identity, their use of other than the primary language of the country of residence becomes a major barrier to education, employment, and utilization of social and health services. In some cases, illegal entry into the country further complicates access to employment, as well as health care and social services (Kiyak 1989).

Ethnicity, as a measure of traditional values, affects individual knowledge, attitudes, and behaviours. These, in turn, affect how symptoms are interpreted and what response is given. For example, sociocultural predispositions of Hispanics in the United States towards the use of the health care system have been proposed as an explanation of low use of services, and consequently, health (Andersen et al. 1986), Also, 'baby bottle caries', frequently found in lower socioeconomic class American Indian and Hispanic populations in the United States, is often attributed to feeding behaviours reflective of prevailing attitudes toward child care (Bruerd et al. 1989). Persons of Asian and Pacific Island backgrounds in the United States appear to rely heavily on non-Western medicine or family support systems for resolution of their health problems. It has been suggested that in these Asian and Pacific Island populations there is some sense of shame in the use of public services which is viewed as an indicator of dependency and inability to care for oneself (Kiyak 1989). In the case of occlusion, where there is some evidence of racial differences, attitudes toward the importance of occlusion and the accessibility to appropriate services result in different definitions of treatment needs.

Patterns of interaction in the family and among peers also may vary by ethnic groups, resulting in differential risks for oral diseases and disorders. All types of head injuries are more common among non-whites in the United States, because of the high prevalence of violent behaviours (Alvarez et al. 1988).

Race and ethnicity are highly correlated with measures of oral health, oral hygiene behaviours, overall use of dental services, and receipt of symptomatic dental care in the United States. Even though the medical and dental care systems have been expanding, poor minority persons (blacks, uninsured groups, people on public assistance) have considerably more unmet needs than do others. The proportion of United States black individuals covered by any private or public insurance has decreased during the 1980s (Andersen *et al.* 1986; Jaynes and Williams 1989).

While race and ethnicity represent cultural and lifestyle orientations reflected by differential knowledge, attitudes, and behaviours, much of the effect on oral health is indirect (Davies *et al.* 1987). Low socioeconomic status and associated maldistribution of, and accessibility to, services appear to explain much of the variance in oral health status (higher rates of caries and periodontal diseases) and unfavourable health-related attitudes and actions among minority groups.

Educational attainment

Level of formal education appears to be one of the most powerful forces in oral health. Dental knowledge, positive attitudes, regular use of services, and continuity of care are highly correlated with formal education. Education appears to reflect an improvement in both orientation and specific oral health knowledge (Gift 1986, 1988; Gift *et al.* 1990).

Individual socioeconomic status

In market-based economies in particular, socioeconomic characteristics are often measures of individual resources, reflecting general current social conditions and previous lifestyle. Socioeconomic status can have either a negative or a positive effect on an individual's oral health status; health promoting knowledge, attitudes, and behaviours; out-of-pocket cost of care; and potential outcome of any oral health promotion activities. A lower socioeconomic status individual usually has less prior and current access to health-sustaining resources in society, such as food, shelter, basic education; a lower level of oral health; health orientations inconsistent with professional norms; and absence of a regular source of care. In contrast, an upper socioeconomic status individual usually reflects adherence to self-care practices and other behaviours reflective of oral health promoting actions.

Socioeconomic status in industrial countries is inversely related to most measures of oral diseases (caries, edentulousness, periodontal diseases) and treatment need. Also, there is a positive relation between income, education, occupation, and oral hygiene behaviours and dental utilization (composite indicators of oral health promotion actions). The impact of socioeconomic forces on oral health status and use of services seems to remain after other confounding factors are controlled (Belangér 1988; Grembowski *et al.* 1989; Petersen 1990).

To a certain extent there has been a compression in the differences among socioeconomic and demographic groups over the years with respect to oral health status and behaviour measures. In all socioeconomic groups there has been a decrease in the proportion of individuals who have lost most or all of their teeth. These changes appear to reflect dynamics in general social–cultural orientations which ultimately affect the individual. Yet, oral problems are often magnified within the increasingly large segment of the population at the low end of the socioeconomic scale which often is culturally separated from the predominant population in the country. This same segment of the population all too often exhibits a higher incidence of chronic and infectious diseases and disabilities (Jaynes and Williams 1989).

Employment and occupational status

Employment status and nature of employment are related to oral health status and use of services. At the most basic levels, type of employment represents a lifestyle, and often determines availability of dental insurance or accessibility of services during non-working hours.

Social inequality in treatment needs has been evident in many adult employed populations. For example, in Scotland manual workers were found to have more treatment needs than did non-manual workers (Vogan 1970). Among Danish industrial workers, individuals in shift work had more untreated dental decay than did those in non-shift work, and workers in the confectionery industry appeared to run a greater risk of diseases than did similar workers in other industries (Petersen 1981, 1983). The findings from the Rand study in the United States did not support these occupational differences when insurance and other social factors were controlled (Davies *et al.* 1987).

Employment appears to be beneficial in providing social contacts and supports, as well as resources to perform health behaviours. Yet even with the benefits of employment, two-income families or working class, single parents may face excessive time-costs or problems of access resulting from occupational regulations which determine pay and absences from work (Lutz 1987; Pill and Stott 1985).

Previous research has indicated that lower-class, unemployed parents with children at home, who are particularly likely to be socially isolated, are at much greater risk for developing poor general health. The unemployed, similar to poor employed individuals, face problems with ability to pay, child-care, and transportation. The extended family in this case, rather than the delivery system, often becomes the major link with the development of preventive orientation and behaviours (Jennings *et al.* 1984; Kessler *et al.* 1987).

Perceived and actual cost of care

Often 'cost of care' is measured by income, availability of insurance or public assistance, or other socioeconomic measures. While clearly related to these factors, perceived and actual costs of health-related activities at the individual level are also measured by time lost, money spent, and social pressures. Both time and social costs associated with dental visits are related to socioeconomic status, ethnicity, and race. In the United States, evidence suggests that black individuals wait longer for health care services and display more displeasure per unit of delay, thus incurring more time and social costs than do other groups. This pattern reduces use of services, particularly among the poor (Schwartz 1978).

Social costs include anxiety, loss of self-esteem, and cost of the search for care. Less familiarity with the system and with kinds of care increases anxiety for individuals of lower socioeconomic class. Departure from middle-class norms of providers, whether racial, ethnic, or socioeconomic, can increase social costs. Since word-of-mouth is a common search approach in dentistry, among lower socioeconomic classes without access to health information, the social cost of finding care probably is greater than for those in more advantaged classes.

A critical social cost related to the dental practice is the discomfort of the patient. Communication between the dental professional and patient is influenced greatly by a patient's socioeconomic status, race, ethnicity, gender, and disability status. These are all factors which most likely reflect a cultural gap between the dental professional and the patient (Dunning 1988). Negative interactions reduce the value of the visit and add to the imbalance of power which already exists. This imbalance is further reinforced since lower class individuals tend to ask fewer questions than do middle or upper class patients (Grembowski *et al.* 1989).

Ability to pay is an important variable for understanding oral health promotion. Income, insurance, state delivery systems, and public assistance influence an individual's ability to pay. Ability to pay is related to probability of participation in organized oral health promotion. The greatest need for preventive services in the United States is among the uninsured at all levels, followed by those with low income and some insurance or those on public assistance, then those with middle-class income even without insurance, and middle class with insurance (Ball 1985).

Individuals on fixed incomes, particularly older adults, may be particularly affected by their ability to pay large dental bills. While economic measures such as income are correlated with use of services, an individual's perception of the ability to pay may be even more important than are the actual costs. If the person believes that he cannot cover the out-of-pocket costs (even though he may have an exaggerated concept of the expenses) care will not be sought.

Nowhere are the differences in access to health care among socioeconomic groups seen more dramatically than in the use of oral health services. Generosity of payment programmes and dental care insurance are both directly related to dental visits and services received. Insurance appears to help equalize access to services across socioeconomic groups, and full coverage dental insurance increases use of dental services, at least initially, and decreases the number of untreated caries (Davies *et al.* 1987).

Evidence suggests that voluntary participation (as opposed to automatically imposed programmes) in a dental plan and selection of a specific type of plan by the individual increases utilization by individuals of lower socioeconomic class. Also, evidence from the Rand Insurance Experiment in the United States illustrates the profound effect on dental utilization and oral health which results from the individual sharing the cost of care with the insurer (co-insurance). Sharing in the cost increases the probability of any use of dental services more than changing the mix of services received once in the dental office (Davies *et al.* 1987).

Location of residence

Current and past residential location are important in interpreting oral health status and needed oral health interventions. Traditionally, concern for location of residence has been related to the rural/urban or inner city/suburban dimensions. Persons living in rural areas appear to have both economic and cultural barriers. Rural residence has been associated with less access to oral health education and services, resulting in higher rates of untreated oral diseases. Also, place of residence determines access to central water supplies which may or may not be fluoridated.

As the population profiles and the distribution of oral diseases change, more emphasis by public health authorities is being placed on populations which are mobile (for example, migrants, immigrants, and the homeless) and those with little mobility (such as the homebound or institutionalized). At both extremes, there is less access to oral health care, less continuity or care, and considerable evidence of untreated oral diseases.

Not only does mobility denote problems in lack of continuity of care, but it also suggests the presence of enhanced risk factors, such as poor nutrition, disruptions in self-care, and physical and emotional stress. Immigrants new to a country have problems with communication and acculturation, and may not grasp essential information about the tools needed for either self-care or professionally delivered care, and due to extended time without care, have higher levels of disease (Ekman 1990; Kiyak 1989; Syme 1986). Additionally, migrants within a country such as the United States are a specifically problematic group since they are both rural and mobile.

Similarly, traditional delivery systems (clinics and private practices) are not well suited to the delivery of dental care to the institutionalized, the homebound, or those in prisons. Residents of institutions face numerous barriers for obtaining oral health services. These people are isolated from normal social supports and routine health care delivery systems. Often they suffer from multiple chronic diseases, disabilities, social or psychological maladies, and/or are taking medications that affect oral health status or compromise their ability to perform oral hygiene procedures.

Implications of micro-level social factors for oral health promotion: targeting programmes and services

Years ago, prior to recent technological advances in prevention, there were more oral diseases than the profession could handle. With the advent of fluorides and preventive oral hygiene regimens, there has been a consequent improvement in oral health at the population level. What is now clear is that certain subgroups in a population exhibit higher rates of oral diseases. Many of these groups are ones which do not have ready access to the delivery system, have inadequate diets, and display low levels of knowledge and negative attitudes regarding oral health. These subpopulations, which, in fact, may be ambivalent about oral health and believe that what they do does not matter, can be reached more directly through specific targeting to counteract the factors which set them at risk. Attempts to determine the best ways to target these groups with specific oral health education or behaviour modification have been moderately successful (Schou *et al.* 1990*a*).

Social factors provide identifiers or markers for individuals and groups which allow for segmentation of the population. This segmentation allows for more effective planning and implementation of programmes for those in most need or at highest risk. This is called targeting. Observable social identifiers (education, income, ethnicity, and age) are used initially to reflect underlying attitudes and knowledge, but they may not do so accurately. It is necessary to refine targeting, beyond social identifiers, to indicate specific individual groups which display knowledge, attitudes, and behaviours needing enhancement. Once determined, these problems can be specifically addressed within the context of the social, cultural environment of those targeted for oral health promotion strategies. Such an approach is more realistic than attempting to change the social factors (education, income, ethnicity, and age) *per se*.

Targeting, using social identifiers, while not explaining why differences exist nor acknowledging wide variations within groups, allows the first cut at limiting the scope of an oral health promotion programme to a high-risk population. There is a cost efficiency in targeting by expending resources where the efforts are needed most. (Some day it will be possible to target risk factors in an individual rather than label an individual by social identifiers. This will provide a less stigmatized method.)

Historically, attempts to alter communication, care delivery locations, hours of care provision, and other characteristics of oral health systems to meet the needs of key targets have been slow to develop. It is too easy to say that everyone is affected by oral diseases, thus there is no need to segment and identify key groups by social factors. Yet, this historical emphasis (that everyone has equal need) has resulted in a very general focus — school-children in formal programmes, or those willing to enter a private or public delivery system. This approach has resulted in groups — such as those not in school or with no knowledge of how to use the system — who have great need but somehow have been missed by the generalized approach to education or care.

Successful oral health promotion activities require that the target groups be defined, their special needs identified as specifically as possible, followed by directed and focused programme planning, implementation, and evaluation (Frederiksen *et al.* 1984). As an illustration, research has repeatedly indicated that 'the absence of perceived need' is correlated with low dental service utilization, yet 'perceived need' has never been clearly defined. A key first step in an oral health promotion plan is not only to assess biologically defined need but also to identify ways to improve perceived importance of oral health. To do that, it is necessary to understand the social factors associated with this perception. If appropriate routes could be used to assist the individual in identifying perceived need, then education and delivery of appropriate services could be tailored to fit that need.

Some very successful targeting has been done in health; one example in the United States has been the emphasis on control of high blood pressure among blacks. Age-graded and socioeconomic targeting designed for school oral health has been successful in some programmes (Schou *et al.* 1990b; Horowitz 1983, 1984). The nature of school-based programmes varies throughout the world, ranging from oral hygiene education, nutritional counselling, and fluoride delivery programmes to actual professional delivery of restorative services. Consistency across school education programmes is minimal, however, and most school programmes have been directed towards young children with less consideration being given to the more difficult problems of older, high-risk teenagers. While evidence suggests that some of these programmes are of positive value for parents and children, many are inadequate because they lack sufficient parental involvement; yet others have not been evaluated for effectiveness. Schools, or selected groups within schools, are still excellent targets for oral health promotion if methods can be found of developing habits for continuity of care when the individual leaves the school. Such an approach would reinforce the goal of the school-based programme for use in adult life.

Other efforts exist, including outreach programmes for migrant, poor, and isolated patients, operated from schools which educate dental professionals, yet these are not uniformly available. Only a few of these programmes have been evaluated, and it appears that there are great gaps in addressing the direct and indirect factors affecting the oral health of these target populations.

Some programmes exist addressing the unique needs of ethnic groups, such as efforts directed towards the issue of baby bottle tooth decay among Native Americans in the United States. These campaigns are attempting to improve awareness among high risk groups through existing facilities, such as prenatal, neonatal, and well-baby clinics. Nurses and nutritionists are being trained to facilitate messages, and educational and behavioural interventions are being tested within the context of the Indian Health Service of the United States Public Health Service (Bruerd *et al.* 1989).

New and expanded efforts to increase targeting for the growing number of 'difficult-to-reach' populations for oral health promotion are needed. These approaches might address factors such as:

(1) location of services which are geographically and culturally convenient;

(2) provision of education and care delivery with cultural sensitivity;

(3) non-threatening organizational climates, e.g. attention to directions within large facilities, instructions and attention during admission, information regarding transportation;

(4) professional and support staff who can communicate within the context of a cultural or socioeconomic group;

(5) recognition of disabilities and medical conditions in providing oral health services;

(6) programmes located in sites in which the targeted individuals reside, work, or routinely attend (appropriate screening, referrals, or care provision in non-dental settings such as nursing homes, prenatal clinics, hospital out-patient clinics, daycare facilities, work settings);

(7) integration of oral health within social and medical programmes located in health care facilities, schools, home, and work sites;

(8) liaison with non-traditional groups for purposes of referral and coordinated treatment (e.g. social workers, nurse midwives, or visiting nurses as case finders for oral diseases, conditions, and trauma) (Kiyak 1989).

Targeting using such approaches requires increasing the priority of *preventing* oral problems within the total social environment.

Institutions, organizations, and social networks at the meso level

Family

An individual's norms for behaviour are established and sustained through social support networks, which vary considerably by socioeconomic status. These social support networks include initially the family and, subsequently, friends, neighbours, and coworkers, among other peer groups. These networks extend from individuals to small groups to larger organizations. In fact, it is very difficult to separate individual and group oral health behaviours from the social context within which they exist. Through interpersonal interaction and networks of social groups of all sizes, the individual receives feedback or reinforcement for individually held knowledge, attitudes, and practices. Practices ultimately manifest themselves in the receipt of preventive services, exposure to oral health promotion interventions, occurrence of specific oral diseases and conditions, and eventually determine oral function or dysfunction and quality of life.

Of the social support networks important in health promotion activities, none is so well documented as the family. The family historically has assumed responsibility for initiating oral health care practices. Yet with increasing changes in family structures and participation of women in the labour force, in tandem with alterations in dental delivery systems, the traditional roles of the family may be changing. With increases in single-parent families, some members may become isolated and removed from the reinforcers which are more characteristic of an extended family structure in which two parents, siblings, and grandparents can provide multiple role-models for healthy behaviours.

It is important to note the feedback within the family: parents influence children, experiences of children influence their parents, and children ultimately become parents who will influence their own children. Family members become an extension of the communication, education, and health care delivery system and can be critical partners of health care providers in sustaining oral health behaviours. This partnership has been used for years in the development of oral hygiene behaviours of young children. Collaboration among dentists, hygienists, school teachers, and parents (in reinforcing contexts) have fostered the child's ability to learn life-long habits to improve oral health.

A child is in a unique situation in regard to oral health promotion; a child is not totally a free agent. Evidence suggests that oral health status and use of dental services by a child are correlated with the dental status of the mother, her age at pregnancy, dental visits during pregnancy, her education, and her current age, among other parental characteristics (Blinkhorn 1980; Gift and Newman 1979; Nowjack-Raymer and Gift 1990).

Ability of a child to act is limited by parental willingness and ability to assist the child through purchase of materials, supply of appropriate food, provision of transportation, and, in many countries, payment of bills. Parental attitudes and perceived need will encourage or discourage the child's use of care as well as affect socialization for future use of services. A child may perceive a need for care and value it (if learned through a school programme, for example), but may not receive care if parents have different values, or lack the resources to obtain care. If a child is raised in an atmosphere where dental care is viewed as a luxury, rather than a necessity, it is likely that the child will not be taken regularly to a dentist, and once grown, may feel that dental care is not essential. At the most negative extreme, parental attitudes and behaviours are reflected in 'dental neglect' — failure or parents or caregivers to seek treatment for visibly untreated caries, oral infections, and pain; or failure to follow through with treatment once informed that such conditions exist (Loochtan *et al.* 1986).

The family network is equally important in the provision of education, hygiene, and services for the older adult. Family members are often the first-line recipient of information about the health complaints of older people, particularly for the homebound or institutionalized individual.

While acknowledging the importance of the family network throughout the life cycle, it is critical to know the nature of changing resources within the individual's family. Some children have only one parent, and many older adults do not have children who can serve in the caregiving capacity. The ethic of the health care provider must be to promote the oral health of individuals in an equitable manner regardless of the level of family resources.

Community

Social-support networks operate within community contexts and reflect both societal and cultural norms. Community structure and processes are important factors to consider in determining which health promotion strategies can be used. The health care system itself exists in a community context which is characterized by constant social change. Not only do the physical and economic resources change, but the composition and density of the population change as well.

The health care system operates within a system of power in the community structure, but in many cases health care providers do not take key leadership roles in this community structure. All too often intense concern of a cross-section of community leaders is not commanded by oral problems, since these are, on the whole, less dramatic and less central to economic interest in comparison to education, crime, and other community issues.

Media are a key institution at the community level. It is a powerful force to communicate oral health issues to the public. All too often, however, the media is disdained by professional groups, and thus not used to its best advantage as a mechanism for social change or education (Frazier 1984).

While it is known that the decision to fluoridate the community water supplies is often a decision made by community leaders, dental professionals have been known to lose the fight for this preventive measure primarily because they failed to understand the power structure and enter into the decision-making process appropriately on behalf of that effort (Frazier 1984). The establishment of an oral health promotion strategy outside the private dental practice sector requires:

(1) recognition that community human and fiscal resources can be mobilized around oral health concerns;

(2) interaction and cooperation with the broad community leadership structure.

The involvement of the community leadership structure and media in oral health promotion are discussed in detail in other chapters.

Delivery system

A great deal of oral health promotion occurs within the context of dental care operatories and practices. Dental practice responds to social factors and, in fact, becomes part of the social structure, affecting oral health promotion. Current delivery systems emerged over time primarily in response to the demands for treating caries and periodontal diseases. The organization of health education along with delivery of oral health services has emerged uniquely in different countries in response to dominant societal pressures, in large part with little directed, advance planning (Davis 1980). In North America, dentistry developed as a separate and distinct profession, while in many European countries it emerged more directly from medicine. Historic development has affected the mechanisms of practice and payment for services provided.

Depending on the nature of the health care system, the impact of socioeconomic factors will be different. For example, in a relatively 'market-based' delivery system, individual socioeconomic factors will have more direct impact on use of services than in a system which has a more centralized tax-financed national health services system, essentially free from direct out-of-pocket costs to all residents. Countries which have systems in between the two extremes, or have mixed types of systems, might exhibit the influence of certain social factors more than others (Davis 1980; Fredericks et al. 1980; Cockerham et al. 1988).

In a predominantly private sector delivery system model, funded through direct out-of-pocket expenditures, private insurance, and public assistance funds (such as in the United States), services from the private practice sector are generally more available to middle and upper socioeconomic status individuals. In contrast, services from public clinics and school programmes are more available to the lower socioeconomic status groups.

The organization of dental services is a result of the interaction of a variety of factors acting on the profession and the community. Policies at the national and state levels affect distribution and structure of practice through the social processes of licensing and credentialling. Social and economic factors (reflected in the standard of living, prevailing social philosophy, the size and distribution of the population, and the incidence of oral diseases) influence the overall supply of dental providers, the ratio of public and private dental providers, and the mix of services provided. These, in turn, influence the availability and functions of auxiliary personnel, ready availability of services (such as full service hours and minimal waiting time which can affect loss of time from school and work site), and whether services are provided in schools, homes, offices, or institutions. Interpersonal relationships, as well as bureaucratic and administrative incentives or barriers, vary between countries and may differ in public and private sector delivery systems even within a single country.

The interface of the delivery system with the general social structure affects the continuity of care. A system with national health services more readily has control oversight of the continuity of care, while continuity of care is left to individual decision-making and initiative in the market-based system.

The social structure of a specific dental practice, whether public or private, has considerable influence on oral health promotion. All evidence suggests that the receipt of dental care is, in fact, a social process that includes the interactions between the dentist, patient, and often family members and insurers (Grembowski et al. 1989). Individual dental practitioners are critical gatekeepers with primary responsibility for transferring information and establishing preventive orientation and programmes. Communication style and orientation of the provider, as well as the availability of services, affect the outcome of the visits. Not all practices have a preventive orientation, nor provide preventive services to appropriate age groups. When preventive auxiliaries (for example, hygienists) are not employed, the dental practice appears to be placing less focus on prevention and health promotion since the use of auxiliaries in practice is associated with higher levels of preventive services provision. This is particularly noteworthy in the case of providing dental sealants, dietary fluorides, and oral health education (Gift et al. 1984). Some strategies of oral health promotion, such as counselling about nutrition or smoking, have been met with resistance and have not been built into the culture of the dental practice (Omenn 1990).

Payment system

In most countries, financial mechanisms are integrally related to the organizational structure of the dental care system, as well as to utilization and accessibility of that system (Gift et al. 1981). In some countries groups have been active and effective in involving local government entities and employers in the financing and delivery of care (Davis 1980). Although variable throughout the world, the structures of payment plans affect the quantity and quality of oral health services, as well as the costs.

While payment assistance (private insurance or public programmes) for oral health care services is not as widespread as for medical care services, many populations have been provided for through local and/or national governmentally administered programmes. These programmes have varying histories of success in reducing oral diseases, in part because appropriate services may not always be matched with needs of specific target groups. Also, sufficient resources may not be available to sustain appropriate services. Additionally, there may be inadequate recognition of the complexity of the biological, individual, professional, social, and cultural factors interacting to determine oral health outcomes. Payment policies in many public and private programmes operate to deny the very health-promoting and preventive services which would have the longest term benefit (for example, payment for dentures in lieu of restorations; non-payment for pit and fissure sealants).

These issues can be illustrated in systems in which public payment is available for individuals to use private dental practices. Utilization rates for children living in poverty covered by state-based Medicaid plans in the United States are far below that of the middle-class child. The less than expected value of public programmes may result, in part, from the lack of reimbursement for comprehensive services at usual and customary fees in this type of programme. (Grembowski *et al.* 1987; Groenewegen and Postma 1984). Additionally, there is evidence of differences in cultural orientation between the provider and the patient. Publicly funded patients may often break appointments and fail to comply with treatment regimens which are designed for patients better equipped to carry out these regimens, by virtue of having norms for self-care practices, and economic resources consistent with professional monitoring (Grembowski *et al.* 1989).

Research on alternative payment systems show some differences in provision of preventive services, but the providers are still limited by what they traditionally perform and their knowledge of preventive services (Davies *et al.* 1987; Coventry *et al.* 1989). For example, in a three-year clinical trial, comparing capitation and fee-for-service among general practice dentists, capitation dentists carried out more preventive services and advice and restored teeth later, yet capitation dentists saw children less often and provided an equally low number of dental sealants. There was no difference in oral cleanliness nor level of oral diseases in the two groups of children (Coventry *et al.* 1989).

Despite problems or inconsistencies, optimal payment models can make an impact, in a positive way, on cost to the patient: reducing disparities of economic status, increasing comprehensiveness of services received, and improving satisfaction with care (Davies *et al.* 1987; Manning *et al.* 1985). Whether such payment models alone have improved oral health status is still unclear.

Implications of provider characteristics, delivery systems, and payment systems for oral health promotion

Availability of *appropriately trained providers* affects the scope and type of services an individual will receive. Successes in oral health promotion will require considerable *reorientation of providers* through their dental school curriculum or through continuing education. The educational system for health care providers has been slow to place emphasis on the preventive and behavioural aspects of practice, which affect social interaction between provider and patient as well as health promotion strategies. Evidence of this lack of focus in education and training is shown in practice characteristics and provider orientation towards prevention and initiation of oral health pro-moting activities.

Attitudes and behaviours of providers are based on a complex web of scientific, experiential, administrative, and legal forces, many of which will need to be addressed to effect change in provider orientation. For example, dentists may be discouraged from learning and applying new skills regardless of reimbursement for them, as has been the case with pit and fissure sealants (Coventry *et al.* 1989).

Preventive services need to be available to a full range of targeted individuals. While preventive services are reported to be available in almost all private dental practices and clinical dental facilities, little data exist to show whether these services are directed to those in most need. In the United States, there is little evidence to suggest that periodontal conditions are routinely examined or recorded, or that dental sealants are applied to other than a very small fraction of newly erupted molars.

Diet, smoking, and other risk behaviours of individuals need to be addressed, and health promotion skills or behaviours to counteract those risks need to be developed. Dentists appear to doubt the importance of some of these risk behaviours, and there is still little in the practice of dentistry that is conducive to altering behaviours (Johns *et al.* 1987). Dentists appear diffident about carrying out interventions focused on changing behaviours. Perhaps lack of knowledge of how to intervene effectively and a perception that the patients might not be receptive to advice or willing to change result in lack of initiative by the oral health care provider (Omenn 1990). Even if oral health care providers see themselves as unskilled or unsuited to provide counselling and education for smoking cessation or nutrition and other health promotion services, conceivably they could serve as facilitators, referring to others who *are* appropriately trained (Brody 1990). Teams of health and social care providers could be developed which could be on-call for individual patients, their families, or could be available in the community to facilitate reduction of risks. Health promotion in areas of uncertainty, for example smoking cessation counselling, for the dental professional is a critical challenge for the future.

Oral health care providers need to develop improved skills to bridge the sociocultural chasm separating themselves from individuals of lower socioeconomic groups. The imbalance in social exchange between dental personnel and these lower socioeconomic individuals, suggested in the literature, is a critical problem for health promotion. Much of health promotion depends on changing values and behaviours through adequate exchange of information. Poor communication exchange reduces the probability of success for any desired outcome. In medicine, guidelines have been developed for treating patients drawn from different racial and ethnic groups than those of providers. Such guidelines are designed to develop cohesiveness between the patient and the provider. Such approaches might be developed for dentistry to help reduce discrepancy in values.

Dentists need to develop enhanced skills in management of 'total oral health' of individuals, since oral conditions are related to systemic diseases and the social conditions in which they present. All medical, dental, allied health, social, and community workers must work together with full recognition of all factors contributing to health.

The dental delivery system is part of the social structure affecting oral health promotion. The combination of vested interests of currently trained professionals working in the system, supporting licensing regulations, traditional and usual hours of practice, and the need for cumbersome dental equipment, altogether make the delivery system difficult to change. Yet, the future success of oral health promotion requires that professionals should be open to new ways to delivery of an appropriate mix of services in settings close to patients in need.

Creative oral health promotion strategies can occur in the existing care system or in alternative settings. In most existing health care systems dentists and physicians operate in a fixed, bureaucratically isolated setting, and they play the central role in prevention of disease and delivery of services. Attempts to reduce system-related barriers to oral health care in private practices and public clinics by expanding office hours, employing preventive and educational auxiliaries, and facilitating assistance in payment for care all can be enhanced. By necessity, such alterations in the system involve the direct participation of individual dentists and professional organizations in problem-solving activities — a challenging exercise, but one that can work if self-interest and reward for change are maximized.

Alternative settings for care delivery can be successful as well. Work site dental programmes in the United Kingdom have yielded substantial reductions in the amount of time spent to receive dental care during work hours. By eliminating both cost and access barriers, overall health has been enhanced, and thus productivity and profitability increased (Silversin and Kornacki 1984). Also, system barriers have been reduced by providing oral health education and preventive and restorative care in school settings. Research which tests methods to promote compliance with preventive health practices in such settings demonstrates that comprehensive and intensive self-care motivation curriculum sessions can result in maintenance of optimal behaviours, particularly in lower socioeconomic groups (Horowitz *et al.* 1987).

While school and work site programmes are excellent examples of system level oral health promotion efforts, their potential is not fully developed in most countries. Providing screening, prevention, and other well-care services (with referrals for therapy) through schools, work sites, or other community-based settings, might encourage the concept of health promotion. Additionally, targeting based on social correlates of oral conditions and diseases within existing school and work site programmes might improve the outcome of these programmes.

For the delivery system to respond better to the factors associated with oral health promotion, it is necessary to develop more flexible approaches. Among the many possibilities, examples might include:

1. In response to significant oral health problems evidenced by migrant children, it is necessary to develop new approaches responsive to mobile

populations. Although the use of mobile clinics and/or mobile records is a challenge to develop and monitor, dental societies and public health departments could develop a programme to ease transfer of records for continuity of care.

2. Community-dwelling elderly individuals, with decreasing autonomy and chronic health problems, are likely to be suffering from solitude and isolation which can aggravate all kinds of problems. Medical and dental interventions might parallel social interventions, thereby reviving a network of social supports, reducing isolation, and providing needed routine and hygiene services. Self-help and support groups could be organized; or, if organized for different purposes, could be enhanced through activities related to oral disorders.

3. Oral health promotion efforts need to reach confined older adults or handicapped individuals. Medical complications, oral conditions, absence of readily available facilities, and the socioeconomic status of the residents in institutions need to be addressed concurrently in such efforts. Oral health education and training for personnel working in institutions needs to be critically evaluated.

4. 'Prevention workers', such as dental nurses, hygienists, or indigenous health care workers in developing countries, could be trained to educate, screen, and refer from settings with high numbers of individuals at risk for oral diseases.

For prevention and oral health promotion to become priorities, both as concepts and a series of actions, the structure of the health care delivery system has to be examined and evaluated. What are the incentives in the existing system? What are the barriers? What barriers can be eliminated? How can they be eliminated? How can the incentives be maximized? Can the current delivery system be structured to produce health rather than treat disease? And if not, can it be enhanced to do so (Bailit *et al.* 1979)?

As discussed above, *payment systems* interact with delivery systems and provider orientations to determine the structure, process, and outcome of oral health promotion activities. The influence of individual and community social factors on payment systems may differ in public delivery system models such as exist in the United Kingdom compared to more market-based models such as in the United States. Systems which offer tax-supported care to all children in schools may delay much of the interaction of micro- and meso-level social factors with oral health until adulthood. In a universal market-based system model, social and cultural differences within the patient pool are magnified. Yet, the interaction of culture, delivery system regulations, and ability to pay are evident across delivery systems. In all economies, the least healthy groups (for example immigrant populations) offer a challenge to oral health promotion planners. Ways must be sought and tested to overcome the inability to access care and to maximize self-care strategies.

Most public systems and private insurance plans world-wide tend to be treatment-orientated. More efforts need to be directed towards prevention, screening, and referral, and to the integration of oral health care with medical care. Financial assistance programmes for oral health care services are not utilized to their maximum possible extent. This under-utilization has been attributed to lack of knowledge of the programmes, difficulties in applying for eligibility, an aversion to accepting public benefits, lack of transportation, linguistic and cultural differences, fear of bureaucracies and health care providers, and lack of faith in the efficacy of health and social service professionals (Kiyak 1989). Also, evidence suggests that once in the delivery system, low income and minority individuals often do not receive the same mix of services. They may not receive comprehensive care; they may receive less expensive services, fewer preventive services, and more extraction services. Assistance programmes need to be developed which broaden their objectives to cover services to meet individual needs. In the end, a well-reasoned prevention plan can serve to reduce unnecessary treatment services and might serve to reduce costs and make care more accessible.

With the exception of dentures, most payment assistance and public delivery mechanisms have been directed towards children. Evidence in the United States suggests that more comprehensive prepaid dental plans for older adults, as a supplement to general medical plans (such as Medicare), can be managed in a cost effective manner (Greenlick *et al.* 1986). Based on what has been learned to date, other experimental payment programmes to increase oral health promotion in all ages might be tried. Even in national oral health or public assistance systems, which provide treatment services for all ages, methods to create an oral health promotion/prevention approach for older adults need to be established. Also, the concept of the family as a unit of care rather than incremental care for isolated age-groups should be developed and tested.

With growing involvement of individuals in their own health care, improved oral health promotion at the meso level may come from the bottom up — from the consumer of services. The consumer may be a strong force in modifying the dental delivery and payment systems to be more health promoting in ways which make these systems more responsive to their needs (Grembowski *et al.* 1989).

Culture and society at the macro level

Culture has both direct and indirect effects on oral health. Cultural taboos may affect acceptability of interventions and thus contribute to illness. Factors at the societal level determine availability of appropriate information through a variety of institutions and organizations.

Change and disruption at either the cultural or societal level (such as droughts, war, fertility control policies, and unemployment) may alter age or economic structures, occupational hazards, or nutritional patterns, and in turn bring about changes in disease status. The climate may affect crops, thus altering availability of foods, and consequently nutrition. Similarly, introduction of refined sugars and other cariogenic foods into developing countries has been shown to be a contributing factor to increased prevalence of dental caries. Societal norms determine the preponderance of cariogenic foods in the market. These norms are clearly evident in the presence or absence of national policy, advertising, or societal restraints on package labels for snack foods (Klepp and Forster 1985).

Cultural norms are seen in social policies. A given culture may emphasize an age-graded structure, or in contrast, a social unit structure (such as family or clan). As the norms are translated to policies, the focus of the culture may determine whether specific age groups are treated differently. In the case of an age-graded society, policies affect whether given age groups benefit from prevention initiatives, how different age groups are treated, what kind of care they receive, and the payment mechanisms associated with the care (Omenn 1990). Attention given to special training of caregivers for specific age groups or special care patients also reflects concern at the societal level. School oral health programmes illustrate the operation of a positive policy regarding children. At the other age extreme, any prejudice against older adults at the cultural level may result in the lack of positive role models for adaptation to ageing. The functional status of older adults may be largely dependent on the types and levels of competence expected or required and the compensatory resources available at the societal level to reduce the effect of any impairments. If institutionalization of older adults, which encourages disengagement from self-care and self-reliance, is a societal norm, this affects expectations for oral health. Societal norms which envision the older adult as a positive part of society make improved oral health status a more likely outcome (Maddox 1990; Roos and Havens 1991).

Societal and cultural norms, reflected in policies and institutions, are not static, yet these are slow to change. Consequently, they may be functioning in response to outdated values. Many institutions and organizations, including the health care delivery system, were developed in times when the norms and values were different from what they are at present. The past few decades have witnessed tremendous technological and social changes and their impacts have been more than economic ones. Changes which are having a clear impact on health care delivery, particularly the health promotion component of the delivery system, are:

(1) the prevailing view that health care is a right;

(2) the increasing responsibility of individuals;

(3) the growing role of community organizations in the assurance of health, through self-help and development programmes (Belangér 1988).

Illustrative of this is the success over the past decades that working class unions have had in obtaining increased private and public funding for health care, across social systems, by emphasizing that it is a right. While the pressure from specific interest groups varies across different countries, the principal outcome has been the greater involvement of people in decisions regarding the financing and organization of oral health services (Davis 1980). Even in the most market-based economies such as the United States and South Africa, there are publicly-funded health programmes as well as private insurance for work-based groups for selected populations.

There are many examples of how the culture and society can influence oral health promotion. Prevailing attitudes towards utilization of services for treatment, rehabilitation, or prevention are key. Societies have different priorities towards health. Many societies are orientated towards the provision of sickness (not wellness) services, resulting in a remedial rather than preventive and promotional approach to professional care delivery. (Health care providers, who dispense curative services to individual laypersons, may not adapt easily to providing health promoting services.) Resources for, and activities related to, oral health will be affected by such policies. Policies creating insufficient reimbursement for preventive dental care affect oral health promotion, as do policies which create programmes with an emphasis on extraction and the provision of dentures.

Observed individual or professional behaviours are often responses to existing social and cultural norms. Thus, changes at the individual level may be difficult without first drawing attention to the macro-level conditions. This impact is usually expressed through individual attitudes and behaviours. In a society where there is considerable emphasis on independence and activity, there may be a tendency not to accept illness easily, while in others loss of health may be seen as a normal part of living (Kiyak 1989). Similarly, different cultures have unique orientations towards immediate or future gratification which will affect the acceptance of preventive activities. Preventive services are underutilized in the United Kingdom, as well as the United States, reflecting underlying societal attitudes that put low emphasis on reducing current risks for future benefit, which prevail irrespective of available payment systems (Blaxter 1983; Omenn 1990).

Water fluoridation is a classic example of an oral health promotion strategy influenced by social factors at the societal (community) level. The society's political and social structures provide the contextual framework within which the fluoridation proposition is processed. These structures also are the major determinants that set the stage for the types and styles of social and institutional actions (including media), as well as individual behaviours which occur (Frazier 1984). Fluoridation, as a public issue, is a complex interrelation among psychological motivators of individual voters, social pressures, and political mechanisms, representing oral health promotion strategies at all levels including the individual, small groups, and the social–political collectivity.

Implications of macro-level social factors for oral health promotion

It is still unclear how demographic changes in the population, economic policies of nations, and changing patterns of oral diseases will affect the oral health sector, patients, and other individuals in the next decades. What is clear is that such changes will occur, and that projection of future needs for appropriate kinds of health care professionals, designs for organizations to provide education and care, and financing of care are greatly influenced by such changes. Effective oral health promotion requires managing changes in social factors by institutionalizing more preventive focus at the sociopolitical level.

For oral health promotion efforts to have an impact at the cultural or societal level, it is necessary to be cognizant of, and responsive to, existing trends. For example, the increasing numbers of older adults suggests that oral health must be viewed over the lifetime and within the context of chronic diseases. In turn, high birth rates in lower socioeconomic groups place a burden of disease prevention for children in traditionally difficult-to-reach populations. Immigration of individuals from other countries introduces cultural and communication issues into otherwise relatively stable societies.

Social factors at the cultural level are changed through education and exposure to new ways. A classic example would be the introduction of oral health education and delivery of care to less developed countries which have no previous exposure to 'modern dentistry'. For example, in Zululand, where milk was a cultural taboo, it was necessary to introduce powdered milk into the food processing chain in order to change the malnutrition status of the population (Fredericks *et al.* 1980). On a less global basis, attempts to change the habits of immigrants from the use of traditional home remedies to current oral hygiene regimens represent a challenge for proponents of cultural change.

Societal changes are most often brought about through legislation, regulations, or alteration in bureaucratic process. The best known of these in oral health are water fluoridation at the community level; the introduction of hygienists, dental health nurses, and other preventive auxiliaries into the care delivery system; and attempts to control health care costs at the national level. Other attempts to reduce barriers at the societal level might include changes in day-care laws and regulations which specify provisions for staff training and administrative procedures for oral hygiene, improved feeding practices, provision of fluoride supplements, and provision for dental emergencies (Nowjack-Raymer and Gift 1990).

Societal changes can occur by organizations working together. Broad-based voluntary organizations such as the Red Cross in specific countries could increase the focus on oral health. Also, programmes can be developed to improve fluoride administration by: establishing negotiations with laboratories to accept reduced fees for testing of water fluoride levels; and developing protocols for use by child health, neighbourhood, and rural health clinics regarding methods of water sample collection and testing for fluoride content (Nowjack-Raymer and Gift 1990). Evidence exists that organizations working together can enhance the interactive effects of micro-, meso-, and macro-level factors on oral health promotion. For example, efforts to improve dental visits through dental awareness campaigns have been more successful when private and public sectors work together (Schou and Blinkhorn 1990).

Social factors at the cultural and system level are difficult to alter. Yet it is essential to address cultural and societal issues rather than shifting all responsibility for social, economic, and environmental forces away from these sources to individuals with their inability to alter these forces. There are simply too many factors beyond the individual's control — poverty, chronic illnesses, and threatening environment — which affect oral health promotion (Morisky *et al.* 1986). Effecting and managing sociopolitical and regulation issues, particularly in critical areas such as payment programmes, availability of health and social programmes, and fluoridation, will be essential if future improvements in oral health promotion are to be seen.

A key factor for additional gains in prevention of oral diseases through sociopolitical changes is enhanced dissemination of information. An unacceptable social barrier to oral health promotion is inadequate science transfer which results in inconsistent professional and public knowledge and values. Of the several factors impeding sound oral health of the population, not least is the lack of accessibility and availability of efficacious methods to prevent and control diseases. Research in science transfer has demonstrated that: newly developed oral health measures are disseminated slowly to the public and the research on the use of such procedures develops even more slowly; use of oral hygiene measures is dependent upon the development and acceptance of techniques that must be justified in terms of time and cost — a form of evaluation which is often slow; and the relative worth of any oral hygiene measure is not common knowledge, and updated information is not routinely and carefully disseminated to the public or professions (Scheirer 1990). Consensus has to be developed first among scientists and health care professionals, followed by the development of strategies to inform the general population and third-party insurers.

Acknowledgement of social factors allows us to communicate using health and social motives more effectively by improving the relevance of the topic to the group being addressed. Thus, science transfer, as a social process, needs to be a major focus of oral health promotion.

Summary

1. Prevention of oral diseases through oral health promotion strategies is the key to reducing inequities in oral health resulting from socioeconomic and political forces.

2. Oral diseases appear to affect all age, racial, and ethnic groups, as well as both genders. The burden of oral diseases concentrates in lower socioeconomic groups, and owing to the cumulative effects of oral diseases and tooth loss, the aged become a most needy target group worldwide.

3. Evidence suggests that lower socioeconomic groups, as well as ethnic and racial minorities, will benefit from oral health promotion. Interventions need to be designed to take account of inter- and intra-cultural, socio-demographic, and economic risk factors associated with specific diseases and disorders.

4. Many individual behaviours and lifestyles are not conducive to oral health. Behavioural interventions and social strategies need to be developed to help change these behaviours and lifestyles to reduce risks and enhance self-care strategies.

5. In many countries, inequities in services, particularly preventive education and care, are associated with the structure of the dental delivery system, characteristics of the professional provider, and administrative elements such as legislation, regulation, and third-party payment systems. Oral health promotion may require changes in the knowledge, attitudes, and behaviours of individual dental care providers towards preventive strategies, as well as changes in the oral health care delivery systems and their associated regulating and payment processes.

6. Basic social, economic, and political forces in society are behind the relationships between poverty, illness, and access to care. National, local, and community policies which promote opportunity for lower classes also may reduce social risk and financial barriers for oral health. Refining policy and updating regulations which govern the supply of appropriate health care services, access, finances, oral health standards, and availability of community or school oral disease prevention strategies, remains critical. Finding ways to reach the family, a key social unit of care, remains a challenge in most existing systems worldwide.

7. The interactions among social factors need to be considered carefully in planning oral health promotion, particularly since there is evidence that focus on only one often does not completely solve a problem.

8. Knowledge of social factors can improve the development of oral health promotion strategies by helping to focus on risk reduction methods which work in real environments. Identifying social factors assists in the selection of communities or populations which can participate in oral health promotion programmes. Social factors, used for targeting, result in increased efficacy, cost containment, and satisfaction by decision-makers and the public at large.

9. Acknowledging social factors and working with strategies within the context of social factors increase the likelihood of successful oral health promotion.

Further reading

The best accounts of social factors in relation to the health care system and disease prevention are Belangér (1988), Cockerham, Kunz, and Lueschen (1988), Hooyman and Kiyak (1988), 'Social determinants of human health' (1976), and Syme (1986).

Good reviews of the social context of dentistry and prevention of oral diseases are in Cohen and Bryant (1984), Davis (1980), Fredericks, Lobene, and Mundy (1980), Gift (1986), Gift, Gerbert, Kress, and Reisine (1990), Grembowski, Andersen, and Chen (1989), Petersen (1990), and Schou (1991).

Good perspectives on health promotion, targeting, and marketing are given by Bausell (1986), Cohen (1985), Frederiksen, Solomon, and Brehony (1984), Gift (1988), Johns, Hovell, Ganiats, *et al.* (1987), McGuire (1984), Morisky, McCarthy, and Kite (1986).

References

Alvarez, W. F., Donis, J., and Larson, O. (1988). Children of migrant farm work families are at high risk for maltreatment: New York State Study. *American Journal of Public Health*, **78**(8), 934–6.

Andersen, R. M., Giachello, A. L., and Aday, L. A. (1986). Access of Hispanics to health care and cuts in services: a state-of-the-art overview. *Public Health Reports*, **101**(3), 238–52.

Antczak, A. A. and Branch, L. G. (1985). Perceived barriers to the use of dental services by the elderly. *Gerodontics*, **1**, 194–8.

Bailit, H. L., Raskin, M., Reisine, S., and Chiriboga, D. (1979). Controlling the cost of dental care. *American Journal of Public Health*, **69**(7), 699–703.

Ball, J. K. (1985). *Stimulating the use of preventive health services: pricing and promotion*. Syracuse University Dissertation.

Bausell, R. B. (1986). Health seeking behaviours: public versus public health perspectives. *Psychology Reports*, **58**, 187–90.

Belangér, J. P. (1988). Sociopolitical perspective on preventive services. In *Implementing preventive services, American journal of preventive medicine, v. 4 (4, supplement)*, (ed. R. N. Battista and R. S. Lawrence), pp. 176–85. Oxford University Press, New York.

Binnie, W. H., Rankin, K. V., and Mackenzie, I. C. (1983). Etiology of oral squamous cell carcinoma. *Journal of Oral Pathology*, **12**, 11–29.

Blaxter, M. (1983). Health services as a defence against the consequences of poverty in industrialised societies. *Social Science and Medicine*, **17**, 1139–48.

Blinkhorn, A. S. (1980). Factors influencing the transmission of the toothbrushing routine by mothers to their pre-school children. *Journal of Dentistry*, **8**, 307–11.

Brody, E. M. (1990). Social factors in care: the elderly patient's family. In *Principles of geriatric medicine and gerontology*, (ed. W. R. Hazzard, R. Andres, E. L. Bierman, and J. P. Blass), pp. 232–240. McGraw-Hill, New York.

Bruerd, B., Kinney, M. B., and Bothwell, E. (1989). Preventing baby bottle tooth decay in American Indian and Alaska Native communities: a model for planning. *Public Health Reports*, **104**, 531–640.

Cockerham, W. C., Kunz, G., and Lueschen, G. (1988). Social stratification and health lifestyles in two systems of health care delivery: a comparison of the United States and West Germany. *Journal of Health and Social Behaviour*, **29**, 113–26.

Cohen, L. K. (1985). Market and community responses to changing demands from the workplace. *Community Health Studies* (supplement), **IX**(1), 18s–24s.

Cohen, L. K. and Bryant, P. S. (ed.) (1984). *Social sciences and dentistry II*. Quintessence Publishing Company, London.

Corbin, S. B. (1991). Oral disease prevention technologies for community use. *International Journal of Technology Assessment in Health Care*, **7**, 327–44.

Coventry, P., Holloway, P. J., Lennon, M. A., Mellor, A. C., and Worthington, H. V. (1989). A trial of a capitation system of payment for the treatment of children in the general dental service. *Community Dental Health*, **6** (supplement 1), 1–63.

Davies, A. R., Allen, H. M., Manning, W. G., *et al.* (1987). *Explaining dental utilization behaviour*. RAND Publication No. R-3528-NCHSR. RAND Corporation, Santa Monica, California.

Davis, P. (1980). *The social context of dentistry*. Croom Helm, London.

Dunning, J. M. (1988). The best is the enemy of the good. *Journal of Public Health Dentistry*, **48**(1), 3–4.

Ekman, A. (1990). Dental caries and related factors — a longitudinal study of Finnish immigrant children in the north of Sweden. *Swedish Dental Journal*, **14**, 93–9.

Frazier, P. J. (1984). Public and professional adoption of selected methods to prevent dental decay. In *Social sciences and dentistry, II*, (ed. L. K. Cohen and P. S. Bryant), pp. 84–144. Quintessence Publishing Company, London.

Fredericks, M. A., Lobene, R. R., and Mundy, P. (1980). *Dental care in society: the sociology of dentistry*. McFarland & Company, Inc., Jefferson, North Carolina.

Frederiksen, L. W., Solomon, L. J., and Brehony, K. A. (1984). *Marketing health behaviour*. Plenum Press, New York.

Gift, H. C. (1986). Current utilization patterns of oral hygiene practices. In *Dental plaque control measures and oral hygiene practices*, (ed. H. Löe and D. V. Kleinman), pp. 39–71. IRL Press Limited, Oxford.

Gift, H. C. (1988). Issues of aging and oral health promotion. *Gerondontics*, **4**, 194–206.

Gift, H. C. (1991). Prevention of oral diseases and oral health promotion. *Current Opinion in Dentistry*, **1**, 337–47.

Gift, H. C. and Newman, J. F. (1979). Socialization and children's use of dental services: the impact of predisposing, enabling, and need factors. Paper presented at the 107th annual meeting of the APHA.

Gift, H. C., Newman, J. F., and Loewy, S. B. (1981). Attempts to control dental health care costs: the U. S. experience. *Social Science and Medicine*, **15a**, 767–79.

Gift, H. C., Milton, B. B., and Walsh, V. (1984). *The role of health professions in the delivery of caries prevention, V. I: dentists*. American Dental Association, Chicago.

Gift, H. C., Gerbert, B., Kress, G. C., and Reisine, S. T. (1990). Social, economic and professional dimensions of the oral health care delivery system. *Annals of Behavioural Medicine*, **12**(4), 161–9.

Greenlick, M. R., Sarvey, R., Lamb, H., Robinson, G., and Pinardi, J. (1986). Prepaid dental care for the elderly in an HMO Medicare demonstration. *Gerondontics*, **2**, 131–4.

Grembowski, D., Conrad, D., and Milgrom, P. (1987). Dental care demand among children with dental insurance. *Health Services Research*, **21**(6), 755–75.

Grembowski, D., Andersen, R. M., and Chen, M. (1989). A public health model of the dental care process. *Medical Care Review*, **46**(4), 439–96.

Groenewegen, P. P. and Postma, J. H. M. (1984). The supply and utilization of dental services. *Social Sciences and Medicine*, **19**(4), 451–9.

Hooyman, N. R. and Kiyak, H. A. (1988). *Social gerontology: a multidisciplinary perspective.* Allyn and Bacon, Inc., Boston.

Horowitz, A. M. (1983). Effective oral health education and promotion programs to prevent dental caries. *International Dental Journal*, **33**, 171–81.

Horowitz, A. M. (1984). The prevention of dental caries and periodontal disease. *International Dental Journal*, **34**, 141–58.

Horowitz, A. M. and Larach, D. C. (1991). *Diet and dental caries: a practice gap.* Paper presented at the 119th annual session of the American Public Health Association, Atlanta, Georgia.

Horowitz, L. G., Dillenberg, J., and Rattray, J. (1987). Self-care motivation: a model for primary preventive oral health behavior change. *Journal of School Health*, **57**(3), 114–18.

Jaynes, G. D. and Williams, R. M. (1989). *Blacks and American society.* National Academy Press, Washington, D. C.

Jennings, S., Mazaik, C., and McKinlay, S. (1984). Women and work: an investigation of the association between health and employment status in middleage women. *Social Science and Medicine*, **19**(4), 423–31.

Johns, M. B., Hovell, M. F., Ganiats, T., Peddecord, K.M., and Agras, W.S. (1987). Primary care and health promotion: a model for preventive medicine. *American Journal of Preventive Medicine*, **3**(6), 346–57.

Kessler, R. C., House, J. S. and Turner, J. B. (1987). Unemployment and health in a community sample. *Journal of Health and Social Behavior*, **28**, 51–9.

King, S. H. (1972). Social-psychological factors in illness. In *Handbook of medical sociology* (2nd edn), (ed. H. E. Freeman, S. Levine, and L. G. Reader), pp. 129–47. Prentice-Hall, Englewood Cliffs, New Jersey.

Kiyak, H. A. (1989). Reducing barriers to older persons' use of dental services. *International Dental Journal*, **39**(2), 95–102.

Klepp, K. I. and Forster, J. (1985). The Norwegian nutrition and food policy: an intergrated policy approach to a public health problem. *Journal of Public Health Policy*, **6**(4), 447–63.

Loochtan, R. M., Bross, DC., and Domoto, P. K. (1986). Dental neglect in children: definition, legal aspects, and challenges. *Pediatric Dentistry*, **8**, 113–17.

Lutz, M. E. (1987). *In sickness and in health: women's employment status and the use of health services by women and children* (dissertation). Columbia University, New York.

McGuire, W. J. (1984). Public communication as a strategy for inducing health-promoting behavioral change. *Preventive Medicine*, **13**, 299–319.

Maddox, G. L. (1990). Sociology of aging. In *Geriatric medicine and gerontology*, (ed. W. R. Hazzard, R. Andres, E. L. Bierman, and J. P. Blass), pp. 115–24. McGraw-Hill, New York.

Manning, W. G., BaiLit, H. L., Benjamin, B., and Newhouse, J. P. (1985). The demand for dental care: evidence from a randomized trial in health insurance. *Journal of the American Dental Association*, **110**(6), 895–902.

Morisky, D. E., McCarthy, W. J. and Kite, E. A. (1986). Targeting primary prevention programs to high-risk populations. *Advances in Health Education and Promotion*, **1**(part A), 23–64.

Newburn, E. (1982). Sugar and dental caries: a review of human studies. *Science*, **217**, 418–23.

Nowjack-Raymer, R. and Gift, H. C. (1990). Factors contributing to maternal and child oral health. *Journal of Public Health Dentistry*, **50**(6, special issue), 370–8.

Omenn, G. S. (1990). Prevention and the elderly: appropriate policies. *Health Affairs*, **9**(2), 80–93.

Petersen, P. E. (1981). *Dental health behaviour, dental health status and dental treatment needs among workers and staff-menbers at a Danish shipyard; a socio-dental industrial investigation*. Odense University Press, Odense.

Petersen, P. E. (1983). Dental health among workers at a Danish chocolate factory. *Community Dentistry and Oral Epidemiology*, **11**, 337–41.

Petersen, P. E. (1990). Social inequalities in dental health-toward a theoretical explanation. *Community Dentistry and Oral Epidemiology*, **18**, 153–8.

Pill, R. and Stott, N. C. (1985). Prevention procedures and practices among working class women: new data and fresh insights. *Social Science and Medicine*, **21**(9), 975–83.

Ripa, L. W. (1988). Nursing caries: a comprehensive review. *Pediatric Dentistry*, **10**(4), 268–82.

Roos, N. P. and Havens, B. (1991). Predictors of successful aging: a twelve-year study of Manitoba elderly. *American Journal of Public Health*, **81**(1), 63–8.

Scheirer, M. A. (1990). The life cycle of an innovation: adoption versus discontinuation of the fluoride mouth rinse program in schools. *Journal of Health and Social Behavior*, **31**, 203–15.

Schou, L. (1991). Social factors and dental caries. In *Dental caries, markers of high and low risk groups and individuals* (ed. N.W. Johnson), pp. 172–97. Cambridge University Press, Cambridge.

Schou, L. and Blinkhorn, A. S. (1990). Combining Commercial, Health Boards' and GDPS' sponsorship in an effort to improve dental attendance for young school leavers. *British Dental Journal*, **169**, 324–6.

Schou, L. and Eadie, D. (1991). Qualitative study of oral health norms and behaviour among elderly people in Scotland. *Community Dental Health*, **8**, 53–8.

Schou, L., Currie, C., and McQueen, D. (1990). Using a `lifestyle' perspective to understand toothbrushing behavior in Scottish schoolchildren. *Community Dentistry and Oral Epidemiology*, **18**, 230–4.

Schou, L., Wight, C. and Wohlgemuth, B. (1991). Deprivation and dental health. The benefits of a child dental health campaign in relation to deprivation as estimated by the uptake of free meals at school. *Community Dental Health*, **8**, 147–54.

Schwartz, B. (1978). Time, patience, and black people: a study of temporal access to medical care. *Sociological Focus*, **11**(1), 13–31.

Silversin, J. B. and Kornacki, M. J. (1984). Controlling dental disease through prevention: individual, institutional and community dimensions. In *Social sciences and dentistry, II*, (ed. L. K. Cohen and P. S. Bryant), pp. 145–201. Quintessence Publishing Company, London.

Smoking and Tobacco Control Taskforce (1991). *Strategies to control tobacco use in the United States: a blueprint for public health action in the 1990's.* U. S. Department of Health and Human Services, Public Health Services, National Institutes of Health, National Cancer Institute. NIH Pub. No. 92–3316.

Social determinants of human health (1976). In *Preventive medicine USA* (sponsored by The John E. Fogarty International Center for Advanced Study in the Health Sciences, National Institute of Health and the American College of Preventive Medicine), pp. 617–74. Prodist, New York.

Syme, S. L. (1986). The social environment and disease prevention. *Advances in Health Education and Promotion*, **1**(part a), 237–65.

Vogan, W. I. (1970). Dental knowledge and attitudes: an investigation. *British Dental Journal*, **128**, 481–6.

4

The role of the decision maker in oral health promotion

SUSAN REISINE

Decisions about health promotion occur at many levels. The individual decides to brush his or her teeth. The state adopts a water fluoridation programme. Professional organizations endorse the use of sealants. As these few examples illustrate, the location of the decision maker will have important implications for the scope and efficacy of oral health promotion programmes.

Oral health promotion decision makers can be situated anywhere along a continuum from the individual who decides to consume less sugar to prevent caries to the level of international organizations, such as the Federation Dentaire Internationale which sponsors oral health promotion activities across member nations. Decision makers who influence oral health promotion activities may or may not be affiliated with the dental health profession. In fact, organized dentistry and members of the profession may have their greatest impact by reaching out to decision makers in the community who have access to populations targeted for oral health promotion activities. Figure 4.1 illustrates the relationships among various levels of decision makers in the oral health promotion process.

Once beyond the level of the individual, decision makers are the people in positions of power in organizations who make the choices to endorse policies, to fund programmes, and to render services to patients. A variety of factors will influence the decision making process for those holding key positions within organizations (Reisine 1985). These include the goals and priorities of the organization, structural constraints, the location of the decision maker within the organization, availability of resources, and the attitudes and beliefs of the person holding the social position.

This chapter will outline the various levels at which decisions are made and the process by which they are reached. Examples from research and demonstration projects will be used to illustrate how the various levels interact to promote oral health in populations.

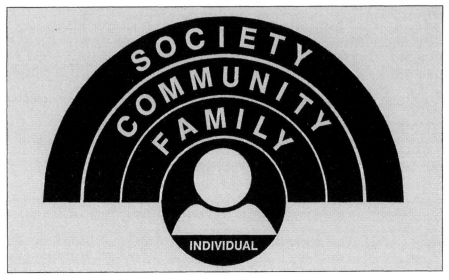

Fig. 4.1 The relationships among decision makers in oral health promotion.

Decision making at the level of the individual

Ultimately, oral health promotion efforts are aimed at preventing disease and improving health status at the level of the individual. For macro-level interventions, it is believed that passive systems where no direct action is required of the individual are most effective in health promotion (Silversin and Kornacki 1984). An example of this is water fluoridation, where the effective agent, fluoride, is added to the community water supply and people are exposed to the caries preventive agent without any personal effort besides water consumption.

However, primary and secondary preventive oral health actions actively taken by the individual are of the utmost importance in any oral health promotion agenda. Primary prevention refers to actions taken before disease onset in order to inhibit the development of the disease. Secondary prevention denotes intervention after the disease occurs in order to halt its progression. The objectives of secondary prevention are to diagnose the diseases as early as possible and to treat promptly (Jong 1988). These include things such as personal oral hygiene and plaque control measures, use of fluoride, avoidance of cariogenic foods, and seeking professional care for primary and secondary preventive services. Previous chapters have discussed theories of health behaviours and the social factors that influence oral health promotion activities, but these will be touched upon again briefly.

Theories on health behaviour, including sick role theory (Parsons 1951), the health beliefs model (Haefner 1974), health locus of control (Wallston and Wallston 1976), and social learning theory (Bandura 1969), for example, are most relevant to modifying the behaviours of individuals. However, interventions based on behavioural principles may be difficult and expensive to implement on a large scale basis. This is because most oral health promotion activities undertaken by individuals require considerably more personal effort, financial expense, and knowledge than required by passive oral health promotion programmes, such as community water fluoridation. Further, research investigating the effectiveness of health promotion interventions based on these theories has demonstrated the difficulty of getting individuals to improve and maintain oral hygiene (Albino et al. 1977; Kegeles et al. 1978; Nikias et al. 1979; Schou 1984; Cipes and Miraglia 1985; Russell et al. 1989).

For example, Nikias et al. (1979) conducted a study assessing the benefits of a plaque control programme implemented in private practices and in urban dental clinics. Patients were trained in the use of disclosing tablets, tooth brushing, and flossing and were counselled in reducing cariogenic elements in their diets. Patients were interviewed and examined in their homes 28 to 36 months later. It was found that about 50 per cent of patients complied with flossing recommendations, although there was little decline in compliance over time.

Kegeles et al. (1978) and Cipes and Miraglia (1985) investigated the use of rewards as a way of improving adolescents' compliance in a fluoride rinsing programme. Both studies found that rewards increased fluoride usage but once they were withdrawn compliance in the programme steadily declined. Cipes and Miraglia (1985) also showed that monitoring the use of the fluoride mouth rinse increased its use and these effects were sustained longer among those in the monitoring group than in the reward group. Kiyak (1988) also found that these methods could be used successfully with older adults living in either the community or in nursing homes.

A notable exception to the studies showing a decline in the effectiveness of health education programmes over time, is Schou's Dental Health Education programme initiated in Denmark (Schou 1985). This programme, founded on the active involvement principle, consists of five procedures carried out at a Danish factory, namely:

1. Teaching was carried out in pre-existing peer group of 5–7 persons.

2. Participants' own goals and needs were included.

3. Traditional dentist–patient barriers were excluded.

4. Traditional dentist–patient roles were changed.

5. Sessions were repeated.

Sixty-eight unskilled workers were recruited into the experimental group. The experimental and matched control group received dental examinations before the educational intervention and 6, 12, and 36 months after the intervention. Gains in oral health status, measured by the Gingivitis Index, and knowledge persisted over time for the experimental group compared to the control group. There were no differences between the two groups in terms of attitudes or self-reported oral hygiene behaviours. A recent follow-up study, comprising in-depth interviews (Schou and Monrad 1989) showed that the participants themselves believed that the long-term effect was caused by the active involvement principle.

The location of individuals in society and their social characteristics can also have a strong impact on their likelihood of undertaking preventive health behaviours. Grembowski's work (1989) on a public health model of the dental care process, suggests that individuals weigh the costs and benefits associated with obtaining professional dental care. If the benefits outweigh the costs, individuals will seek professional care. However, other structural factors will have large effects on the decision to seek care. These included features of the health care delivery systems, such as accessibility, availability, and financing mechanisms; cultural factors such as attitudes towards health promotion and social norms about dental care; features of the social system, such as social class factors and income; and, finally, sociodemographic characteristics of the individuals themselves, such as age and sex (Reisine 1981).

Gift's review (1986a) of oral hygiene practices of individuals suggests that tooth brushing and use of fluoride dentifrices is nearly universal in developed countries. However, the quality of tooth brushing in the community, and hence its health promotion benefits, is probably not at the level characteristic of clinical caries trials. Use of floss and other plaque control techniques are less common in the general population. She concludes that beyond these few facts, relatively little is known about home oral hygiene care and the factors that contribute to health practices. She also suggests that the professional dental care providers play an important role in teaching patients about oral hygiene techniques and in encouraging their use.

Although the decision to engage in oral health promotion activities ultimately takes place at the level of the individual, many factors related to both the individual and the larger social structure come to bear on that decision. This section has discussed some characteristics of the individual such as perception of need, cost–benefit appraisals, and perceived access and availability of care. Also discussed were behavioural interventions to enhance compliance. The remaining sections will present material on how elements of the social structure, including the health care delivery system, impinge upon the decisions of individuals to promote oral health.

The dental health professional as decision maker

Dental health professionals, including dentists, hygienists, and dental assistants, have their greatest effect on oral health promotion through the preventive and restorative services they provide on a one-to-one basis. Most important in the delivery of dental care is the role of the dentist as the gatekeeper to the therapeutic and preventive measures (Gronroos and Masalin 1990; Silversin 1989). In addition, a decision maker (usually the dentist) in the dental practice establishes oral health promotion policy (Grembowski *et al.* 1988). The policy may include standards not only about how and when to provide primary and secondary preventive services, but also about furnishing patient education in caries and plaque control and in nutritional and diet counselling. These policies are critical to oral health promotion activities in the private practice setting. Without such a policy in the dental practice, primary preventive care will not be provided in a systematic way.

In most cases, the person establishing such a policy is the dentist. In the case of the United States, where the organization of dental practise is characterized primarily by fee-for-service private practices, the dentist is the sole decision maker within the confines of professional licensure. The dentist's power and authority are based both on ownership of the practice and on the dentist's training and expertise in clinical dentistry (Parsons 1951; Freidson 1970). In other countries characterized by publicly funded programmes, such as that in the United Kingdom, decisions about eligibility for care, and the remuneration for different treatments provided, are made by people holding positions within the health care bureaucracy. However, the oral health promotion policy is still the province of the individual general dental practitioner, the only exception being the salaried community dental service who treat special groups of patients. In this case, overall policy decisions will usually be made by a specialist in dental public health.

Dentists' decisions about treatment can have a large effect on patterns of care and oral health promotion. Gift (1983) surveyed the preventive measures used and advocated by dental practitioners in the United States and their willingness to expand their roles in delivering caries preventive services: 3500 general practitioners and 500 specialist completed mailed questionnaires about their attitudes towards preventive services and provision of such services.

The study found that most dentists used topical fluorides on children in their practices (80 per cent), provided oral prophylaxis (96 per cent), and offered education on plaque control. The majority (56 per cent) of dentists did not use pit and fissure sealants, primarily because they believed they were not effective in preventing caries, despite the large literature documenting their efficacy. Other studies (Glasrud *et al.* 1987; Gift 1986*b*) agree that although the number of dentists using sealants is increasing, a majority of practitioners in the United States still do not use them.

The case of sealants in the United States illustrates clearly the pivotal role dentists play in primary prevention of occlusal caries, particularly among children. The decision to provide this service and other oral health promotion programmes is sensitive to several factors, including economic constraints, beliefs and attitudes about the service, and availability of knowledge about the efficacy of health promotion techniques (Rubenstein and Dinius 1986).

Silversin (1989) also suggests that dentists can influence oral health promotion programmes in other ways. They can take a leadership role in influencing public policy and creating legislation to promote preventive health programmes. Another approach for individual dentists is to work with physicians and other health professionals to develop oral health programmes as part of other health programmes. For example, dentists in a Boston hospital have intergrated information about fluorides, tooth development, and bottle caries into prenatal education classes. Conversely, the dental practice can be the focal point for the development of general health promotion plans, such as smoking cessation clinics, general nutrition programmes, or childhood development instruction.

Therefore, dentists have an important role to play as decision makers in their own practices, in organizing local dentists into programmes directed towards oral health promotion activities, and in influencing legislation at a local and national level.

State and local agencies

Strategically placed individuals in local community and state public and private organizations can have a large effect on oral health promotion efforts in local communities. For example, Schou (1989) has described work site oral health programmes and their efficacy. Several investigators (Sweeney 1983; Schou 1987) have shown how mass media can be used to effectively transmit oral health promotion information to large populations. Two examples of the effects of state and local political influences on oral health promotion will be discussed in detail, including community water fluoridation in the United States and the United Kingdom and an international survey of school-based oral health promotion programmes.

Water fluoridation in the United States

Newbrun (1980, p. 243) states that communal water fluoridation is an axiom of caries prevention; it is effective, inexpensive and nondiscriminatory. Children of all sexes, all races and all socioeconomic classes benefit thereby, and its dental benefits extend throughout the lifetime of residents of optimally fluoridated communities. Given the overwhelming evidence of the efficacy of fluoride in the prevention of caries, the ease of administration, and its low cost, universal adoption of community water fluoridation would be expected. However, only 55 per cent of Americans (Harris and Christen 1987; Jong 1988) benefit from optimally adjusted or naturally fluoridated water: approximately 77 million Americans live in communities that do not have fluoridated water systems.

By and large, community fluoridation is a public health issue managed at the local community level. In the United States, state and municipal governments rather than the federal government control these public health issues. The state of Connecticut was the first to mandate statewide water fluoridation. Other states require an election to authorize fluoridation of community water supplies, while other states still have 'option out' laws where municipalities must indicate within a specified period whether they *do not* wish to fluoridate. In Massachusetts the state board of health may order water fluoridation, but local communities can vote to reject fluoridation.

Depending upon the political structure in states and municipalities, the public health officer, if empowered to mandate fluoridation, can hold a crucial position to influence oral health promotion efforts. The public health officer may be the person to convince on the decision to evaluate the benefits of fluoridation, on budgets for the costs of such a programme, and on implementation of a plan.

State and local politicians are also crucial to community water fluoridation programmes. These people are involved in the process of writing and passing legislation to mandate the fluoridation of public water supplies. Politicians must be assured that the initiation and support of such measures will not alienate their constituents or divert funds and support from other high priority programmes. Finally, leaders in local communities must support fluoridation of the public water supply in order for the passage of laws to initiate the programme.

Antifluoridationists have come to understand the importance of decision makers in the political process of passing fluoridation programmes. The Center for Health Action was recently formed out of a merger of the National Health Federation (NHF), the Safe Water Foundation, and the National Health Action Committee. The NHF was founded to help defeat fluoridation of community water supplies. More recently, these organizations have advocated the use of non-traditional medical therapies, such as the use of laetrile in the treatment of cancer. These groups also criticize many accepted health practices, such as pasteurization of milk and polio immunization.

Yiamouyiannis, a biochemist, founded the NHF and based much of his publicity on the supposed health risks of water fluoridation, particularly the excess risk of cancer in communities with fluoridation programmes. His work has been criticized extensively (International Association for Dental Research 1990) on methodological grounds. Yet, members of the Center for Health Action and other antifluoridationists have exploited the data from his studies to defeat referenda on water fluoridation and to lobby politicians and public health officers on fluoridation legislation (Easly 1985).

Fluoridation activists stress the importance of focusing oral health promotion activities at crucial decision makers and of avoiding popular elections. This strategy will avoid public debate of scientifically technical issues on the benefits of fluoride and the politically sensitive one regarding the unfounded excess risk of cancer in previously fluoridated communities (Margolis and Cohen 1985).

Fluoridation in other countries

At present, about 215 million people outside the United States have drinking water that is either naturally or artificially fluoridated (Ekstrand *et al.* 1988). Arguments against the implementation of water fluoridation programmes in other countries are similar to those found in the United States, namely safety, civil rights, and cost–benefit ratios. Yiamouyiannis has been active throughout the world in arguing against fluoride legislation and in legal proceedings challenging existing fluoridation programmes.

Some countries have passed national legislation mandating fluoridation of national water supplies. Interestingly, some countries, such as the Netherlands, passed such legislation, then repealed the law because of legal challenges. The case of Scotland and the United Kingdom also illustrates the effectiveness of the organized antifluoridation groups and the importance of judges in the decision making process.

In 1978, Strathclyde Regional Council, as a statutory Water Authority, agreed to a request from four Area Health Boards to fluoridate the regional public water supplies. However, the plans for large scale fluoridation in the Glasgow area were halted by legal action, by a citizen of Scotland, which challenged fluoridation on the grounds of legality, safety, and risks to health. Many expert witnesses gave testimony in a trial which lasted from September 1980 to July 1982. The Court of Sessions sat on 201 days, making it the longest and costliest civil action in Scottish legal history (Fluoridation Society 1983*a*, 1983*b*). The judge spent a further 11 months preparing a lengthy judgment 'Lord Jauncey, 1983'. The major part of the judgment covered the verdict that fluoridation of water supplies was beneficial, safe, and carried no risk to health whatsoever. However the judge also found that water fluoridation was *ultra vires* and it was beyond the legal powers of Strathclyde Regional Council to add fluoride to the public water supply. Although all other arguments were rejected in the judgment, many believed wrongly that the judge found for the petitioner on the principle that fluoridation was an infringement of personal rights and restricted freedom of choice.

As a result of the finding that there was no legal mechanism allowing fluoridation of public water supplies, fluoridation ceased in Scotland in 1983. As no legal action has been taken in England and Wales, water fluoridation continues.

This Scottish judgment led Parliament to review the Water Scotland Act in order to clarify the legality of artificially fluoridated water supplies. As a result, a bill legalizing water fluoridation received the Royal Assent in November 1985, 'Water (Fluoridation) Act, 1985'.

However, although it appeared that water fluoridation could start again in Scotland, an indemnity and guidelines had first to be agreed by the Scottish Office and the Confederation of Scottish Local Authorities (COSLA). The .

guidelines and indemnity were not published until June 1991, finally allowing Health Boards to begin the consultation process to reintroduce fluoridation of public water supplies to Scotland. The guidelines confirmed the government view that water fluoridation was a safe and effective means of reducing tooth decay.

School-based oral health promotion programmes

Elementary and secondary schools provide an effective forum for the delivery of health promotion programmes (Kenney 1979; Loupe and Frazier 1983; Flanders 1987). Schools have access to large numbers of children and adults and health promotion activities, particularly health education, can be integrated into the regular curriculum. School boards, administrators, and teachers play important roles as decision makers since they control the content of the curriculum, participation in health promotion activities, and compliance with health regimens (Cons 1979).

Frazier *et al.* (1979, 1983) conducted a survey of 79 member nations of the FDI to assess the current programme activities in dental programmes for school-aged children. They received 119 responses from 34 countries. The results showed that 75 per cent of programmes were separate oral health programmes with 50 per cent serving more than 10 000 children in each. Further, over half of the programmes served parents as well as children. Programmes consisted primarily of instructions, although more than half also provided primary and secondary prevention treatment services by dentists or hygienists. Two questions were asked about sources of influence on the programmes. One concerned influences on policy decisions and the second sources of influence on daily operation.

The investigators identified three major sources of influence on policy decisions, including programme and executive director and supervisory personnel. Parents were considered one of the least important actors in these decisions, suggesting that once the programme is in place in the school, most children participate. Persons considered most influential in the daily operation of programmes were programme directors, supervisory personnel, and other staff, such as teachers and school board officials. In evaluating the programmes, respondents stated that the existing programmes could be improved by adding more primary prevention services.

The five most frequently mentioned barriers to programme development were finances, manpower, public acceptance, policy-maker attitudes, and facilities. The authors conclude that an important factor in building effective school-based programmes is the extent to which health professionals, politicians, and the public can achieve consensus on the value of competing service programmes. These decisions are generally based on the perceived benefits of dental programmes compared to the social value of .other programmes.

The political organization and historical development in local communities can have a significant affect on the potential to reach consensus on these issues. Riska (1984) studied two communities in the United States, analysing their ability to meet district health care needs as a function of community power structures. The two communities had similar health status and economic and sociodemographic characteristics. However, one community, when faced with an impending shortage of hospital beds, rallied local support to increase the number of beds in local hospitals and increased public expenditure for health care. The second community also had a considerable shortage of hospital beds and relatively little public spending on health care.

The first community was characterized by a centralized power structure founded on a longer history of economic development and shared cultural values. This community had several large business corporations in the area providing a cadre of area-wide leadership validated by a common social legacy. The leaders also were a part of an integrated and extensive network and worked together on many boards of voluntary agencies in the community. This power structure fostered shared values that could lead to consensus on the need for hospital beds and the allocation of resources for this need.

In contrast, the second community under study was a newly developed suburb on the fringes of a powerful economic urban centre. The community itself had branches of major corporations, but no headquarters that could provide the elite economic leadership found in the first community. Further, the pattern of housing growth in the community contributed to fragmentation and little shared cultural traditions across the community that formed the political organization governing the district. Thus, the second community was characterized by smaller municipalities and townships making up the larger district with local leaders drawn from small business and middle management. The political structure limited the growth of social networks. Leaders often generated power in their own municipalities by emphasizing the different values, priorities, and political needs within their district. Parochial concerns of the leaders prevented agreement on the need for more hospital beds and the allocation of resources to this effort in the larger community.

Health promotion advocates should have an understanding of the power structure in local communities in order to achieve their aims. In the case of decentralized political power hierarchies, strategies should be aimed at local leaders; where power is centralized the efforts should be focused on the key decision maker for the community at large.

Scheirer's analysis (1990) of the discontinuation of school-based fluoride mouth rinse programs also stressed the importance of the organization of programmes within the school and its relationship to the external political and power structure within the community. She found that of 409 school districts studied in 1981 who had a mouth rinse programme, 21 per cent had discontinued the programme in 1985. Few districts actually made a formal decision to end the programme, but continued support for the programme relied on three factors: continued support from the political process that initiated the programme; continued involvement from external administrators in a higher position of authority within the education bureaucracy; and favourable attitudes among key administrators.

Once into larger organizational structures, particularly local political parties and school boards, it is critical to the strategy of developing programmes to gain an understanding of the power structure and identify the person who is the decision maker. For example, in terms of school programmes, efforts at initiating a school mouth rinse programme should be aimed at administrators rather than at parents, who are the least influential in programme funding and implementation.

Workplace programmes

Oral health promotion at the workplace offers many of the advantages of school-based programmes, in that workplace programmes can potentially reach large numbers of individuals with relatively small effort (Towner 1988). Although the advantages of health promotion at the workplace is clear, most health promotion programmes in both the United States and other countries have focused on alcohol and drug abuse and cardiovascular disease as their targets. Few such programmes have included an oral health component with the general health promotion efforts. Schou (1988) discusses several barriers to the implementation of workplace oral health promotion programmes, including national health insurance mechanisms, lack of proper evaluation, the overall state of the economy, and the dental profession.

The health insurance reimbursement mechanism can exert a marked effort on oral health promotion, as it greatly influences the likelihood of establishing work site programmes and the type of programme that will be initiated. Decision makers at a factory or other workplace will be less willing to begin an oral health promotion programme if it is funded through company funds rather than state or insurance funds. Workplace decision makers are faced with competing priorities for scarce resources and must be convinced that oral health promotion programmes will not be costly, will reduce worker absenteeism, will improve productivity, and will give the company a competitive edge either in acquiring good workers or in producing goods and services. A major problem facing health promotion workers is the difficulty in demonstrating the benefits of an intervention programme, particularly in dentistry where clinical changes occur slowly. Efforts should be aimed at developing oral health status indicators that are more sensitive to changes over time (Reisine 1985).

A report by Petersen (1988) on an oral health promotion programme in the Danish confectionery industry illustrates the importance of legislation and key decision makers in initiating and implementing a successful oral health promotion campaign. The Act on Working Environment was passed in 1975 in Denmark. This act was aimed at assuring a safe working environment. Enforcement of the act was provided for under the guidance of the Labour Inspection and the act required the formation of a safety committee at companies with more than nine employees. In 1982 the safety committees at two Danish chocolate factories became concerned with oral health of employees. A clinical assessment of the workers exposed to a high level of sugar dust found that 33 per cent were edentulous compare to 11 per cent in a matched comparison group. The safety committee concluded that the chocolate workers were at a high risk of oral disease because of exposure to high levels of sugar dust at work.

The safety committee worked with the health personnel to reduce the risk of oral diseases by helping to reduce the level of sugar dust and to remove organizational constraints that could adversely affect oral health promotion programmes. In 1984 an oral health promotion programme was implemented that consisted of four visits to a dental hygienist in the first year and two visits in the second year. The workers also were allowed to brush their teeth at work and could participate in dental health education programmes. All parts of the programme were available to employees without the loss of wages. Evaluation of the programme at 12 and 24 months showed that oral hygiene practices improved, awareness of the risk of dental diseases improved, oral hygiene was better, and the number of decayed surfaces declined. The success of the programme can be attributed to the cooperation of management, the safety committee, and labour representatives, and to the support of the health personnel. Most important was the development of a corporate policy favourable to the implementation of the programme, primarily that workers could participate in the programme during working hours without loss of wages.

National programmes

Oral health promotion activities can be effected at the national level from many locations. Three major structures will be discussed: national governments, national professional organizations, and health services reimbursement organizations.

National governments

National governments make policy and pass laws that directly influence allocation of resources to oral health promotion activities. It is a common feature of national governments to have a national level health officer and/or a bureau governing health affairs for the country. Key decision makers at this level include the national leaders of countries, such as presidents and prime ministers, who establish a political philosophy about the role of government in the provision of health services. The national health officer and administrators that supervise the management of dental care in a particular country are of key importance because they establish the regulations that influence the day-to-day operation of health programmes.

The organization of the health care delivery system and the role of national government in the delivery of dental services have a critical effect on oral health promotion activities. National governments have a more indirect effect on oral health promotion activities in systems characterized by private practices with self-employment and direct payment systems. Governments with this kind of decentralized structure can issue guidelines and health objectives for the population that constitute recommendations to be carried out by health care professionals and organizations. Governments also can pass legislation requiring insurance coverage for certain services. For example, insurance companies may be required to include coverage for oral prophylaxis but not for orthodontic care. However, decentralization can cause problems of consistency across local programmes. For example, in the United States, Medicaid legislation has mandated funding for health care for the poor. However, level of services, eligibility for care, and types of services provided are decided individually by each state. Many states do not include dental services in their health care financing plans.

Health care systems that are financed in part or entirely by public funds, such as those in New Zealand and Japan, will be affected more directly by government policies and regulation. For example in Japan, under the current school health law, students in compulsory education schools and senior high schools are required to receive an annual oral examination. In the United States, people covered by Medicare or Medicaid (publicly funded programmes) who are in nursing homes also must receive an annual oral exam in order to become eligible for reimbursement under these financing programmes (Arnljot et al. 1985).

Lobbying efforts can greatly influence the passage of laws at all levels of government. This is clearly illustrated by the efforts of the sugar industry that has adeptly avoided food labelling requirements about the risks of sugar consumption on caries. The tobacco industry in the United States has successfully prevented efforts at banning the use of tobacco products. However, health advocates have been able to help pass legislation requiring health warning labels on tobacco products. One particular accomplishment in the United States has been passage of Public Law 99–252, the Comprehensive Smokeless Tobacco Health Education Act of 1986. Capwell (1990) has outlined the ways in which local authorities can implement the provisions of the act which are aimed at reducing smokeless tobacco use in the United States. Chen and Schroeder (1990) have tried to evaluate the effects of the Act and found that both the industrial production of smokeless tobacco and per capita use among adults has declined since 1986. Prevention and reduction of smokeless tobacco use may affect relatively few people, but the consequences of this habit for oral health are serious in terms of increasing the risk of oral cancer and other types of soft tissue lesions. These efforts also illustrate how effective national legislation can be on oral health promotion.

National professional organizations

Cohen (1990*a*, 1990*b*) has developed guidelines for dental associations defining their roles in promoting oral health. She argues that dental associations, regardless of their structure, can play a pivotal role in influencing national health policy. This can be accomplished through lobbying for legislation, health planning, developing insurance benefits programmes, defining standards of care for dental practice, evaluating cost and quality of care, identifying oral health promotion research issues, and defining criteria for dental education (Kress 1984; Loupe *et al.* 1988; Nakata *et al.* 1989; Cohen and Sheiham 1990).

Reimbursement mechanisms

The system for reimbursing or financing dental care costs can have a profound effect on the use of primary and secondary preventive dental services. The ways in which benefits are defined, and eligibility criteria for those covered by insurance plans, are critical to fostering use of dental services. In countries where dental care is financed through public funds, decisions about who and what services are covered will determine the priorities placed on health promotion versus disease treatment. For example, in Japan, where 98 per cent of the population is covered under the government dental plan, preventive services are not included in the insurance scheme for adults. An oral examination is covered only when a patient has a complaint and not for a routine visit. This type of system fosters treatment rather than prevention of disease.

Decisions about services and eligibility for care are made at fairly high levels in the organizational bureaucracy. In the case of insurance companies, benefits are negotiated when costs of premiums are discussed between the companies, the beneficiaries, and the premium payer (Bailit 1980, 1985; Bailit *et al.* 1985). In countries where national publicly funded programmes exist, the decision about eligibility and coverage are determined by cultural norms and values, and the political priorities placed on a particular health problem (Hobdell and Sheiham 1981).

The structure of insurance schemes can also affect an individual's decision to seek dental care. People who have coverage for preventive services are more likely to seek routine or regular care. People who are not covered for such services are less likely to make these decisions.

International programmes

Several international organizations have had an effect on policy decisions about oral health promotion. They included the Federation Dentaire Internationale (FDI), the World Health Organization (WHO), and the International Association for Dental Research (IADR) (Chesters *et al.* 1987). These three organizations have worked together and separately to foster research and treatment programmes aimed at improving the oral health status of nations. They have worked to establish guidelines for the development of oral health promotion programmes, conducted needs assessments, and evaluated the effects of health care delivery systems on the oral health status of nations.

The chairmen of the WHO advisory committees on oral health promotion and the presidents of the FDI and IADR are in important decision-making positions. They provide leadership roles for defining the direction of these organizations and establishing the priorities for oral health promotion activities. These organizations have been effective in helping member nations to establish priorities for oral health promotion activities throughout the world.

Summary and discussion

Oral health promotion decisions occur at many levels. This chapter has described the various levels at which decisions are made. Three major points from the foregoing discussion should be stressed:

1. Decisions are made at many levels. Even personal decisions about oral health promotion can serve as model behaviour to influence the behaviour of others.

2. In order to initiate and implement oral health promotion programmes it is important to identify the position that controls the policy for the target organization. In the dental practice, it is the dentist. To influence insurance schemes, the dentist is not the person to target — rather, insurance administrators should be targeted in order to change health promotion policies and reimbursement of services.

3. Local and national legislation can have a large effect on the legitimacy and perceived importance of oral health promotion activities. Politicians should be challenged to take a stand on health promotion issues and to support programmes that call for these kinds of activities.

References

Albino, J. E., Juliano, D. B., and Slakter, M. J. (1977). Effects of an instructional motivational program on plaque and gingivitis in adolescents. *American Journal of Public Health Dentistry*, **37**, 281–8.

Arnljot, H. A., Barmes, D. E., Cohen, L. K., Hunter, V., and Ship, P. B. (1985). *Oral health care systems, an international collaborative study*. Quintessence, London.

Bailit, H. L. (1980). Issues in regulating the quality of care and containing costs within private sector policy. *Journal of Dental Education*, **44**, 530–6.

Bailit, H. L. (1985). The prevalence of dental pain and anxiety to quality of life. *New York State Dental Journal*, **53**, 27–30.

Bailit, H., Newhouse, J., Brook, R., Duan, N., Goldberg, G., Hanley, J., *et al* (1985). Does more generous dental insurance coverage improve oral health: a study of patient cost sharing. *Journal of American Dental Association*, **110**, 701–7.

Bandura, A. (1969). *Principles of behavior modification*. Holt, Rinehart, and Winston, New York.

Capwell, M. (1990). P. L. 99–252 and the roles of state and local governments in decreasing smokeless tobacco use. *Journal of Public Health Dentistry*, **50**, 70–76.

Chen, M. and Schroeder, K. L. (1990). An epilogue to evaluating the impact of P. L. 99–252 on decreasing smokeless tobacco use. *Journal of Public Health Dentistry*, **50**, 101–4.

Chesters, R. K., Dexter, C. H., Life, J. S., Smales, F. C., and Van der Ouderaa, F. (1987). Periodontal awareness project in the United Kingdom: CPITN and self-assessment. *International Dental Journal*, **37**, 218–21.

Cipes, M. and Miraglia, M. (1985). Monitoring versus contingency contracting to increase children's compliance with home fluoride mouthrinsing. *Pediatric Dentistry.*, **7**, 198–204.

Cohen, L. and Sheiham, A. (1990). Influence of dental school experience on sealant use by British dentists. *International Dental Journal*, **40**, 249–52.

Cohen, L. K. (1990a). Leadership role of dental associations: oral health promotion. *International Dental Journal*, **40**, 48–53.

Cohen, L. K. (1990b). Promoting oral health: guidelines for dental associations. *International Dental Journal*, **40**, 79–102.

Cons, N. C. (1979). Using effective strategies to implement a program administrators goal. *American Journal of Public Health Dentistry*, **39**, 279–85.

Easley, M. W. (1985). The new antifluoridationists: Who are they and how do they operate? *American Journal of Public Health Dentistry*, **45**, 133.

Ekstrand, J., Fejerskov, L., and Silverstone, L. M. (1988). *Fluoride in dentistry*. Munksgaard, Copenhagen.

Flanders, R. A. (1987). Effectiveness of dental health educational programs in school. *Journal of American Dental Association*, **114**, 239–42.

Fluoridation Society Ltd (1983a). *Comments on the case Mrs. Catherine McColl v. Strathclyde Regional Council held in the court session, Edinburgh*. London.

Fluoridation Society Ltd (1983b). *Supportive statements for the fluoridation of water supplies*. London.

Frazier, P. J., Jenny, J., and Johnson, B. G. (1979). Preventive dental programs for school-age children in 8 countries: pilot survey, 1979. *International Dental Journal*, **32**, 204–13.

Frazier, P. J., Johnson, B. G., and Jenny, J. (1983). Health education aspects of preventive dental programs for school age children in 34 countries — final report of FDI international survey. *International Dental Journal*, **33**, 152–70.

Freidson, E. (1970). *The profession of medicine*. Dodd, Mead, New York.

Gift, H. (1983). *The role of the health professional in the delivery of caries prevention, Vol. 1: Dentists*. Final Report, National Institute of Dental Research, NIH, RO1-DE-02424, Bethesda, MD.

Gift, H. C. (1986a). Current utilization of oral hygiene practices: State-of-the-science review. *Dental plaque control measures and oral hygiene practices*, (ed. H. Löe, D. Kleinman), pp. 39–71. IRL Press Ltd, Oxford.

Gift, H. C. (1986b). Sealants: changing patterns. *Journal of American Dental Association*, **112**, 391–2.

Glasrud, P. H., Frazier, P. J., and Horowitz, A. M. (1987). Insurance reimbursement for sealants in 1986: report of a survey. *Journal of dentistry for Children*, **54**, 81–8.

Grembowski, D. (1989). *A public health model of the dental care process*. Final Report to The American Fund for Dental Health and the National Center for Health Services Research and Health Care Technology Assessment (HS 5789).

Grembowski, D., Milgrom, P., and Fiset, L. (1988). Factors influencing dental decision making. *American Journal of Public Health Dentistry*, **48**, 159–67.

Gronroos, C. and Masalin, K. (1990). Motivating your patients: marketing dental services. *International Dental Journal*, **40**, 18–23.

Haefner, D. P. (1984).The Health Belief Model and preventive dental behavior. *Health Education Monographs*, **2**, 420–32.

Harris, N. O. and Christen, A. G. (1987). *Primary preventive dentistry*. Appleton & Lange, Norwalk, CT.

Hobdell, M. H. and Sheiham, A. (1981). Barriers to the promotion of dental health in developing countries. *Social Science and Medicine*, **15A**, 817–23.

International Association for Dental Research (1990). Panel discussion on *The safety of fluoride in the public water supply*. 1990 Annual Scientific Session, Cincinnati, OH, March 1990.

Jong, A. W. (ed.) (1988). *Community dental health*. C. V. Mosby Co., St Louis.

Kegeles, S. S., Lund, A., and Weisenberg, M. (1978). Acceptance by children of a daily mouthrinse program. *Social Science and Medicine*, **12**, 199–209.

Kenney, J. B. (1979). The role and responsibility of schools in affecting dental health status — a potential yet unrealized. *American Journal of Public Health Dentistry*, **39**, 262–7.

Kiyak, H. A. (1988). Recent advances in behavioral research in geriatric dentistry. *Gerodontics*, **7**, 27–36.

Kress, G. C. (1984). The impact of professional education on the performance of dentists. Chapter 6 in *Social sciences and dentistry*, (ed. L. Cohen and P. Bryant), Vol. 2, pp. 323–88. Quintessence, The Hague.

Loupe, M. and Frazier, P. J. (1983). Knowledge and attitudes of schoolteachers toward oral health programs and preventive dentistry. *Journal of the American Dental Association*, **107**, 229–34.

Loupe, M. J., Frazier, P. J., Horowitz, A., Kleinman, D., Caranicas, P., and Caranicas, D. (1988). Impact of NIDR education programs on teaching caries prevention in dental hygiene. *Journal of Dental Education*, **52**, 149–55.

Margolis, F. J. and Cohen, S. N. (1985). Successful and unsuccessful experiences in combating the antifluoridationists. *Pediatrics*, **76**, 113.

Masalin, K. (1988). Finnish examples of oral health promotion in the workplace. In *Oral health promotion at the workplace*, (ed. L. Schou), pp. 32–45. Scottish Health Education Group, Edinburgh.

Nakata, M., Kuriyama, S., Mitsuyasu, K., Morimoto, M., and Tomioka, K. (1989). The transfer of innovation for advancement in dentistry: a case study on pit and fissure sealants' use in Japan. *International Dental Journal*, **39**, 263–8.

Newbrun, E. (1980). Achievements of the seventies: community and school fluoridation. *American Journal of Public Health Dentistry*, **40**, 234–47.

Nikias, M. K., Budner, S., Agatstein, N., and Budner, N. (1979). Compliance over time with preventive oral care regimens, paper presented at IADR, New Orleans, March 29, 1979.

Parsons, T. (1951). *The social system*. Free Press, Glencoe, Ilinois.

Petersen, P. E. (1988). Oral health promotion in the workplace — experiences from a programme in the Danish confectionery industry. In *Oral health promotion in the workplace*, (ed. L. Schou), pp. 45–60. Scottish Health Education Group, Edinburgh.

Reisine, S. T. (1981). Theoretical considerations in sociodental indicators. *Social Science and Medicine*, **15A**, 745–50.

Reisine, S. T. (1985). Dental health and public policy: the societal impacts of dental disease. *American Journal of Public Health*, **75**, 27–31.

Riska, E. (1984). *Power, politics and health: forces shaping American Medicine*. Finnish Society of Sciences and Letters, Helsinki.

Rubenstein, L. K. and Dinius, A. (1986). Dental sealant usage in Virginia. *American Journal of Public Health Dentistry*, **46**, 147–53.

Russell, B. A., Horowitz, A. M., and Frazier, P. J. (1989). School based preventive regimens and oral health knowledge and practices of sixth graders. *American Journal of Public Health Dentistry*, **49**, 192–200.

Scheirer, M. A. (1990). The life cycle of an innovation: adoption versus discontinuation of the fluoride mouth rinse program in school. *Journal Health and Social Behavior*, **31**, 203–15.

Schou, L. (1985). Active-involvement principle in dental health education. *Community Dentistry and Oral Epidemiology*, **13**, 128–32.

Schou, L. (1987). Use of mass media and active involvement in a national dental health campaign in Scotland. *Community Dentistry and Oral Epidemiology*, **15**, 14–18.

Schou, L. (1988). Obstacles and benefits of oral health promotion in the workplace. In *Oral health promotion at the workplace* (ed. L.Schou), pp. 19–31. Scottish Health Education Group, Edinburgh.

Schou, L. (1989). Oral health promotion at worksites. *International Dental Journal*, **39**, 122–8.

Schou, L. and Monrad, A. (1989). A follow up study of dental patient education in the workplace: participants' opinions. *Patient Education and Counselling*, **14**, 45–51.

Silversin, J. (1989). Communicating with each other. *International Dental Journal*, **39**, 258–62.

Silversin, J. B. and Kornacki, M. J. (1984). Controlling dental disease through prevention: individual, institutional and community dimensions. Chapter 3 in *Social sciences and dentistry*, (ed. L. Cohen and P. Bryant) Vol. 2, pp. 145–201. Quintessence, The Hague.

Sweeney, E. (1983). The effects of television advertising on children. *Journal of Dentistry*, **11**, 175–81.

Towner, E. (1988). Brush up your smile — a United Kingdom workplace dental health education programme. In *Oral health promotion at the workplace*, (ed. L. Schou), pp. 61–72. Scottish Health Education Group, Edinburgh.

Wallston, B. S. and Wallston, K. (1976). Development and validation of the Health Locus of Control Scale. *Journal of Consulting and Clinical Psychology*, **44**, 580–5.

5

The role of oral health promotion in oral health policy

MARTIN C. DOWNER

Introduction

Policy is a plan for action adopted or pursued by an individual, government, political party, commercial enterprise, or any other organization. The nub of the definition is 'plan for action' and this implies action towards a specified objective or goal. In many places in the world examples may be found of governments, professional organizations, or other groups prescribing broad aims for their communities' dental services or adopting goals for oral health. In those countries where health care and related systems are most highly developed, action towards these goals is generally supported by a strong statutory framework. Nevertheless, while some countries have a long history of slow and gradual development of their dental services underpinned by networks of laws and regulations, health promotion has been included in oral health and related legislation only relatively recently. In countries at the opposite end of the spectrum health promotional activities, where they exist, have arisen haphazardly mostly from the initiative of local authorities or professional groups. These countries have not yet come to rely on formal legislation.

Laws and regulations do not of themselves define strategies for health promotion. This is the domain of programme planning and management, and prevailing laws and regulations are only one of a variety of parameters within which these processes take place. In countries with a well developed health infrastructure built on a statutory foundation a variety of agencies may be involved in promoting oral health and may contribute to the formation of policy aimed at improving the oral health of the public through education, disease prevention, and other relevant activities. An examination of the way in which central decision making is shaped and influenced provides insight into how the various agencies involved interact, both with government and among themselves.

In order to optimize effectiveness and efficient use of resources in health promotion, the tenets of management science would prescribe that it should take place within a planned programme incorporating a cycle of situational analysis, objective setting, implementation of strategies, evaluation, and review; all stages being supported by appropriate management information. The planning and management process forms a useful model for examining the structure and process of health promotional activities and their outcome systematically. It is used in parts of this chapter in discussing examples of oral health promotion in the context of overall policy.

For more in-depth analysis of a particular system, the United Kingdom experience is taken as an example for illustrative purposes. The UK is a country with comprehensive, largely publicly financed health care services, a variety of agencies involved in oral health promotion, a well motivated professional dental association, good communication networks, and a strong applied research base.

Health promotion may be considered as any combination of educational, organizational, economic and environmental supports for behaviour conducive to health (Cohen 1990). Providing learning opportunities designed to facilitate voluntary adaptations of behaviour towards a healthy lifestyle is a necessary ingredient. However, health promotion includes a far wider range of activities than just health education. These attempt to alter the environment in which people live and work in order to improve their health despite possibly adverse lifestyles or to enable them to take advantage of preventive services. Health promotion depends on science transfer which is the practical application of knowledge gained from research. Education is the medium through which science transfer takes place and is required to initiate, implement, and maintain ideas, procedures, and programmes. Promotion is needed to reinforce positive behaviour over time and to create opportunities for improving health in the environment. Nowadays it is widely accepted that for success to be achieved, the consumer's viewpoint should always be taken as the starting point in health promotion — yet this is not always recognized in practice.

Oral health promotion embraces a variety of established intervention strategies. These cover three broad areas:

(1) disseminating knowledge to both individuals and groups to encourage appropriate personal behaviour;

(2) providing access to high quality preventive oral health care services;

(3) modifying the environment to mitigate known hazards to oral health while implementing measures aimed at controlling disease on a population scale.

Thus there are elements which relate to the primary prevention of oral disease in individuals on the one hand and to mass application procedures on the other. However, with regard to the provision of oral health care services, it should be noted that the vast majority of dental expenditures in European countries — and the same would apply elsewhere — are for secondary prevention, that is to say early diagnosis and surgical treatment to arrest disease progression rather than primary prevention (Pinet 1987).

In order to keep the material presented within manageable bounds, no attempt is made to analyse exhaustively all the policy initiatives in the field that have occurred either in the industrialized world or in developing countries. This would be an altogether impossible task within a text of limited length. The concern rather is with presenting illustrative examples of policy processes which have led to successful outcomes and some which have failed. In this way it is hoped that useful general conclusions can be drawn about those approaches which are likely to succeed and those which would be better avoided. In looking at achievements it is also pertinent to consider whether oral health promotion should comprise an explicit, formulated part of national or local policy or whether improvements can be attained just as readily without its being integrated into policy. In other words, are there circumstances where, paradoxically, 'no policy' can also be policy?

The stakeholders and their role in policy

The term 'stakeholders' is borrowed from a concept used in the field of management studies in a technique known as communication audit. Stakeholders are all those interested groups, parties, organizations, individuals, and institutions, both internal and external to an undertaking, who affect and are affected by its policies and activities. An enumeration of those agencies which contribute to or will benefit from the success of the undertaking, together with those whose interests will be constrained by its success, leads to an identification of stakeholders in the undertaking's activities. In examining oral health care systems, for example, the stakeholders have sometimes been grouped conveniently and simply into those who commission or administer the services, those who provide them, and those who receive them (Downer et al. 1983). However, in applying the concept to oral health promotion, the list must be expanded to include a far larger intercommunicating network of agencies and groups. Some stakeholders have an explicit involvement in action plans and make a direct contribution to promoting oral health. Others do not have an explicit role but, as a by-product, their operations none the less have a potent effect on the oral health of the population. Stakeholder groups may have either a stated or implicit policy towards oral health promotion or no policy as such. Either way, their stance will inevitably be determined by their own explicit or implicit organizational aims and objectives.

The main stakeholder groups in oral health promotion are listed in Table 5.1. Those with a specific involvement may include departments of central government, governmental agencies, regional or local government, education authorities and schools, national dental associations and their constituencies, and specialist dental societies, community groups, and consumer organizations. Those generally without an explicit policy interest but whose activities have a substantial positive or negative influence on oral health promotion and who may be affected in one way or another by its success include the mass media, manufacturers and marketers of oral hygiene products, the dental education and research institutions, the sugar industry and its marketing outlets, and antifluoridation groups.

While these represent the main stakeholders the list is not necessarily exhaustive. In the particular area of oral cancer, evidence indicates that the tobacco and liquor industries generate environmental risk factors. They are therefore stakeholders whose activities, albeit legitimate in the eyes of society, stand to suffer from a successful health promotion undertaking.

Table 5.1   The main stakeholders in oral health promotion

Explicit policy interest	Implicit policy influence
Central government	Consumer
Governmental agencies	Communications media
Regional and local government	Dental education and research institutions
Education authorities	Manufacturers of oral hygiene products
National dental associations	Sugar industry
Specialist dental societies	Tobacco and liquor industries
Consumer organizations	Marketers and retailers
Community groups	Antifluoridationists

Evaluating policies: SWOT

A rapid rule-of-thumb checklist useful to decision makers in evaluating a proposed policy and its potential consequences is known by the acronym SWOT. This stands for **s**trengths, **w**eaknesses, **o**pportunities, and **t**hreats. The policy of fluoridating public water supplies is a good example to illustrate the application of the SWOT principle in determining the likely outcome of a policy and its impact on external stakeholders (Table 5.2). The *strengths* of fluoridation are that it is an effective, efficient, and safe method of reducing the incidence of dental caries in the population, with concomitant benefits, and is favoured by the majority of consumers. Its *weaknesses* are possible technical difficulties where the water supply network is complex giving rise to questions about its feasibility, its marginal benefit over cost in less densely populated areas or in populations with low caries prevalence, and the political

Table 5.2   SWOT applied to water fluoridation policy

Strengths	Weaknesses	Opportunities	Threats
Effective	Possible technical difficulties	Improved oral health of population	To anti fluoridationists
Efficient			
Safe	Reduced cost-effectiveness in some situations	Reduced treatment costs	As perceived by some dentists
Concommitant benefits (reduced pain, exodontia, general anaesthesia; improved appearance, oral function)	Political difficulties		As perceived by water suppliers in absence of specific legislation
Consumer support			

difficulties of introducing it. The *opportunities* presented are for greatly improved oral health in all sections of the population, and reduced demands and possible cost savings in the primary care sector. It will be perceived as a *threat* by, and will evoke a negative reaction from, politicians opposed to fluoridation, antifluoridation lobbyists, less enlightened dental professionals who may fear for their livelihood, and perhaps by water supply undertakers who may regard it as the imposition of an added unnecessary burden, lying outside their contractual responsibilities in the absence of a specific statutory obligation to fluoridate.

In general terms the question of whether or not a policy is worth pursuing will depend on a favourable balance between its strengths and the opportunities it offers on the one hand and its weaknesses and the threats it poses on the other. Alternative policies will be weighed in the same way. Although all sorts of management tools such as cost-effectiveness analysis and market research can aid the decision maker in refining choice, the adoption or rejection of a policy will depend in the end on value judgements made in a political climate.

Irrespective of whether stakeholders consciously apply the SWOT principle in formulating their policies or attitudes towards oral health promotion, bearing the principle in mind helps to elucidate and explain how they interact and communicate with one another and the complex way in which the thrust of overall policy is determined.

By taking a selection of the main stakeholder groups and analysing what motivates their policies, determines their postures, and guides their internal and external relations, it is possible to gain an understanding of the complicated, dynamic 'life-world' within which oral health promotion takes place and the pressures which both facilitate and constrain it.

Policy formation

What most organizations do can be conceived of as the product of five basic component elements (Table 5.3). These are task, structure, processes, reward systems, and people. In this model *task* comprises the fulfilment of the organization's goals, objectives, or 'mission statement'. *Structure* embraces its organizational framework together with the resources (monetary, human, and physical) at the organization's disposal, where the financial resources come from, and how they are deployed. *Processes* are the activities and day-to-day operations which take place in performing the task. *Reward systems* are the monetary and other incentives used to motivate and satisfy the workforce. *People* are those who work in or for the organization at all hierarchical levels and in all functional groupings.

Table 5.3   The component elements of an organization

Task	Goals and objectives
Structure	Organizational framework and resource
Processes	Strategies and operations
Reward systems	Monetary and other motivating incentives
People	Management and workforce

It may be helpful to broaden the latter component to include in the case of a professional organization, for example, its members, and in the case of a commercial enterprise, its shareholders. However these, like patients, consumers, or customers, should perhaps more properly be regarded as external stakeholders in their own right. Where these groups are placed will in fact depend on the viewpoint of the observer. While classically the model is applied to commercial enterprises, whatever the business of an organization it is generally possible to look at it in terms of these five components or analogues of them.

National dental associations, central governments, and the mass media represent three major stakeholder groups with diverse interests in oral health promotion. An examination of their explicit or implicit policy roles and their relationships with other stakeholders, using elements of the communication audit approach, will help to provide an overall picture of the dynamic processes of policy formation.

National dental associations

The essential task of a national dental association is to protect and further the interests of its members. An activity central to this task is likely to be a continuing dialogue and regular process of collective bargaining with government or third-party insurance providers in order to improve the income and working conditions of the members. The association will seek to maintain its prestige, influence, and span of control by being the arbiter of professional standards and by preserving professional exclusivity. It may therefore have official registration, licensing, and disciplinary functions although, in the assumed public interest, these responsibilities may be separated off and vested with a more independent body.

No two national dental associations are exactly alike. The extent to which they are actively involved in oral health promotion in addition to their more fundamental perceived tasks varies enormously worldwide. There are numerous examples of national associations having a coherent and explicit policy towards oral health promotion. However, many others still need to develop one. In a detailed and comprehensive exposition of the role of national dental associations in oral health promotion, a Working Group of the Federation Dentaire Internationale (FDI) has prescribed four conditions to be met as a prerequisite to an association's developing a constructive policy (Cohen 1990). First, it should acknowledge a collective commitment to improving oral health; secondly, it should form a view as to the relative roles of the private and public sectors in delivering dental services; thirdly, it should form an attitude towards the relative priorities of diagnosis, prevention, and treatment; and finally, it should have a willingness and capacity to invest in oral health promotion programmes and evaluate their outcome.

In accordance with its essential functions, the main thrust of a dental association's policy is likely to aim at promoting oral health through communication with its professional constituency and the public in order to encourage utilization of the preventive services which its members can offer. It may also act as a gatekeeper to information, ensuring that other stakeholders receive correct and appropriate messages.

Association policy may be established from the top down, in which case ideas generated by a policy-making body are delegated to designated agencies or committees within the association for implementation. Alternatively it may be established from the bottom up so that ideas generated by individuals or groups within the association are transmitted upwards to the policy-making body. Cohen (1990) has illustrated a suitable model structure to accomplish the making and implementing of policies and decisions for an oral health promotion plan based on the organizational chart of the American Dental Association. She has also enumerated a wide range of activities relevant to oral health promotion with which an association should be concerned. Among these are advocating policies to governmental bodies for incorporation into legislation; health planning; developing and evaluating benefit programmes; identifying cost-effective preventive procedures; quality assurance; fostering research and disseminating its findings; making recommendations on the content of professional education; developing health education material; marketing the services provided by members; maintaining an up-to-date library; and organizing appropriate scientific sessions.

It is apparent that national dental associations will need to relate to and communicate with most of the other main stakeholder groups in fulfilling these tasks. While their policies will be geared primarily to expanding the opportunities for their members — for it is the members who furnish an association's resources and for whom axiomatically it exists — in the most favourable instances these policies will be motivated by an ethical desire ultimately to improve the dental health of the public.

Governments

The role of governments in oral health promotion ranges from minimal direct involvement through to tenure of the key position as orchestrator and coordinator of action plans. Where government does not actively involve itself in oral health promotion, it may choose to delegate the task to a governmental or some non-governmental agency.

The policy of governments towards oral health promotion depends on a complex interplay of geographical, cultural, and social factors, the political flavour of the ruling administration, the way in which the administrative system is organized, and not least the economic resources at a country's disposal. It is possible to select examples from both industrialized and developing countries that broadly typify the prevailing approaches to policy.

In some developing countries the World Health Organization (WHO) has assisted governments to devise policies suited to their limited resources by providing expert help to set up model demonstration projects based on the primary health care concept (Sardo Infirri 1990). This concept is supported by a strong commitment from WHO and has a high health promotional content.

However, the very use of the term 'developing countries' calls for a word of caution since these countries show great variation in their stages of development and degrees of prosperity. In discussing the complex relationship of oral health, and in particular dental caries, to economic levels and standards of living in the industrialized and developing world, Pinto (1990) grouped countries into three broad categories:

(1) the poorest nations in which traditionally low levels of caries have started to rise in line with industrialization;

(2) those developing countries that have made definite economic progress but which are, in general, undergoing a period of severe economic crisis and which are top of the world caries statistics;

(3) the most affluent nations which have reached high levels of caries in the past but which have gradually managed to control the disease.

Based on average per capita gross national product (GNP) and standard of living, and broken down into broad geographical aggregations, the first group of countries comprised nations of Africa and Asia with a per capita GNP averaging US$528; the second group; Latin American countries with an average per capita GNP of US$1699; and the third group industrialized countries of both East and West whose average per capita GNP amounted to US$9416. It should be noted, however, that the first geographical group included a collection of more prosperous countries of the Middle East and Asia with GNPs averaging over US$3000. From a policy point of view, the monetary resources at a country's disposal are an important factor in determining its ability to choose and invest in health promotional enterprises. At the same time, the income accruing to individual citizens influences the breadth of choice they can exercise in their personal lifestyle options.

Many countries have a strongly regional system of administration, and oral health promotion is dependent on initiatives by regional governments. Among the industrialized nations Spain is an example. In 1988 the Pais de Vasco introduced its own water fluoridation programme. Elsewhere, the regional health department of Murcia undertook a population based survey of children in 1989 (Navarro Alonso 1990) and embarked independently on a fluoridation programme. Parts of Andalusia are also fluoridated. However, by the beginning of the 1990s not all regions of Spain had plans that had reached a comparable stage of development and the national picture of oral health promotion was patchy. Canada has a federal system of government with a degree of central monitoring and coordination of oral health promotion. At the same time each province has autonomous responsibility for implementing its own programmes. Patterns of provision which vary in their content and comprehensiveness have developed. Most provinces have, as a minimum, dental health education and group fluoride prophylaxis programmes for schoolchildren. In addition a number of the major cities, such as Calgary and Toronto, have water fluoridation.

In contrast to this are countries like Denmark and Finland which are highly centralized. In the industrialized world, centralized systems of government tend to be a characteristic feature of countries with relatively small populations, limited size, or both. In these two Nordic countries it is noteworthy that the health education and preventive components of the free dental care services provided for children stem from specific primary national legislation. In Denmark a law on child dental care, enacted in 1971 and modified by subsequent amendment, set up clinics for the preventive and therapeutic care of children. This resulted in comprehensive health educational and preventive services being provided by both dentists and auxiliary personnel for the individual child at the chairside and for groups of children in a school setting (Schwarz 1987). In Finland the Primary Health Care Act of 1972, and successive supplementary directives, provided the cornerstone for similar health centre based primary preventive activities for school children which also extend to preschool children and expectant mothers (Tala 1987).

At the lower end of the economic scale, Tanzania, one of the poorest countries in the world, has a planned oral health care programme under government auspices which is designed to reach the majority of the population in rural areas. One of its main objectives is to promote lifestyles conducive to oral health and to change the prevailing approach of the basic treatment services which exist from curative to preventive. A pyramidal organizational structure has been adopted, based on the primary health care concept, and most of the services are implemented by the government, by government-owned companies and corporations, or by voluntary agencies (mainly religious organizations). A primary task has been to develop individual awareness of oral diseases and of the changes in behaviour needed to reduce self-imposed risks such as frequent sugar and confectionery intake and tobacco chewing. The key field personnel in this health education strategy are rural medical aides and other primary health care workers, with school teachers also being heavily committed (Lembariti 1990). The use of auxiliary personnel with minimal essential training who instruct local teachers and enlist their aid, as well as providing health education and oral hygiene instruction as part of the care they offer to rural communities, is a mainstay of government policy in a number of developing countries.

Governments in many countries at the transitional stage of economic development and industrialization, where the availability of dental services to the mass of the population is limited, have also implemented oral health promotion programmes suited to their limited resources. Singapore, Malaysia, and Hong Kong have water fluoridation schemes with the achievement of virtual total coverage of the population in the latter. In Brazil also, preventive and curative treatment services are complemented by extensive water fluoridation. Millions of people in the vast conurbations of São Paulo and Rio de Janiero benefit from fluoridated water supplies. In the remoter areas of Brazil the progressive introduction of piped water has been accompanied by the installation of fluoridation equipment so that population coverage by this public health measure continued to increase during the 1980s. Many developing countries are major producers of cane sugar and global economic pressures tend to encourage them to consume their own produce. In these countries, government-sponsored mass fluoride prophylaxis programmes, where feasible, are likely to be the most effective and realistic policy for containing escalating caries levels.

So far the policy role of governments has been considered mostly in relation to two external groups of stakeholders, namely, the providers and consumers of services. However, within governments there are powerful groups of internal stakeholders who have their own goals and objectives and who are involved in their own networks of communication with other outside interest groups. The most influential department of a civil government is likely to be its treasury which has a financial overview of all facets of policy and controls the flow of resources. The treasury is usually close to the ultimate decision-making processes and forms an integral part of them. One of the tasks of treasury departments is to ensure that sources of revenue, an example being money raised from taxes on tobacco products, are safeguarded. At the same time the treasury has to keep a tight control on public expenditure and balance the competing demands of all sectors of government, including health ministries. Both the generation of revenue and the way in which resources are deployed can work adversely against health promotion.

In another area of government, those ministries responsible for agriculture and food can have strong vested interests in sponsoring and protecting farmers and the food industry. Attractive subsidies may be offered to farmers in particular, which may encourage the growing, processing, and distribution of products whose consumption is not always conducive to health. Therefore policies supported by these ministries can also run counter to health promotional interests.

On a day-to-day basis the tensions which inevitably arise within the government machine are usually resolved through negotiation and compromise between officials, in the light of the overriding goals and objectives of the administration and the dictates of existing laws and regulations. However, policy decisions of sufficient importance or precedent will be taken at ministerial level. All decisions should ultimately be made in the name of government. Outside pressure groups constantly seek to influence policy making and their effectiveness will depend on their prestige and authority, the monetary resources they control, and the degree of access they have to politicians. In order to further their interests, influential organizations often sponsor politicians, or cultivate them, to work behind the scenes of government or act as their spokesmen in the legislative assembly.

In order to foster and retain popular support, governments (like many other organizations) often devote considerable energy to public relations whereby they can create goodwill and a favourable image in the outside world. The demonstration of a keen interest and effective policy in health promotion is a public relations opportunity that many governments are not slow to exploit.

It is clear that in those countries where government adopts an interventionist policy, exercises a high degree of central control, and is generally benevolent in posture, it can hold the pivotal role in oral health promotion.

The mass media

The mass media comprise a very large, heterogeneous collection of broadcasting and news publishing organizations engaged worldwide in communicating and diffusing information to the public. The communications industry is a powerful and influential force in modern society. Public opinion and attitudes are shaped by the media, they affect policy making at every level, and permeate all aspects of life. Through their role in advertising or simply presenting information the media can provide enormous opportunities for promoting oral health. Equally they can also, often unwittingly, represent a strong negative influence. These seemingly contradictory positions will be considered in turn.

Taking first a very positive contribution to oral health promotion to the credit of the media, there is little doubt that in many Western industrialized countries competitive television advertising by the leading dentifrice manufacturers has played a major part in increasing both the volume of sales of fluoride dentifrices and the share of the market which they command with consequential benefits for oral health. This advertising has also had secondary benefits by boosting sales of toothbrushes especially and generally encouraging better standards of oral hygiene. The role of fluoride dentifrices in the improvement in dental health observed in many industrialized countries over the last two decades can scarcely be disputed. The opinion of a Working Group of the Federation Dentaire Internationale (1985) was that while these products had not necessarily been wholly responsible for the dramatic reductions recorded in caries prevalence, it seemed likely that the sudden surge of improvement during the 1970s could be ascribed to the marked increase in their use. This has been fully discussed elsewhere (Downer 1991a).

A further secondary benefit of toothpaste advertising campaigns has been to make 'fluoride' a household word with generally favourable connotations in the public mind. This has probably served to assist consumer acceptance of water fluoridation as a beneficial measure. Overall the value of the advertising of fluoride dentifrices in oral health promotion has been very considerable.

Apart from advertising, the broadcasting of documentary television programmes and publication of informative articles in newspapers and magazines on matters related to oral health promotion serves to increase public knowledge and awareness. However, the dissemination of ill-informed or scientifically inaccurate material can be counterproductive and will tend at the very least to confuse recipients. On the negative side also, the mass media provide a vehicle to promote their wares for those industries whose products, consumed in excess, may be injurious to health.

From a policy viewpoint, this highlights the dual role of the mass media in health promotion in those countries with a capitalist or mixed economic system. Advertising is the principal means by which the media operating in the commercial sector generate their financial resources, so advertisements form a significant proportion of their broadcast or printed output. However, the main business of the communications industry is to disseminate news, entertainment, features, editorial comment, and all the other material that the various organs making up the industry provide. The policy implications of these two spheres of activity are distinct and separate.

Thus although the content of advertising may be subject to regulation, such as in the UK where a quasi-independent authority scrutinizes television advertising material, for example, to ensure that it is legal, honest, and decent, generally speaking it is the policy of the media to advertise products without fear or favour. An exception applies to certain tobacco products. Thus in many industrialized countries the direct advertising particularly of cigarettes is proscribed on television on grounds of risk to health. However, even this policy may depend only on a fragile voluntary agreement arrived at with government.

On the other hand, the style, flavour, and policy of the essential bulk of material produced by the communications industry will depend on the aims and motives of controllers, proprietors, and editors, or individual producers, broadcasters, and journalists. Thus there is almost unlimited scope for the diffusion of material which can either serve or undermine the interests of health promotion.

It would be out of place to pursue this topic through an exhaustive examination of case histories, but in passing it is worth remarking on one rather curious phenomenon. Local newspapers not infrequently adopt an antifluoridationist stance as part of their editorial policy and it is interesting to speculate as to why this should be so. There would appear to be two reasons. Possibly the proprietor or editor is giving vent to a personal conviction or mere whim. Alternatively the newspaper may see itself as the champion of the 'little man' defending the rights of the individual against the juggernaut of authority. Students of the history of water fluoridation will instantly recognize this scenario.

It is clear that those stakeholders whose mission is to promote oral health must seek to ally the media to their cause and exploit every opportunity to influence and use these potent public information sources in pursuance of their policies.

The United Kingdom experience

In foregoing sections of this chapter, the role of various stakeholders in determining oral health policy has been analysed in general terms. It would be instructive at this juncture to examine the development of policy in one particular country in more detail. To this end the United Kingdom is selected as an example since it has a multiplicity of organizations with a stake in oral health promotion which interact in a fairly sophisticated way. In recent years this has led to action plans with a clear oral health promotional content developing on several fronts.

The UK is a centrally governed Western industrialized country which is composed of the territorial regions of England, Wales, Scotland, and Northern Ireland, and is part of the European Community. The population, of over 57 million, is concentrated most densely in England. There is a comprehensive National Health Service (NHS) which is financed mainly through general taxation and devolved operationally to controlling regional and district health authorities which are upwardly accountable to ministers through a central

NHS Management Board. The health authorities are evolving into purchasers and commissioners of services within an internal market structure. The organization of the NHS in the four territorial regions varies in detail but the arrangements are parallel and broadly similar. England will be taken as the definitive model for illustrative purposes.

The organization of the dental services within the NHS has been described elsewhere (Downer 1988). Suffice it to say here that the great majority of primary dental care is provided, in response to demand, by independent contractor practitioners in the General Dental Service (GDS). A complementary salaried Community Dental Service (CDS) acts as a safety net responding to the needs of priority groups. These include children, expectant and nursing mothers, and lately all groups who experience difficulty in obtaining treatment elsewhere. In all branches of the NHS dental services, children are offered free care.

Staple industries in the UK of immediate relevance in the context of oral health promotion include the refining of domestic and imported sugars, giving rise to an annual per capita net consumption of the order of 45 kg, and the manufacture of oral hygiene products, the biggest producers being UK divisions of multinational companies. Sales of toothpaste by the late 1980s amounted on average to over 400 g per person per year, 95 per cent of which contained fluoride. In addition, over 65 million toothbrushes are marketed per year (Downer 1991a). This amounts to a little over one toothbrush on average per dentate individual though there will be considerable variation in the pattern of purchasing among the different socioeconomic groups.

A framework of laws and regulations underpins the provision of public dental services in the UK, including their preventive functions, and also covers many other spheres of activity which bear on oral health promotion (Downer 1987). The main primary legislation guiding the development of the dental services since the late 1970s has been the National Health Service Act 1977 and amendments. The 1977 Act places on the Secretary of State for Health, the minister responsible, the duty to promote a comprehensive health service designed to secure improvement in the physical and mental health of the population, and in the prevention, diagnosis, and treatment of illness. The Secretary of State's functions under the Act include the duty to provide dental services to such extent as he considers necessary to meet all reasonable requirements. He is also empowered to do any other thing which is calculated to facilitate, or is conducive or incidental to, the discharge of his duties. Most importantly, this includes the provision of facilities for the prevention of illness. In the context of oral health promotion, a notable piece of primary legislation in relation to the latter responsibility was the Water (Fluoridation) Act 1985. This placed beyond doubt the existing legal powers of statutory water undertakers to implement fluoridation schemes at the behest of District Health Authorities after conducting certain publicity and consultation procedures.

It is fair to say that until the 1980s, no specific aim for the dental services, as a foundation for action plans to promote oral health, had ever been made explicit (Downer 1988). In 1980 a working party composed of leading members of the profession, and known as the Dental Strategy Review Group, was formed by the Government to advise on the future direction of the dental services. Its terms of reference were to review the development of dental health policy and in particular a preventive strategy and the future function of the Community Dental Service. The principal professional stakeholder interests were represented on the group, which proposed in its report that the aim should be that of 'providing the opportunity for everyone to retain a healthy functional dentition for life, by preventing what is preventable and by containing the remaining disease (or deformity) by the efficient use and distribution of treatment resources' (Department of Health and Social Security 1981). Implicit in the fulfilment of this aim was a strong commitment to oral health promotion and this was reflected in the report's main recommendations. These were accepted by the Secretary of State and many have since been implemented.

In structural terms the principal stakeholders in oral health promotion in England are the Government, and in particular the Department of Health (DH); the Health Education Authority (HEA), a quasi-independent body sponsored by government; the British Fluoridation Society, a profluoridation pressure group also supported by government; the British Dental Association (BDA); sundry other professional interest groups, including the British Association for the Study of Community Dentistry (BASCD); the local health and education authorities; and various consumer organizations. Manufacturers of oral hygiene products also sponsor health promotional activities including the dissemination of health education material and, on a limited scale, the distribution of products free to schools. In addition, university dental hospitals make a continuing important contribution through their professional education and research roles.

An example of cooperation between different interest groups, including the Department of Health, HEA, BDA, dental schools, and local health and education authorities, was a collaborative effort initiated in 1988 to implement a number of experimental demonstration projects in dental health education in different parts of the country. This was a consequence of an increasingly visible commitment towards all aspects of health promotion on the part of the Government. The projects involved central expenditure of over £1 million in the three financial years following their commencement. The main purpose of the projects was to investigate ways in which uptake of dental services by the public might be increased. However, one project in the north of England targeted towards mothers of young children, also emphasized strongly the dangers to the infant dentition of sugar abuse.

Applied research plays an important part in oral health promotion, first by enabling science transfer to take place, and secondly by providing the means for decision makers to evaluate different operational strategies objectively and thus make informed choices when selecting from among possible alternatives. In this connection, the role of the pragmatic clinical trial as a technique which allows health care planners to both innovate and collect appropriate information concurrently has become acknowledged in the oral health field (Lennon *et al.* 1981).

The largest and most ambitious pragmatic clinical trial in dentistry has probably been the multistage capitation experiment conducted in the UK in the 1980s. This followed from a recommendation of the Dental Strategy Review Group. The project commenced in 1983 and culminated in a three-year randomized controlled trial among children treated in the GDS (Coventry *et al.* 1989). The objective of the trial was to test capitation against the prevailing fee-for-service method of remuneration in as near as possible real-life conditions.

The concept of capitation as a method of paying dentists is closely allied with the principles of oral health promotion. Thus among the theoretical benefits claimed for it are that it should encourage dentists towards a pattern of treatment which emphasizes continuity of care, prevention, and innovation. Capitation should also promote better dental health through patient education and self-help. It should increase patient and professional satisfaction, and should encourage dentists to enlarge their clientele of patients. At the same time capitation should tend to discourage over-prescription of treatment.

In fact, over its limited duration, the trial failed to support most of the hypotheses and also failed to establish capitation as a more suitable means of paying dentists for treating children than fee-for-service. Nevertheless, while there was little evidence either to support or oppose a change to capitation, at the conclusion of the trial the BDA felt able to commend it to their members as a practical way of paying for children's dental care. They believed that it offered significant advantages to dentists in terms of clinical freedom and a stable income. Government was firmly committed to capitation in principle and following intensive negotiation with the profession, a system of payment for the care of children based mainly on capitation was incorporated into the general dental practitioners' contract in 1990.

One of the most notable features of the capitation experiment was the close cooperation throughout between the various stakeholder interests which consisted of the Department of Health and various other agencies administering the GDS, the BDA representing the profession, and the university team commissioned to undertake the research.

Apart from the capitation experiment, a number of other significant events occurred in the UK during the 1980s each of which tended in some measure to promote better oral health in the community. The contribution of these developments was either by promoting the evolution from a restorative to a preventive philosophy in dental care and directing dental professional education into more consciously health promotional channels, or by assisting consumer choice so as to enable individuals to increase control over the determinants of their health and thereby improve it. Various stakeholder groups were involved in bringing the events to fruition with the Government taking the policy lead. Two of the more important developments will be briefly mentioned.

In 1984 the Minister for Health set up a Committee of Enquiry into Unnecessary Dental Treatment in response to media, consumer, professional, and parliamentary concern (Department of Health and Social Security 1986). Certain recommendations in its report provided a powerful stimulus in orientating dental professional education towards a less interventionist approach, and led in due course to a great enhancement of continuing postgraduate education and training. Among specific initiatives, a programme of distance learning via videos delivered free to all dental practices was launched in 1988 under Government financial sponsorship (Downer 1990b). The educational content of these strongly emphasized the practitioner's role in oral health promotion.

On a different theme, the Government's Committee on Medical Aspects of Food Policy (COMA) convened a panel in 1986 to inquire into and report on health aspects of the consumption of sugars in UK diets (Department of Health 1989). The panel reaffirmed that extensive evidence suggested that sugars were the most important dietary factor in the cause of dental caries. A number of important recommendations were made in the report aimed at reducing the amount and frequency of sugars intakes particularly among infants, older children, and the elderly. For people on long-term medication the panel advised that sugar-free liquid medicine formulations were the preferred alternative and should be made more widely available. It also recommended that food manufacturers should produce low-sugar alternatives to existing sugar-rich products and label products to indicate their total sugars content. The COMA report provided the most unequivocal advice promulgated by any authoritative UK body on the direction which future policy in this area should take.

A number of separate strands of oral health promotion policy that had been developing during the 1980s were drawn together when, after comprehensive review and widespread formal consultation, which included most importantly national consumer groups, the Government published its proposals for improving all aspects of primary health care in the form of a 'White Paper' (Cm249 1987). Entitled Promoting better health, this document set out among other things the next stages for implementing prevention in the UK dental services. The general objectives were to make the services more responsive to the needs of the consumer; to raise standards of care; to promote health and prevent illness; and to improve value for money. A whole range of proposals of relevance to oral health promotion were made which covered such issues as the extension of water fluoridation, initiatives in health education, a change in the role of the CDS, an increased preventive component in treatment provided by the GDS, and improved provision for the continuing education and training of practitioners.

In its response to the White Paper the BDA produced its own practical proposals for the introduction of capitation for children and a continuing care contract to cover adults. This formed the basis for subsequent negotiation with the Department of Health which led to the introduction of a new GDS contract in 1990. As a result, an estimated 20 per cent of central expenditure on the GDS was moved from treatment under fee-for-service to a capitation element. At the same time, a shift in approach in the CDS, stemming from legislation and central guidance which followed from the White Paper, reinforced its complementary role to the GDS and strengthened its responsibilities in monitoring the dental health of the population, providing health education and group preventive programmes, screening susceptible target groups, and delivering treatment services selectively on the basis of agreed priorities. The White Paper represented an important landmark in the development of health services in the UK.

The critical question that remains to be addressed is what has been the outcome of oral health promotion in the UK and to what extent can any achievements in terms of the improving oral health of the population be attributed to explicit policy?

The dramatic decrease in caries prevalence since the early 1970s in UK children has been extensively documented. While this appeared to have stabilized for the time being at a relatively low level in the majority of young children by the mid-1980s (Downer 1989), the decline continued in adolescent and young adult cohorts of the population and accelerated in the second half of the decade (Downer 1990a). Among older adults, steady and substantial improvements in dental health occurred throughout the 1970s and 1980s as measured by progressive reductions in edentulousness, increases in proportions of the working-age population remaining substantially dentate, and higher average numbers of sound untreated teeth in all sections of the population. These encouraging national trends were accompanied by increasingly positive public attitudes towards the value of securing and maintaining a healthy natural dentition (Downer 1991b). It seemed that ten years down the road, the aim for the dental services proposed by the Dental Strategy Review Group, although perhaps appearing Utopian to some at the time, was in sight of fulfilment. By the 1990s a realizable goal for the dentate population (virtually all children and some 80 per cent of adults) was to retain sufficient teeth to have a functional dentition, with or without the help of prosthesis but without the provision of extensive dentures.

The contribution of policy to improvements in oral health

As national policy in the 1980s began to focus increasingly on health promotion, much of its thrust, as far as oral health was concerned, was directed at modifying the activities of the dental services to embrace more health education and primary prevention. However, this only reflected a trend that had been advocated well before the advent of the Dental Strategy Review Group. It would be tempting to suppose that the gradual evolution of the dental services from a restorative to a preventive philosophy accounted in a major way for the demonstrable improvements in the oral health of the population, but this is unlikely to have been the case. The factors determining the distribution of dental caries in industrialized countries of Europe and the reasons, postulated by a number of authorities, for the observed decline in disease levels, was the subject of a previous examination (Downer 1991a). The general conclusion was that exposure of populations to fluoride in various forms, and particularly fluoride dentifrices, probably accounted for most of the reduction in caries which, nevertheless, remained the main disease responsible for tooth loss. Thus it was surmised that improvements in oral health had arisen from factors largely outside the control of the profession. The evidence reviewed also gave little support to the notion that mass dental health education, intended to change individual behaviour, worked as it was generally practised. Therefore, although better oral health might represent in some part an achievement of formal health education, more importantly perhaps, it stemmed from the general rise in public aspirations and expectations, and the continual reassessment of personal priorities witnessed in recent years.

It would appear that the contribution of explicit Government policy to improved oral health must remain indeterminate for the time being. Taking specific aspects of policy, the Government's long term support for water fluoridation, for example, has undoubtedly had a measurable effect on oral health. Yet this has nevertheless been comparatively minor overall. By 1990 only a little over 10 per cent of the population enjoyed the benefit of a fluoridated water supply. On the other hand, the policy of the toothpaste companies in manufacturing and marketing fluoride dentifrice nationally has had a strikingly positive effect. Apart from selling toothpaste, the advertising mounted by these companies may well also have contributed substantially to raising public awareness of the value of good dental health. The policy interest of the Government here was only in the matter of regulating and licensing the products. Yet despite the reservations expressed about the role the dental services in improving dental health, the constant drip-feeding of health education messages to individual patients by many dentists and their staff must have played a significant part in moulding public attitudes. This in turn feeds back and changes the expectations that people have of what type of dental treatment they should receive. In an indirect way, therefore, Government policy for the dental services has helped to promote oral health, albeit the contribution of this and the policy of other stakeholders is virtually impossible to quantify and apportion with precision (Downer 1991a).

Concluding commentary

Oral health promotion embraces a range of diverse activities operating within an involved dynamical system. Straying into the terminology of mathematics, it can be said that its outcomes are subject to the influences of a complexity of interacting variables many of whose effects cannot be modelled by simple linear relationships. Forecasting the likely result of policies in any but the broadest of generalities is highly problematic because of the sensitive dependence of trends on initial conditions.

With these reservations in mind, what can then be learned from an analysis of oral health policy in relation to oral health promotion? By looking at the international picture a few conclusions can probably be drawn with a reasonable degree of confidence.

In industrialized countries dental caries is the most important oral disease in public health terms. It accounts directly or indirectly for most dental service expenditure and remains the major cause of morbidity and tooth loss. Periodontal diseases and occlusal anomalies represent an important though lesser challenge. Oral cancer has a high mortality rate and appears to be increasing, but the incidence amounts to only a handful of new cases annually in every 100 000 of the population. It is therefore in a different category in so far as it is a great deal more serious yet at the same time far more rare than the main burden of oral disease. The countries that have been most successful in reducing and controlling caries levels and therefore, by extension, the most successful in oral health promotion, have a number of features in common. Among these are:

(1) a framework of laws and regulations relating specifically to oral disease prevention and health education;

(2) public health programmes such as water or salt fluoridation or organized group prevention in the school system, together with commercial availability and mass advertizing of fluoride toothpaste, or combinations of these;

(3) regular surveying of population dental health and the systematic collection and use of other relevant management information;

(4) independent professional advice provided to government by dentists in government service who are trained in public health;

(5) a forward-looking and enlightened national dental association;

(6) a well established research base in prevention and dental public health which recognizes the importance of behavioural sciences.

Switzerland is a country which exemplifies most of these characteristics and demonstrates convincingly the combined effect of legislation and information leading to acceptance and support of public health measures. These have been demonstrably successful in improving dental health. Fluoride-based caries prophylactic programmes for schoolchildren were introduced as early as the 1950s but have been adapted over the years to suit changing conditions. Thus tablet distribution in schools has been discontinued upon the introduction of fluoridated table salt as a domestic commodity. Also in Switzerland, as in Finland, the manufacture and marketing of sweets and chewing gum made with sucrose substitutes is well developed. These products are prominently labelled as being 'safe for teeth' and such claims are subject to official regulation. Explicit policies in Switzerland have been crowned with solid success.

Pinet (1987) analysed the reasons for success and failure in the implementation of caries prevention in European countries and it is worth reflecting briefly on some of the failures she highlighted as well as on successful action plans. West Germany was cited as a place where there was no mechanism established to stimulate dental patients to demand prevention nor for professionals to give it. There was said to be a lack of initiative from public authorities to educate and motivate the population, so that public demand failed to match the services available. In West Germany caries levels during the 1980s remained high. Pinet also quoted examples of spectacular failures in oral health promotion, in relation to fluoridation in particular, from which there were lessons to be learned. In Greece, lack of coordination between separate government ministries and their failure to resolve opposing views prevented the implementation of water fluoridation in the 1980s. The political stalemate, it was said, was not helped by professional inertia. By prevailing Western European standards caries levels in Greece remained high throughout the 1980s. In the Netherlands lack of an adequate legal base led to the unfortunate discontinuance in 1973 of the country's well established fluoridation programme. History is littered with examples of proponents of fluoridation consistently underestimating the strength and resilience of the opposition and its ability to exploit legislative inadequacies. It brings into prominence the importance of legislation as a tool for efficient action in this programme area as in many other aspects of oral health promotion.

References

Cm 249 (1987). *Promoting better health*. Her Majesty's Stationery Office, London.

Cohen, L. K. (1990). Promoting oral health: guidelines for dental associations. *Int. Dent. J.*, **40**, 79–102.

Coventry, P., Holloway, P. J., Lennon, M. A., Mellor, A. C., and Worthington, H. V. (1989). A trial of a capitation system of payment for the treatment of children in the General Dental Service. *Commun. Dent. Health*, **6** (Supplement 1), 1–63.

Department of Health (1989). *Dietary sugars and human disease*. Her Majesty's Stationery Office, London.

Department of Health and Social Security (1981). *Towards better dental health — guidelines for the future*. DHSS, London.

Department of Health and Social Security (1986). *Report of the Committee of enquiry into unnecessary dental treatment*. Her Majesty's Stationery Office, London.

Downer, M. C. (1987). Dental caries prevention in the United Kingdom and its statutory basis. In *Strategy for dental caries prevention in European countries according to their laws and regulations*, (eds. R. M. Frank and S. O'Hickey), pp.37–49. IRL Press, Oxford.

Downer, M. C. (1988). Expectations for oral health in Great Britain and the response of the dental care system. *J. Public Health Dent.*, **48**, 98–102.

Downer, M. C. (1989). Time trends in dental decay in young children. *Health Trends*, **21**, 7–9.

Downer, M. C. (1990a). Caries data from Western Europe. In Caries status in Europe and prediction of future trends. Symposium Report, (ed. T. M. Marthaler). *Caries Res.*, **24**, 381–96.

Downer, M. C. (1990b). Change towards prevention in the UK. In *Evolution in dental care*, (ed. R. J. Elderton), pp. 70–3. Clinical Press, Bristol.

Downer, M. C. (1991a). Description and explanation of the distribution of caries in the populations of Europe. In *Risk markers*, Vol. 1, (ed. N. W. Johnson), pp. 101–32. Cambridge University Press, Cambridge.

Downer, M. C. (1991b). The improving dental health of United Kingdom adults and prospects for the future. *Brit. Dent. J.*, **170**, 154–8.

Downer, M. C., Davies, G. N., and Holloway, P. J. (1983). The Danish oral health care service for children: an evaluation. *Int. Dent. J.*, **33**, 231–7.

Federation Dentaire Internationale (1985). Changing patterns of oral health and implications for oral health manpower: Part 1. Technical Report No. 24. *Int. Dent. J.*, **35**, 235–51.

Lembariti, B. S. (1990). Tanzania — the development of an oral health care service. In *Evolution in dental care*, (ed. R. J. Elderton), pp. 60–2. Clinical Press, Bristol.

Lennon, M. A., Downer, M. C., O'Mullane, D. M., and Taylor, G. O. (1981). The role of community clinical trials in public health decisions in preventive dentistry. *J. Dent. Res.*, **59** (Special Issue D), 2243–7.

Navarro Alonso, J. A. (1990). *Encuesta de salud bucodental en escolares de la Region de Murcia*. Serie Informes 6. Direccion General de Salud, Murcia.

Pinet, G. L. (1987). Analysis of laws and regulations related to caries prevention in Europe: a synthesis. In *Strategy for dental caries prevention in European countries according to their laws and regulations*, (ed. R. M. Frank and S.O'Hickey), pp. 243–62. IRL Press, Oxford.

Pinto, V. G. (1990). *Saude bucal panorama internacional*. Ministerio da Saude, Brasilia.

Sardo Infirri, J. (1990). Oral health for all — a realistic goal? In *Evolution in dental care*, (ed. R. J. Elderton), pp. 53–5. Clinical Press, Bristol.

Schwarz, E. (1987). Dental caries prevention and legislation in Denmark. In *Strategy for dental caries prevention in European countries according to their laws and regulations*, (ed. R. M. Frank and S. O'Hickey), pp. 89–102. IRL Press, Oxford.

Tala, H. (1987). Strategy of dental caries prevention in Finland according to the health legislation and other legal regulations. In *Strategy for dental caries prevention in European countries according to their laws and regulations*, (ed. R. M. Frank and S. O'Hickey), pp. 103–17. IRL Press, Oxford.

6A

National campaigns

CLIVE WRIGHT

Behavioural theory

Where the prevention or early cure of a health disorder is facilitated by voluntary changes in behaviour, population based campaigns are often used to heighten public awareness and stimulate health action (Schou 1987). Oral health campaigns focus public attention on specific oral conditions and promote the contact of message recipient with health agent. National campaigns form one aspect of strategies aimed at information dissemination and raising the level of awareness of disease and its prevention and are most effectively employed as part of a multi-faceted approached to changing life-styles and health behaviour (McAlister et al. 1982).

The basic elements for conducting national oral health campaigns involve organizations, coordination, resources, targeting, and evaluation. Consequently it is only through large agencies such as national professional associations, governments, or national corporations that a readily available infrastructure exists to support such a broad approach to promoting community oral health.

National oral health campaigns may or may not be linked into the planned oral health delivery system of a country (Frazier et al. 1974). Usually, however, they fall into one of three categories depending upon the auspicing agency:

(1) campaigns organized and conducted by the dental profession, such as a national 'dental health week' or 'dental health month';

(2) campaigns operated through government instrumentalities such as a School Dental Programme, Headstart, or Community Dental Service which contain both educational and service delivery components;

(3) campaigns conducted by the oral health product industry promoting the marketing and sale of dentifrices, toothbrushes, and mouthrinses.

Dental association campaigns

Many national professional organizations from as diverse delivery systems as the United States of America to the People's Republic of China, have embarked on nationally coordinated dental health campaigns.

The American Dental Association's (ADA) National Children's Dental Health Month (NCDHM) traces its origins back to a one-day public dental health campaign in 1941 (Association Reports 1987). The annual campaign is now held in February each year and involves state and local dental societies, hygienist associations, state and country health departments, TV and sporting personalities, educators, and business leaders across the US (Association Reports 1985). The Federal ADA through its Division of Communications formulates policy and planning directions annually, and provides some resourcing to state and local groups. Since 1984 the coordinated activities of the NCDHM have centred on a 'Smile America' theme and logo and comprised four basic elements:

(1) media activities and special promotions undertaken on the national level by the ADA;

(2) activities designed for state and local dental society implementation;

(3) activities to be undertaken in cooperation with related dental groups, the dental industry and other special interest groups;

(4) development of materials for in-office use by ADA member dentists. (Berry 1989).

The thematic approach 'Smile America' provides both continuity between campaign years and an easily recognizable focus. Table 6.1 summarizes some of the principal activities undertaken by the 'Smile America' campaign, at a national level, in 1990.

The Canadian Dental Association (CDA) first launched a national dental health campaign in 1985, and by 1988 had extended its campaign into a

Table 6.1 National programme activities sponsored by the American Dental Association's National Children's Dental Health Month, 1990

Activity	Description
Media outreach	Press releases, magazine supplements on technological and scientific advancements in dental research
Media tours	ADA spokespersons featured on news, interviews, and talk-back programmes
Media conference	Leading dental experts as part of an annual dental news conference
Video news releases	Televised press releases on dental topics distributed by satellite to TV stations across the US
Public service announcements	Radio and television spot announcements
Dental health columns	ADA-written material for distribution to small-circulation newspapers nationwide
Dental IQ quiz	National dental IQ quiz for cable TV and national print media

dental health month (News Update 1989a). The CDA provided resources such as professional materials, background information, and media relations tips to provincial and local dental societies. The local dental societies then tailored their activities to specific community and audience groups and issues. In Newfoundland interest and awareness of dental issues was stimulated in the public arena through dental health messages being placed on milk cartons and grocery bags. In contrast, the Manitoba dental group conducted a province-wide survey estimating the public's attitude to dental care. Results of their survey were published on the front page of the province's largest newspaper, the *Winnipeg Free Press*.

Some national professional groups identify strengths and weaknesses in the dental professions' perceptions and practices, prior to mounting public national campaigns. For example in Finland, a national dental health campaign launched publically in 1987 with the goal of increasing public demand for dental services, was preceded by a separate campaign aimed at Finnish dentists to improve their understanding of prevention of dental diseases and the importance of the family dentist in maintaining regular dental visits for their patients (Murtomaa and Masalin 1984). The New Zealand Periodontal Awareness Campaign (Croxson 1987) is a further example where the education of dentists prior to a public campaign was integral to the national promotion of public periodontal health.

In general terms all dental association campaigns have two broad objectives: an improvement in community oral health and increasing the frequency of dental visits. Although evaluation of campaigns is frequently undertaken as part of the total process (News Update 1989b), the outcomes measuring level of achievement, for example attendance patterns, use of dental floss, and knowledge of disease, are often influenced by numerous other factors outside the direct influence of the campaign itself. For example, the Minnesota periodontal awareness campaign which found that TV advertisments achieved the highest levels of stated viewer intention to attend a dentist in the future (Bakdash *et al.* 1983) did not measure the number of people who actually consulted a dentist. In addition, most dental association evaluation efforts lack control group comparisons and the rigorous scientific methodology to reduce sample bias and take account of variation in response rate.

Another significant weakness of national campaigns occurs in the content and activities with the delegation of decision-making to state and local dental societies. Although coordinated centrally, and provided with guidelines and materials, there is often a loss of control in the content of the dental health messages being communicated to the public, and a lack of focusing on the promotion of primary preventive strategies (Corbin 1985). For example, in the three years 1985–7 of the NCDHM, in more than 100 reports published on local activities only three or four reports referred to programmes involving public promotion of fluoridation, topical fluorides, or fissure sealants. Programmes and activities conducted by local groups included: jogathons;

indentification of dentures; promoting child safety seats; visiting dental offices; participating in toothbrush exchange programmes; and gaining free coupons to MacDonald's restaurants for participating in a dental IQ quiz. While many projects showed great initiative, and addressed important issues such as oral cancer screening, the use of smokeless tobacco, and managing avulsed teeth, the very diversity of activity tended to dilute the importance of support for simple, effective, and scientifically based primary preventive programmes (United Kingdom Health Education Council 1979).

The weakness of many dental association campaigns in effectively changing health behaviours has been recognized by numerous workers and organizations (Jones and Glennon 1984; Gift 1988; Federation Dentaire Internationale (FDI) 1989). In 1989 the FDI published the findings of its Working Group on Oral Health Promotion of the Commission on Oral Health, Research, and Epidemiology. These guidelines for dental associations and ministries of health identify both the processes involved in effective preventive programme organization and implementation and the range of *effective interventions* appropriate to the predetermined goals for the improvement of oral health (Cohen 1990*a*, 1990*b*). The principles which influence the effectiveness of dental health campaigns include:

(1) a simple message, scientifically accurate and supportable;

(2) understandable to the target audience;

(3) frequently repeated;

(4) consistently presented in all media statements, for example, leaflets, TV, and magazines.

Government sponsored campaigns

Not all nations lend themselves to increasing the public awareness of oral health through organized professional efforts. In many developing countries especially, acute shortage of trained dental health personnel proscribe nationwide activities through coordinated dental association networks (Saparamadu 1986). In addition, the historical development of public dental health services in the industrialized nations (Dunning 1986) has invariably included organized and coordinated health education campaigns delivered through either a school-based delivery system or specifically targeted programme (e.g. the US Headstart Programme and the UK Natural Nashers Programme).

The survey by Frazier *et al.* (1983) on the health educational aspects of preventive programmes for school-aged children in 34 countries reported that over three-quarters of the programmes were supported by public funds. Further, the principal components of these programmes were directed toward voluntary changes in health behaviour through dental health education.

Government sponsored campaigns, being firmly linked to the delivery of public dental services, differ in a number of respects from dental associations' campaigns. For example, government campaigns provide an ongoing rather than sporadic focus for dental health issues, tend to focus more specifically on the prevention of dental caries rather address diverse issues in oral health, rely more on classroom and one-on-one communication than mass media, and place less emphasis, as an outcome, on increasing dental visitations.

School-based dental health education campaigns demonstrably increase dental health knowledge and change recipients' attitude toward oral health (Laiho et al. 1987; Søgaard and Holst 1988). However, few of these intensive, nationally coordinated programmes have been effective in long-term changes in oral health behaviour or decreasing oral disease (Wright 1990; Frencken et al. 1990). The elements of government-based programmes which are effective in improving oral health are those which bring the individual in direct contact with a preventive agent (for example, fluoride or fissure sealant) or directly prevent contact with high sucrose diets (for example, in restricting access to sugar containing foods) (Nitzel 1981; Dooland and Kelly 1984; Burt 1985).

Campaigns advertising dental products

The role that organized, coordinated, corporate advertising plays in influencing oral health behaviour and dental health has not been widely researched, yet its impact appears self-evident. The psychology of advertising is to familiarize potential product consumers with a specific product, such that, all else being equal (for example there not being a marked cost barrier to selection), the consumer purchases that product recognized (Emery 1981). In addition, there is evidence that children influence their parents in the purchase of advertised products. For example, the study by Longstreet and Orme (1967) reported that 70 per cent of children asked their parents to buy products advertised on television and 89 per cent of these parents bought the product. In both these situations, where advertising campaigns lead to the increased consumption of a particular dental product, if the product contains a known primary preventive agent, such as fluoride, then an inferred link between advertising and dental health improvement can be drawn. Clearly, the influence of fluoride-containing toothpaste on the decreased prevalence and severity of dental caries (Spencer 1986) is an important example of the power of commercial marketing and improvement in oral health. In the USA fluoride toothpastes have been on sale since 1955 with an annual sales figure of US $500 million in the mid-1980s (Renson et al.1985). In 1990, the toothpaste industry in the United Kingdom was estimated to have spent £20 million on advertising campaigns and sold more than 98 per cent of fluoride toothpaste in its total market sales (Kemsley Pers. Comm.).

While there is no clear relationship yet observed between the sale of toothbrushes and periodontal health, the potential exists for anti-plaque agents to be used effectively by the consumer in the future for the prevention and improvement of periodontal health.

References

Association Reports (1985). Bureau of Health Education and Audiovisual Services [American Dental Association] National Children's Dental Health Month. *J. Am. Dent. Assoc*, **111**, 315–19.

Association Reports (1987). Department of Public Information [American Dental Association] National Children's Dental Health Month 1987. *J. Am. Dent. Assoc.*, **115**, 625–9.

Bakdash, M. B., Lange, A. L., and McMillan, D. G. (1983). The effect of a televised periodontal campaign on public periodontal awareness. *J. Periodontal*, **54**, 666–70.

Berry, J. H. (1989). ADA launches Smile America campaign. *J. Am. Dent. Assoc.*, **118**, 690–2.

Burt, B. A. (1985). The prevention connection: linking dental health education and prevention. *Int. Dent. J.*, **33**, 189–95.

Cohen, L. K. (1990a). Leadership role of dental associations: oral health promotion. *Int. Dent. J.*, **40**, 48–53.

Cohen, L. K. (1990b). Promoting oral health: guidelines for dental associations. *Int. Dent. J.*, **40**, 79–102.

Corbin, S. B. (1985). PHS directions in oral health: health promotion and disease prevention. *J. Public Health Dent.*, **45**, 234–7.

Croxson, L. (1987). The New Zealand Periodontal Awareness Campaign 1: preliminary awareness by dentists and the public. *J. N. Z. Soc. Periodont*, **64**, 6–12.

Dooland, M. B. and Kelly, P. (1984). School canteens menus in metropolitan Adelaide. *Aust. Dent. J.*, **49**, 230–3.

Dunning, J. M. (1986). *Principles of public dental health*, 4th edn. Harvard University Press, Cambridge, Mass.

Emery, M. (1981). The role of the mass media in nutrition education. *Proceedings of the Nutrition Education Conference, 29–30 January 1981*. Australian Commonwealth Department of Health, Canberra.

Federation Dentaire Internationale (1989). *Promoting oral health. Guidelines for dental associations*. Rank Xerox Communicatie Service.

Frazier, P. J., Jenny, J., Ostman, R., and Frenwick, C. (1974). Quality of information in mass media: a barrier to dental health education of the public. *J. Public Health Dent.* **34**, 244–57.

Frencken, J. E., Kalsbeek, H., and Verrips, G. H. (1990). Has the decline in dental caries been halted? Changes in caries prevalence amongst 6 and 12 year-old children in Friesland, 1973–1988. *Int. Dent. J.*, **40**, 225–30.

Gift, H.C. (1988). Awareness and assessment of periodontal problems among dentists and the public. *Int. Dent. J.*, **38**, 147–53.

Jones, E. and Glennon, S. (1984). Changing attitudes and behaviour through public health promotion campaigns. *Ann. Roy. Aust. Coll. Dent. Surg.*, **8**, 43–50.

Laiho, M., Honkala, E., Milén, A., and Nyyssonen, V. (1987). Oral health education in Finnish schools. *Scand. J. Dent. Res.*, **95**, 510–15.

Longstreet, B. and Orme, F. (1967). The unguarded house. In *Children and television: television's impact on the child*, (ed. S. Sunderlin), pp. 45–9. Association for Children's Television Internationale, Washington, DC.

McAlister, A., Puska, P., Jukka, T. S., Tuomiletho, J., and Koskela, K. L. (1982). Theory and action for health promotion: illustration from the North Karelia project. *Am. J. Public Health*, **72**, 43–50.

Murtomaa, H. and Masalin, K. (1984). Effects of a national dental health campaign in Finland. *Acta Odontol. Scand.*, **42**, 297–303.

News Update (1989*a*). Dental Health Month: community activities that work. *J. Canad. Dent. Assoc.*, **55**, 161–3.

News Update (1989*b*). Highlights of the CDA's 1988 Gallup Poll — Canadians are getting the message and acting on it. *J. Canad. Dent. Assoc.*, **55**, 241–3.

Nitzel, A. E. (1981). *Nutrition in preventive dentistry: science and practice*, (2nd edn), pp. 53–81. W. B. Saunders, Philadelphia.

Renson, C. E., Crielaers, P. J. A., Ibikunle, S. A. J., Pinto, V. G., Ross, C. B., Sardo-Infirri, S., et. al. (1985). Changing patterns of oral health and implications for oral health manpower: Part 1, *Int. Dent., J.*, **35**, 235–51.

Saparamadu, K. D. G. (1986). The provision of dental services in the Third World. *Int. Dent. J.*, **36**, 194–8.

Schou, L. (1987). Use of mass-media and active involvement in a national dental health campaign. *Community Dent. Oral Epidemiol.*, **15**, 14–18.

Spencer, A. J. (1986). Past association of fluoride vehicles with caries severity in Australian adolescents. *Community Dent. Oral Epidemiol.*, **14**, 233–7.

Søgaard, A. J. and Holst, D. L. (1988). The effect of different school based dental health education programmes in Norway. *Community Dent. Health*, **5**, 169–84.

United Kingdom Health Education Council (1979). The scientific basis of dental health education. *Brit. Dent. J.*, **146**, 51–4.

Wright, F. A. C. (1990). Oral health promotion in schools: a case study. *Health Educ. Q.*, **18**, 87–90.

6B

General dental practice, health education, and health promotion: a critical reappraisal

R AY C ROUCHER

This chapter will discuss factors influencing the value of health education and health promotion in general dental practice. Four key areas are reviewed, namely:

(1) the role that general dental practice could play in health education and health promotion;

(2) criticisms of the current practice of health education in general dental practice;

(3) the role of chairside health education and health education materials in general dental practice;

(4) developing an oral health promotion strategy for general dental practice.

The role of health education and health promotion in general dental practice

It has become popular to emphasize the potential role of general dental practice as a base for health education, both in terms of the prevention of disease and the promotion of a healthy lifestyle. The reasons for this are fourfold. First, general dental practice has been recommended as a 'natural setting' for health education even though it provides services for a minority of the population who are more likely to be recruited from the middle class. However, as Weinstein (1986) comments, while the alternatives, such as the workplace or schools, have been long recommended as locations for oral health education programmes (Rayner and Cohen 1971), initiatives in these settings are more likely to have the status of demonstration projects with problems of funding and continuity. Only in general dental practices will oral health education be available for a greater proportion of the population over an ongoing period of time. Second, new initiatives are being introduced in which it is assumed that general dental practices will adopt a greater role in health promotion. One example is the current changes within the United Kingdom general dental service which offer new opportunities for the prevention of dental disease. The patient has become entitled to a 'treatment plan' which could serve as an aid to discussion about treatment options and their cost. In addition the requirement that practices develop patient leaflets containing core items of information may help the adult patient to gain knowledge and choose between alternative courses of action. The new general dental service contract has as its primary objective 'to secure and maintain the oral health of the patient', which is potentially wider and more positive in scope than the existing minimal concept of 'dental fitness'. Third, there has been a recognition of the value of multiple risk factor approaches which will result in an expansion of the role of the general dental practice to have a greater responsibility for preventive care. One example is the promotion of smoking cessation measures among patients. Giving up smoking will not only improve periodontal health but also reduce oral cancer and heart disease rates (Fried and Rubinstein 1990; Frazier 1992). Fourth, and perhaps most importantly, current definitions of health education and health promotion regard health professional–patient contacts as an opportunity for the health professional to help the patient by improving knowledge, offering health risk advice, and promoting self-esteem and self-empowerment (Catford and Nutbeam 1984).

Criticisms of the current practice of health education in general dental practice

Despite the theoretical and practical opportunities for health education offered within the setting of general dental practice, a series of criticisms have been made of current activity. These are:

1. There has been little change in emphasis in the debates within the profession about the objectives of health education, which is seen as a straightforward and unitary activity emphasizing the issue of prevention and changing patient behaviour. In 1966 an expert committee, considering the status of oral health care for the prevention and control of periodontal disease, reported the need to motivate the individual to follow a prescribed effective oral health care programme throughout life. Corah (1974) argued that there was no evidence that the efforts of dentists were effective in inducing preventive behaviour in their patients. Sheiham (1977), having reviewed the status of oral health education, concluded that the issue was not lack of knowledge but rather one of a failure of that knowledge to be

diffused through the dental profession. He quotes Young's (1970) arguments that the initial professional preparation of dentists emphasizes therapy and repair rather than education, and that the most common method of education used is the KAB (knowledge, attitudes, and behaviour) concept. This assumes a straight-line relationship between information inputs, changed subjective feelings, and practices.

2. As a result, the literature argues that the knowledge and practice base of current health education outside oral health education has been ignored (Frazier and Horowitz 1990; Young 1970; Søgaard and Holst 1988; Sheiham 1977). These debates outside oral health about alternatives for health education (Beattie 1983, 1991; Ewles and Simnett 1985; Tones 1990; Tones *et al.* 1990; Draper *et al.* 1980) show a developing consensus built around the intersection of two factors. First, who owns health education knowledge (professional or lay person) and second, the degree of focus of this knowledge (individual or group).

All these identify a paramedic advice model, which has been long dominant (Cust 1979). This expert-led, individually orientated approach features persuasive, behaviour-changing communication and is based around the KAB (knowledge, attitudes, and behaviour) concept. The status of this model has been criticized by several authors (Rayner and Cohen 1974; Frazier 1978; Søgaard and Holst 1988). Its concern is unambiguous — centring on behavioural outcomes such as improving oral hygiene and reductions in the intake of extrinsic sugars. Rodmell and Watt (1986) summarize the many criticisms which have been made of this model:

(a) The prescriptive and expert led nature of this 'medical model' is victim-blaming (Crawford 1977).

(b) It can cause ill-health by making people feel guilty.

(c) It is elitist. Being expert-led it assumes that the individual has a limited amount of knowledge.

(d) It operates separately from the people it serves, with little if any attempt to find out what they need.

A second emphasis within theories about health education may be termed 'educational', which aims to equip individuals with knowledge and understanding about the cause and effects of ill-health. This emphasis may be further divided between a naïve, passive approach, which would merely supply information, and an active approach. The passive approach neglects the impact of the environmental and political determinants of health, which might limit the ability of individuals to use this new knowledge. On the other hand the active approach would seek to supplement any cognitive input by including the exploration and clarification of beliefs and values and the development of decision-making skills. Such an approach complements the third emphasis upon the environmental and political determinants of health. The concern of this emphasis is to encourage the development and introduction of healthy public policy, such as water fluoridation. This emphasis may be directed at the decision-making elite or develop from the concerns of community groups about local issues of concern. It requires an educated empowered population, and indicates the complementary nature of the educational and political approaches to health promotion. The process of introducing a public policy on health requires a population which understands the need for these policies and is prepared to argue for them.

It also follows from these emphases that alternative evaluative criteria will be used. While all are seeking health-related behaviour change measured in terms of changing adherence to medication regimes, smoking reduction, or improved oral hygiene and eventual positive health outcomes, the time span for these changes and the adoption of other evaluative measures will vary. In the preventive model this outcome will often be the only priority, which should be achieved within a short period of time. Its definitions of success are behavioural outcomes such as adopting a healthy lifestyle and using preventive services appropriately. Other emphases seek changes in levels of self-esteem, decision-making skills, and active participation in campaigns for changes to public policy which will improve health, such as water fluoridation. These may be alternatives to the personal health-related behaviour changes outlined above. An important theme dividing these emphases is the origins of need that are used. The preventive emphasis employs the professionals' definition of need, while, for example, the radical/political emphasis assumes that the community's definitions of need can be the origins of action. Models of self-empowerment are driven by the underlying assumption that individuals or communities should be helped to develop an awareness of their needs and the way these can be articulated (Freire 1968). Despite these debates Gjermo (1986) states that the goals of the dentist remain behavioural — good oral hygiene, use of fluorides, reduced sweets, self-examination, and regular check-ups. In the control of periodontal disease the concern is to encourage the adoption of mechanical oral hygiene practices by the population (Frandsen 1986), and behavioural scientists have not disagreed with this professionally directed agenda (Gift 1986; Kiyak and Mulligan 1986).

3. The content of health education is not consistent with the known scientific basis of prevention (Levy and Gilbert 1984). They note that the perceived effectiveness of preventive regimes can be inconsistent with the scientifically demonstrated measures of their effectiveness. Health care providers are not well informed about the relative value of appropriate measures to prevent oral diseases, often apparently being unable to discriminate between strategies to prevent caries and periodontal disease (Glavind and Nyvad 1986).

4. There is confusion and ambiguity in the encouragement of personal behaviour change on the one hand, and the model of health adopted on the other. Birn and Birn (1985) distinguish between a 'defect–apparatus' model of health based on curative and mechanistic interventions and illness avoidance and a 'social–medical' model emphasizing positive health and well-being (WHO 1984). While positive health, well-being, and empowerment may be adopted as principles, the practice of oral health education continues to emphasize behaviour change with its theoretical origins in the illness avoidance model of health (Frazier 1992). The transfer of the principle of positive health into action would need the development of alternative approaches (Rawson and Grigg 1987).

5. There is a neglect of the needs of the patient (Steuart 1969; Sheiham and Croucher 1989). Need is usually conceptualized in three different ways: 'normative', 'felt', or 'expressed'. Bradshaw (1977) has described 'normative' need as the expert's definition of a situation. If experts' standards are not met there is a need. An example is about minimum standards of oral hygiene. Standards such as these are measured with reference to evidence such as plaque scores. Wilding (1982) argues that normative need involves the imposition rather than agreeing of definitions. As a result expert definitions may well be very different from the ideas of lay people. Sheiham (1990) notes that the person defining need acts in a god-like capacity, passing judgement upon a society's needs. In contrast 'felt' need reflects what people want. It is often linked with past experience, which can lead to either restricted or over-inflated expectations. 'Expressed' need is what people say they want. It is a request or demand for a service or information. 'Felt' need is not automatically 'expressed' if the individual feels there is no easily available solution. 'Expressed' needs may also conflict with 'normative' need — the individual may demand more information about a dental condition than the dentist is able or willing to give.

The current practice of oral health education

A recent investigation of oral health education practices in a sample of general dental practices demonstrated the current validity of these criticisms (Croucher 1989). The context within which health education took place in the Croucher study was individualistic, and associated with dental treatment provided on a fee-for-item basis. The approach adopted within the practices could be characterized as either 'formal' or 'opportunistic'. This would depend on whether the health education was provided by either a dentist or a dental hygienist. 'Opportunistic' advice would often be provided by a dentist in between other clinical procedures. An example of the 'formal' approach is provided below:

She gave me a talk as to what it can lead up to if you don't brush your teeth regularly, methods of brushing your teeth, different mouthwashes, things like that...

A normative definition of need was used. The professional agenda appeared to be primarily information giving:

The way to brush my teeth, the proper way to do it, the best kind of toothbrush to use...brushing up and down...

This agenda was presented in a uniform and simple but incomplete way. A diagnosis was often omitted. The felt needs of patients were different. They wanted more information on the mechanics of prevention, information on anatomy and pathology, and the issues of treatment and cost. Clearly many adult patients wanted more information on their oral health, and simple messages missed the point. Respondents perceived no negotiation about the need for treatment:

I didn't ask to see the hygienist, I was told to, I just expected that was the normal thing.

This quotation illustrates the differing definitions of need used in this situation. Dentists would use their stricter definitions to advocate a particular approach to prevention. An opportunity to create awareness and knowledge of the issues in periodontal health, to create a demand (expressed need) was overlooked.

The concern to prevent disease also resulted in an undue emphasis upon technique and problem solving:

She showed me a way to brush the backs of them which I hadn't thought of before, and to really get down and to push the brush down instead of sideways, and to really go right the way down into the gums.

The information given could be perceived as providing a negative evaluation element:

That's how she made it sound, ticking you off because you hadn't made the effort to clean your teeth properly, and if you didn't do it properly your teeth would fall out.

The emphasis on clinical technique in the health education also contributed to these negative feelings.

She gave me a toothbrush and showed me how to brush my teeth. I mean, I've only been brushing my teeth thirty-odd years, the way she showed me I'd been doing it wrong the majority of that time...

The information giving followed a 'passive' educational model, with no attempt to empower the patient by developing skills of assertiveness. This resulted in a lack of recognition of the wider circumstances which may prevent the following of advice. The emphasis on the individual in the health education meant that the circumstances of family life were often overlooked by the educator:

Unless they have similar experiences, I think they find it difficult to understand, I think sometimes they say you should be spending x minutes, five minutes a day doing it, but that five minutes could be spent doing something slightly more important on the priority list...

It was not unusual for mothers with young children to report that the length of their working day could be up to 18 hours, with its content devoted to family work and leaving little time for the respondent to look after her own health needs.

I'd love to take more care and I will make an effort, but being a mother, especially to four children, it would be demanding...I think it does affect, not the performance of the way I clean my teeth, but how often I clean them.

Another example of the circumstances of the individual being ignored involved the negative impact of marriage:

Recently I'd been rushing a bit more because we'd only just got the place and when I was at home with Mum and Dad I had a bit more time... Now I don't have the time, with a full-time job and coming home to do housework as well.

The finding that respondents with partners and children had more problems in following self-care advice was also of clinical significance:

If she's around fiddling and pulling the toothpaste I don't do a full job because last time I left her it was all over the carpet and everywhere...if she's fiddling I have to stand watching her and neglect myself.

One outcome of these features of the health education was that feelings of guilt and rebelliousness could develop, with the demands made by the dental practices being perceived as unrealistic and inappropriate:

What they [dentists] call clean is not what the man in the street calls clean.

Respondents resented being turned into 'maintenance engineers' which they perceived as being 'narcissistic'.

The lack of negotiation about whether health education was needed resulted in inefficient outcomes. The demands of the dental practice were often perceived as unrealistic. Few gains in knowledge were reported, with a minority being able to successfully define plaque and gum disease after they had received their health education.

Health education materials in general dental practice

Teaching materials such as leaflets are used extensively in the practice of oral health education. However, the value of these leaflets has been questioned for reflecting the criticisms of conventional health education which were outlined earlier (Farrant and Russell 1986). This section will examine 'ingenious' new initiatives (Kiyak and Mulligan 1986) in the development of health education materials for general dental practice:

(1) a self-instruction manual (Glavind et al. 1979, 1981, 1984, 1985);

(2) an oral self-inspection manual (Baab and Weinstein 1983, 1986). Both incorporate the principle of 'active learning' (Schaub 1986).

The Glavind self-instruction manual was developed initially from a study to evaluate periodontal self-examination. The background to this development was as follows:

1. Mechanical tooth cleaning is the preferred method for personal oral hygiene, which in turn is crucial for maintaining periodontal health.

2. Motivation, that is, behaviour change, by the patient can be achieved through activity and involvement.

3. Conventional oral hygiene instruction is time consuming, repetitive, and tedious for skilled dental staff to follow.

4. A standardized approach to the patient was possible, not dependent on the possibly varying quality of individual instruction.

The aim of the manual was to help individual patients examine the effectiveness of their toothbrushing, evaluate where the technique was insufficient, and improve the present tooth cleaning technique. This was achieved by an assessment of the present level of tooth cleaning skill, providing suggestions to improve the tooth cleaning technique and the provision of 'troubleshooting' guidance.

A similar rationale to Glavind's manual was adopted in the Baab and Weinstein oral self-inspection manual:

1. Poor observation of certain areas of the mouth may be a factor in poor patient cleaning.

2. Patients may be instructed to competently examine their own mouths, using an intra-oral light source and mirror.

3. Routine oral hygiene instruction takes considerable professional time and manpower.

4. Oral self-instruction would reduce professional time, allowing the patient to learn at their own pace and receive immediate personal feedback.

These two sets of materials may be evaluated using a framework proposed by Farrant and Russell (1985). This framework asks the following questions:

1. What are the materials for?

2. Why are they produced?

3. Who are they for?

4. Are they effective?

They were innovative in emphasizing 'self-evaluation' and 'activity' by the patient. However, both manuals were produced to effect a behaviour change among their recipients, being designed to assist adult dental patients in the development of more efficient tooth cleaning, and the prevention of periodontal disease. This normative emphasis is reinforced by the response to the second question, why were the materials produced? Both sets of materials were produced to satisfy a professional need, which arose because of the characterization of individual behaviour as the primary cause of periodontal ill health, and the perceived necessity for continual reinforcement of the need for efficient oral hygiene when treating patients. Their origins were fourfold. First, to prevent the inefficient use of professional skills. Secondly, to maintain professional morale by removing the need for constant repetition of the same message. Thirdly, to motivate the patient to improve their tooth cleaning skills. Fourthly, to switch resource time from the professional on to the patient. Glavind suggests that the individual should spend approximately 30 minutes every day completing the exercises in his manual, and that the exercises be completed every day for six days. The materials were designed to be used by adults already receiving treatment for periodontal conditions.

With respect to evaluation, both manuals were evaluated at differing stages of their development with an emphasis upon clinical indices. Opportunities to develop alternative evaluative outcomes were overlooked. Glavind *et al.* (1985) also evaluated their manual with patients from a general dental practice using a questionnaire. Patients reported learning something useful, appreciated participating actively in their treatment, and perceived the importance of cleaning their teeth. No data is presented on whether the recipients of the materials wanted to try them out before taking part. Clinically there were improved plaque scores.

Baab and Weinstein evaluated their manual on two separate occasions. Initially they found that the time spent on self-assessment decreased during the study from a mean of 6.8 minutes to 3.3 minutes. However, more positively, half of the study group were willing to continue inspecting their mouths on a weekly basis after the six-week experimental period and decreased levels of plaque were recorded. In a second evaluation use of the manual by a group was compared with a group receiving 'traditional' instruction from a dental hygienist. After six months tooth cleaning skills were similar for both groups. The average time spent tooth cleaning by both groups, nine minutes, suggested that both groups were more motivated in general than most dental patients. Rugg-Gunn and MacGregor (1978) reported that uninstructed young adults spend less than one minute on tooth cleaning.

The incorporation of novel approaches such as activity and self-evaluation into these materials suggests a growing commitment to involving the patient in their treatment. However, an examination of the background issues in their development shows there had been little change from the fundamental normative objective of achieving patient compliance, with little consumer input. In practice lay people participated in activities designed for them by the professional expert. Thus the fundamental criticisms of oral health education outlined earlier are still valid. Additionally, the possibility of these initiatives developing beyond demonstration projects has to be questioned.

Developing an oral health promotion strategy for general dental practice

The following proposals are priorities for development. They are not intended to be comprehensive, focusing upon increasing lay participation and decreasing inequity. The framework for their development has been provided by the primary health care approach, which, in summary, has the basic principles of equitable distribution, lay participation, a focus on prevention, the use of appropriate technology, and a multi-sectoral approach (Walt and Vaughan, 1981).

From these principles the following perspectives on health education and health promotion have been used. Health education is any planned combination of learning experiences involving knowledge provision and the promotion of self-esteem and self-empowerment, while health promotion is any planned combination of educational, political, regulatory, and organizational support to improve health (Catford and Nutbeam 1984). The intention of this support may be either to alter the environment in which people live (e.g. water fluoridation) or to enable individuals to take advantage of opportunities by removing barriers (e.g. finance). Both health education and health promotion, it should be emphasized, are interdependent.

The practice of health education in general dental practice should reflect the developing challenge to the preventive approach current in general health care contexts. Fahrenport (1987) has proposed that the features of the preventive model, emphasizing compliance and behaviour change, adherence, planning for passive patients, the creation of dependence, and the normative determination of need, should be replaced by a patient-centred model. This emphasizes the desirability of patient autonomy, participation, planning with active, independent patients, and the use of lay defined needs. Of these, the use of lay defined needs is the most important.

Accompanying this should be the development of ideas about the relationship between health professional and patient. Szasz and Hollender (1956) have argued that in addition to the traditional guidance-cooperation model of this relationship which uses the preventive model of health education there is also a mutual participation model which places a greater emphasis upon issues of co-operation between professional and patient. The need to adopt this model in general dental practice has been argued for some time (Ayer and Corah 1984). However little progress in achieving this goal is apparent. More recently, Tuckett et al. (1985) have argued that the consultation is a 'meeting between experts'. Both parties bring differing but equally valid perspectives to the consultation. In this context an understanding of the patient perspective is important.

A similar approach can be adopted in the development of patient materials. Farnes (1988) has argued that it is necessary to encourage individuals to reflect upon their experience, become aware of alternatives, decide what they want, and take action to achieve this. This would be realized through the use of ideas about 'open learning' (Lewis and Spencer 1986; Lewis 1986), individually orientated materials which are designed to remove barriers and focus on the learner's own needs. Rather than domesticating, these materials will be emancipatory (Farnes 1988), bringing an improved self-confidence, knowledge, and skills. As has been noted earlier, oral health education has ignored much of the successful development of these ideas in other areas of health education (Ballard 1987; Heathcote 1987).

Providing information in general dental practice should therefore be a priority, with the aim of improving health literacy (Frazier 1992). The aim should be to move beyond awareness of an issue, such as toothbrushing, to a deeper understanding of the alternative methods and timing of toothbrushing and the issues associated with the design and shape of a toothbrush. Such a commitment to information giving in general dental practice would also bring a reduction in information inequity, whereby members of minority or disadvantaged populations are penalized.

In the context of general dental practice other policies may also contribute to the reduction of inequity by improving access to the services offered. Jacob and Plamping (1989) have noted that while access has features relating to national health care planning these can also be applied to individual dental practices. Penchansky and Thomas (1981) argue that access has the specific dimensions of availability, accessibility, accommodation, affordability, and acceptability. Their application would contribute to the development of practice-based health promotion strategies.

A more available service refers to the adequacy of the supply of dentists, but at the individual practice level adequacy can also relate to the provision of specialized services such as emergency out-of-hours care. Accommodation relates to the manner in which practices are organized to accept patients in terms of their appointment systems, hours of opening and telephone services. Affordability relates prices to services offered. Patients should have clear knowledge about pricing schedules, the cost of treatment, and methods of paying. Finally, acceptability refers to the appearance of the practice and whether patients are made to feel welcome.

There are other specific opportunities for health promotion within general dental practice. In addition to providing tobacco risk information, it is also necessary to develop tobacco control policies in general dental practice. This is only one example of the combining of information with a specific organizational and environmental support designed to promote health. Others would be:

(1) the provision of healthy snack facilities, to support information about diet;

(2) the selling of toothbrushes and dental floss at discount prices, to support information about oral hygiene;

(3) the routine use of patient needs and satisfaction assessments, to evaluate the appropriateness and performance of general practice services;

(4) the implementation of policies for the prevention and control of cross-infection;

(5) providing facilities for use by self-help and pressure groups.

These groups might have personal concerns, such as dietary control and caries reductions, or a more collective agenda, such as promoting water fluoridation or voluntary codes of practice with respect to the positioning of confectionery in supermarkets. Many practice-based health promotion policies would have an impact upon both patient participation and the reduction of inequity. In addition they would have an impact upon the health of staff as well as patients.

A final point is appropriate. As individual general dental practices develop their health promotion strategies, adequate provision should be made to establish procedures of accountability. The success or otherwise of these strategies can only be monitored if goals have been stated prior to their introduction. These goals should move beyond the traditional issues of finance and number of patient contacts to include measures of participation and equity in the provision of care.

Conclusions

In this chapter the current and potential role for health promotion in general dental practice has been examined. I have deliberately ignored the possibility of looking beyond the dental practice to initiatives which are more collective or community orientated, and concentrated upon the current emphasis within general practice of giving advice. An immediate concern has been the discrepancy between rhetoric and reality. There is no lack of activity within general dental practices, but such activity appears to be often inconsistent, fragmented and inappropriate. The longstanding criticisms of current oral health promotion practice — that it is professionally dominated, individualistic, behaviourally orientated, and prescriptive — still retain their validity when current practice and examples of innovation are reviewed.

Strategies for change will involve the following factors. Firstly, the contribution of current organizational arrangements in general dental practice to health promotion should be examined. These organizational arrangements may prevent the wider introduction of opportunities for health promotion. Secondly, if the target for change is within general dental practice, then there is a need for a fundamental change in the nature of the relationship between dentists and their patients. For both of these factors the primary health care approach provides an appropriate framework for developing strategies. Finally, the roles of social scientists associated with oral health education and promotion should be examined. It would seem that some have been too easily prepared to accept the agenda provided by dentists without considering the possibility of an alternative provided through an exploration of the needs of lay people. In doing so they have failed to move the general dental practitioner's perception and practice of health education away from its current limited content and method towards the development of a more coherent contribution to health promotion.

References

Ayer, W. A. and Corah, N. L. (1984). Behavioural factors influencing dental treatment. In *Social Sciences and Dentistry. A Critical Bibliography, Vol. II*, (ed. L. K. Cohen and P. S. Bryant), pp. 267–323. Quintessence, Kingston upon Thames.

Baab, D. and Weinstein, P. (1983). Oral hygiene instruction using a self-instruction plaque index. *Community Dent. Oral Epidemiol.*, **11**, 174–9.

Baad, D. and Weinstein, P. (1986). Longitudinal evaluation of a self-inspection plague index in periodontal recall patients. *J. Clin. Perio.*, **13**, 313–18.

Ballard, A. (1987). Meeting community needs — community education at the Open University. In *Open learning for adults*, (ed. M. Thorpe and D. Grugeon), pp 117–26. Longman, Harlow.

Beattie, A. (1983). *Directions in the development of health education in relation to the prevention of coronary heart disease*. Paper prepared for DHSS/HEC Workshop on 'Action to prevent coronary heart disease'.

Beattie, A. (1991). Knowledge and control in health promotion: a test case for a social policy and social theory. In *Sociology of the Health Service*, (ed. J. Gabe, M. Caulan and M. Bury), pp. 162–202. Routledge, London.

Birn, H. and Birn, B. (1985). Education for wellness. *Community Dental Health*, **2**, 51–6.

Bradshaw, R. (1977). The concept of social need. In *Welfare in action*, (ed. H. Fitzgerald, P. Halmos, J. Mincie, and D. Zeldin), pp. 33–7. Routledge and Kegan Paul, London.

Catford, J. and Nutbeam, R. (1984). Towards a definition of health education and health promotion. *Health Education Journal*, **43**, 36.

Corah, N. (1974). The dental practitioner and preventive health behaviour. *Health Educ. Monog.*, **2**, 226–35.

Crawford, R. (1977). You are dangerous to your health: the ideology and politics of victim blaming. *International Journal of Health Services*, **7**, 636–80.

Croucher, R. (1989). *The performance gap: patients' view about dental care and the prevention of periodontal disease*. Research Report No. 25. Health Education Authority, London.

Cust, G. (1979). A preventive medicine viewpoint. In *Health education: perspectives and choices*, (ed. I. Sutherland), pp. 64–92. Allen and Unwin, London.

Draper, P., Griffiths, J., Dennis, J., and Popay, J. (1980). Three types of health education. *Brit. Med. J.*, **281**, 493–5.

Ewles, L. and Simnett, I. (1985). *Promoting health: a practical guide to health education*. John Wiley and Sons, Chichester.

Fahrenport, M. (1987). Patient emancipation by health education: an impossible dream. *Patient Education and Counseling*, **10**, 26–37.

Farnes, N. (1988). Open University community education: emancipation or domestication. *Open Learning*, **3**, 35–40.

Farrant, W. and Russell, J. (1985). *Health Education Council publications: a case study in the production, distribution and use of health information.* Health Education Publications Project, University of London Institute of Education, London.

Farrant, W. and Russell, J. (1986). *Beating heart disease: a case study in the production of Health Education Council publications.* Bedford Way Paper, University of London Institute of Education, London.

Frandsen, A. (1986). Mechanical oral hygiene practices. In *Dental plaque control measures and oral hygiene practices*, (ed. H. Loe and D. V. Kleinman), pp. 93–116. IRL Press, Oxford.

Frazier, J. (1978). A new look at dental health education in community programmes. *Dental Hygiene,* **52,** 176–9.

Frazier, J. (1992). Research on oral health education and promotion and social epidemiology. *J. Public Health Dent.,* **52,** 1, 18–22.

Frazier, J. and Horowitz, A. (1990). Oral health education and promotion in maternal and child health: a position paper. *J. Public Health Dent.,* **50,** 6, 390–5.

Freire, P. (1968). *Pedagogy of the oppressed.* Seabury Press, New York.

Fried, J. L. and Rubinstein, L. (1990). Attitudes and behaviours of dental hygienists concerning tobacco use. *J. Public Health Dent.,* **50,** 3, 172–7.

Gift, H. C. (1986). Current utilisation patterns of oral hygiene practices. In *Dental plaque control measures and oral hygiene practices*, (ed. H. Loe and D. V. Kleinman), pp. 39–71, IRL Press, Oxford.

Gjermo, P. (1986). Summary of groupwork and plenary discussions. In *Promotion of self-care in oral health*, (ed. P. Gjermo), pp. 197–206. Scandinavian Working Group for Preventive Dentistry, Oslo.

Glavind, L. (1979). *Rene Taender? Renere Taender en selvinstruktion.* Aarhus Tand Laegehojskole.

Glavind, L. and Attstrom, R. (1979). Periodontal self examination: a motivational tool in periodontics. *J. Clin. Perio.,* **6,** 238–51.

Glavind, L. and Nyvad, B. (1986). Scientific basis for oral health: recommendations for self-care. In *Promotion of self-care in oral health*, (ed. P. Gjermo), pp. 77–92. Scandinavian Working Group for Preventive Dentistry, Oslo.

Glavind, L., Zeuner, E., and Attstrom, R. (1981). Oral hygiene instruction by adults by means of a self-instructional manual. *J. Clin. Perio.,* **8,** 165–76.

Glavind, L., Zeuner, E., and Attstrom, R. (1984). Oral cleanliness and gingival health following oral hygiene instruction by self-educational programs. *J. Clin. Perio.,* **11,** 262–73.

Glavind, L., Christenson, A., Pedersen, E., Rosendahl, H., and Attstrom, R. (1985). Oral hygiene instruction in general dental practice by means of self-teaching manuals. *J. Clin. Perio.,* **12,** 27–34.

Heathcote, G. (1987). Promoting health education. *Open Learning,* **3,** 13–16.

Jacob, M. C. and Plamping, D. (1989). *The practice of primary dental care.* Wright, London.

Kiyak, H. A. and Mulligan, K. (1986). Behavioural research related to oral hygiene practices. In *Dental plaque control measures and oral hygiene practices*, (ed. H. Loe and D. V. Kleinman), pp. 225–39. IRL Press, Oxford.

Levy, G. F. and Gilbert, R. A. (1984). The status of fluoride in oral health education in Head Start programs. *J. Dent. Child.,* **51,** 66–70.

Lewis, R. (1986). What is open learning? *Open Learning,* **1,** 5–11.

Lewis, R. and Spencer, D. (1986). What is open learning? Open Learning Guide No 4. Council for Educational Technology for UK, London.

Penchansky, R. and Thomas, J. W. (1981). The concept of access. Definition and relationship to consumer satisfaction. *Med. Care*, **19**, 127–40.

Rawson, D. and Grigg, J. (1987). *Purpose and practice in health education*. Summary Report of the South Bank Health Education Research Project. Polytechnic of the South Bank, London.

Rayner, J. F. and Cohen, L. K. (1971). School dental health education. In *Social sciences and dentistry*, (ed. N. D. Richards and L. K. Cohen), pp. 275–307. Federation Dentaire Internationale, London.

Rayner, J. F. and Cohen, L. K. (1974). A position on school dental health education. *Journal of Preventive Dentistry*, **1**, 11–23.

Rodmell, S. and Watt, A. (1986). Conventional health education: problems and possibilities. In *The politics of health education*, (ed. S. Rodmell and A. Watt), pp. 1–16. Routledge and Kegan Paul, London.

Rugg-Gunn, A. and MacGregor, I. (1978). A survey of toothbrushing behaviour in children and young adults. *J. Perio. Research*, **13**, 382–9.

Schaub, R. (1986). Models and assumptions for changing oral health behaviour. In *Promotion of self-care in oral health*, (ed. P. Gjermo), pp. 125–37. Scandinavian Working Group for Preventive Dentistry, Oslo.

Sheiham, A. (1977). Prevention and control of periodontal disease. In *International conference on research in the biology of periodontal disease*, (ed.), pp. 308–87. College of Dentistry, Chicago, Illinois.

Sheiham, A. (1990). Controversies in periodontics. In *Contemporary periodontics*, (ed. R. Genco, H. Goldman, and D. W. Cohen), pp. 705–9. C. V. Mosby, St. Louis.

Sheiham, A. and Croucher, R. (1989). *Barriers to improving periodontal health — professional and lay perspectives*. Paper prepared for British Society of Periodontology Symposium on the role of supragingival plaque in the control of progressive periodontal disease.

Søgaard, A. J. and Holst, D. (1988). The effect of different school based dental health education programmes in Norway. *Community Dental Health*, **5**, 169–84.

Steuart, G. V. (1969). Planning and evaluation in health education. *International Journal of Health Education*, **10**, 171–9.

Szasz, T. S. and Hollender, M. (1956). A contribution to the philosophy of medicine: the basic models of the doctor–patient relationship. *Archives of Internal Medicine*, **97**, 585–92.

Tones, K. (1990). *The power to choose: health education and the new public health*. Health Education Unit, Leeds Polytechnic, Leeds.

Tones, K., Tilford, S., and Robinson, Y. (1990). *Health education: effectiveness and efficiency*. Chapman and Hall, London.

Tuckett, D., Boulton, M., Olson, C., and Williams, A. (1985). *Meetings between experts: an approach to sharing ideas in medical consultations*. Tavistock, London.

Walt, G. and Vaughan, P. (1981). *An introduction to the primary health care approach in developing countries*. Ross Institute of Tropical Hygiene Publication No. 13; London School of Hygiene and Tropical Medicine, London.

Weinstein, P. (1986). Response to review, behavioural research related to oral hygiene practices. In *Dental plaque control measures and oral hygiene practices*, (ed. H. Loe and D. V. Kleinman), pp. 240–9. IRL Press, Oxford.

WHO (World Health Organization) (1984). Health promotion: a discussion document of the concept and principles. *Health Promotion*, **1**.1, 73–6.

Wilding, P. (1982). *Professional power and social welfare*. Routledge and Kegan Paul, London.

Young, M. (1970). Dental health education: an overview of selected concepts and principles relevant to program planning. *International Journal of Health Education*, **13**, 2–26.

6C

Oral health promotion with children and adolescents

EINO HONKALA

Summary

This chapter emphasizes the population strategy planning in oral health promotion programmes for children and adolescents. The developmental framework of a child and the socialization process should be considered as a basis for all behavioural enterprises targeted towards children. Empowerment of a child for adopting favourable dental health habits demands a practical and educational approach. The concepts proposed by Sheiham (1990) could form the general guidelines for programme planning. Oral health for children and adolescents cannot be reached without the efforts for healthy environment, which would support healthy choices and healthy behaviour of the individuals.

Introduction

The growth and development of a child is a continuous process leading to an independent and self-reliant individual. Of course, no individual is ever totally independent, because he or she needs a social context for his or her existence and social networks and friends for his or her social and psychological well-being. The continuous development of a child can be categorized into different phases of childhood and adolescence (Fig. 6.1). These seven stages are intrauterine (from conception to birth), neonatal (from birth through to the fourth week), infant (from the fourth week to the second year), preschool (years 2 to 6), early school (years 6 to 10 for females and 6 to 12 for males), prepubescent (years 10 to 12 for females and 12 to 14 for males), and adolescent (years 12 to 18 for females and 14 to 20 for males) (Kolbe 1984). Those in the first stages of puberty are more like children than adults. They are just beginning to resemble adults physically, but psychological, social, and cognitive development lags behind. Middle adolescents are those we most often

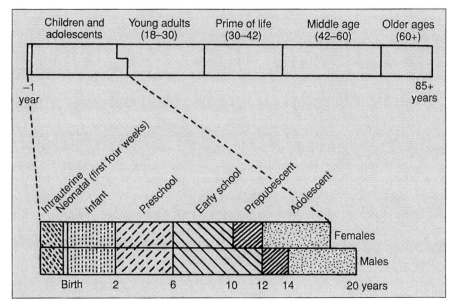

Fig. 6.1 Life cycle development (McHale *et al.* 1979).

associate with the term 'teenagers'. Older adolescents are more like adults than children in all developmental aspects (Petersen 1982).

Childhood and adolescence also includes behavioural development, which can be classified into different phases (Table 6.2). The process of developing coping capacities must be considered when planning the improvement of childrens' learning and the adoption of new behaviour. Each individual has specific physiological and psychological requirements, which will have evolved over the course of time and will enable a person to process information and to consider different behavioural options (Hurrelmann 1989). Some of the important information-processing variables have been described clearly by Ulich (1987):

1. Awareness orientation: it appears that a high degree of self-awareness may well lead a person to pay greater attention to physical and psychological reactions when confronted with critical life-events and to plan and undertake corrective measures earlier. This in turn results in their being less susceptible to disease of a behavioural origin.

2. Self-esteem: various forms of self-esteem play a decisive role in the process of assessing the relative danger of a particular situation, in dealing with difficulties, and in the extent to which a crisis affects the future development of personality. The negative effect of continuous stress and critical life-events may result from the fact that such events lead one to develop a negative view of oneself. The individual experiences restrictions in self-develop-

Table 6.2 Developmental coping capacities and developmental tasks during the life course (Hurrelmann 1989)

Phase of life	Example of developmental behaviour demands
Early childhood	Development of 'basic trust' Formation of social ties Sensomotoric intelligence Preconceptual thinking Basic sensory and motor skills Symbolic and verbal expression
Late childhood	Ability to deal with peers Adequate gender-specific behaviour Basic skills in reading, writing, and calculation Establishment of conscience, morals, and values Positive attitude to oneself as a growing organism
Early adolescence	Formal intellectual operations Scholastic achievement Establishment of relationships with both sexes Acquisition of male or female role Acceptance of own physical appearance Effective use of physical prowess
Late adolescence	Reappraisal of relationship to one's own body Abstract intellectual operations Emotional independence from parents and other adults Preparation for marriage and family life Preparation for occupation System of values that serve as a guideline for behaviour Stable self-image and sense of identity Use of consumer market

ment, satisfaction of basic needs, self-assertion, perseverance, and the potential to organize his or her own life. Positive self-assessment and self-esteem can be influential in diminishing the effects of external influences and crises on psychological health. On the other hand, negative self-assessment and self-esteem can actually magnify problems.

3. Confidence in locus of control: this variable is formed during the process of coming to a decision with respect to the extent to which one feels able to anticipate a particular situation or its consequences, or to the extent to which one feels able to influence or at least interpret them adequately. Here we are dealing with the cognitive realization of wishes, conceptions, and chances of success with regard to an individual's capacity to exert any real influence.

4. Causal attribution: this refers to a person's attempt to explain causality in environmental events. These subjective interpretations are not only manifestations of norms and previous experiences; they are also related to immediate impressions concerning the cause of a problem and the possible desired or undesired changes in one's own situation or state of mind.

When oral health promotion is planned for children and adolescents, the development of the individual needs to be taken into account and activities must be formulated according to the framework of human development.

Lifestyles conducive to oral health

The most common oral diseases, caries and periodontal disease, could well be seen as behavioural diseases, because the adoption of healthy behaviour is crucial for their control. Traditionally, healthy oral health behaviour has been considered to consist of the continuous implementation of those measures which have been scientifically proven to have a positive effect on oral health. A habit with a documented positive relationship to health could be called a health habit. Four distinct oral health behaviours are commonly accepted as being of value in controlling oral diseases:

(1) effective oral hygiene;

(2) restriction of foods containing sugar;

(3) continuous use of fluorides;

(4) appropriate use of oral health services.

The first three behaviours can be seen as habits when they are categorized as regular, frequent, learned, automatic, and self-perpetuating measures by which people consciously try to maintain oral health. After frequent repetition, the consciousness of the subject will be transferred from the control of the actual procedure into the conceptual goals of the action, and the control of the behaviour moves from the grey substance of the brain cortex to the lower level of the central nervous system. Oral hygiene and most fluoride practices fulfil these characteristics very well, but restriction of sugar depends on the frequency with which the many and various sugar-containing food products are consumed.

Use of oral health services does not fulfil the repetitive characteristic of a habit and it never becomes an automatic behaviour, but otherwise the custom of regular dental check-ups has been established in most population groups. This behaviour depends on social influences, as an acceptable frequency reflects the generally adopted norms of the community. Normative behaviour in this respect could mean six-monthly check-ups in Britain (Elderton 1985), annual check-ups in the Nordic countries (Milen et al. 1986), and check-ups according to perceived pain in most of the developing countries (Lembariti 1990). Sheiham (1984a) has proposed a change from this current custom by suggesting that the interval between dental check-ups be increased to two years or more.

Environmental factors play a dominant role in the adoption of these dental health habits. Individual habits cannot be separated from a subject's whole behaviour, but are integral parts of his or her lifestyle. Lifestyle can actually be seen as a composite of all the individual habits. The determinants of a person's lifestyle are consequences of environmental factors, although heredity also plays a role (Fig. 6.2). The main environmental factor is often called social heredity, which includes the environment children usually inherit from their parents. The goal of oral health promotion is the adoption of the appropriate dental health habits at the population level as socially acceptable behaviour, i.e. normative habits. Therefore it is crucially important that the development of these habits is monitored at the population level. It is much easier to facilitate the adoption of these habits early in life than to try to change detrimental oral health behaviour later in a child's development. Therefore, considerable effort needs to be directed towards young children in order to enable them to adopt appropriate dental health habits.

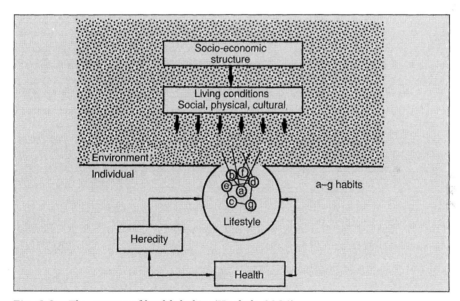

Fig. 6.2 The context of health habits (Honkala 1984).

Effective oral hygiene

Oral hygiene practices are those practices employed personally or professionally to prevent the establishment of pathogenic flora or their disease-causing products in the oral cavity. The ultimate objective is to prevent disease initiation, progression, or recurrence (Sheiham 1986a). For oral health promotion the most effective practices are those performed by individuals themselves. It is commonly accepted among the dental profession that tooth-brushing, as a mechanical measure for removing dental plaque, is the most appropriate oral hygiene habit. The recommended frequency has been twice a day (Frandsen 1986), brushing the whole dentition after breakfast and before going to bed. The effectiveness of plaque removal is more important than the frequency of brushing (Löe and Kleinman 1986). The length of time spent brushing has been shown to be more related to the effectiveness of plaque removal than frequency (Honkala *et al.* 1986).

There is as yet little scientific evidence to indicate that any one type of toothbrush is better at maintaining gingival health. Although no brushing method has been shown to be clearly superior to any other, the scrub technique is the most popular, has been shown to be reasonably effective, and requires the least amount of time. Therefore, it should be encouraged (Frandsen 1986). Regular toothbrushing is important, because the other aspects can have an effect only if the brushing habit is well established. Toothbrushing does not clean interproximal areas effectively, and therefore interdental cleaning should be a fundamental part of personal oral hygiene (Löe and Kleinman 1986). Contradicting views have been expressed about the age at which use of dental floss should begin, but it probably could be recommended that flossing begins in early adolescence, when the grooming aspects of oral hygiene may motivate the adoption of this practice, which demands practical dexterity and time. There are great differences between countries in this respect, which may reflect different cultural norms (Fig. 6.3).

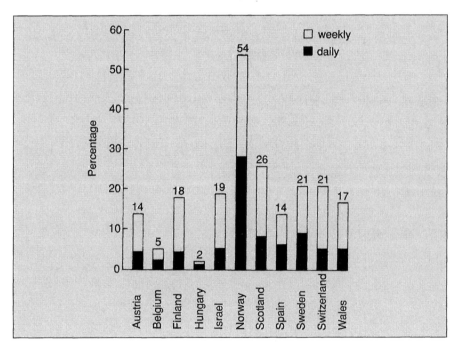

Fig. 6.3   Use of dental floss among 11-year-olds in some European countries (Honkala *et al.* 1990).

Restriction of foods containing sugar

Since the Vipeholm study the main concern in caries prevention has been concentrated on restricting the frequency with which sugar products are consumed, especially between meals. Studies concerning the frequency of intake of different sugar-containing foods have not confirmed any unidimensional pattern of consumption of various sugar products. Therefore in preventive dentistry dietary patterns have been studied by determining the frequency of consumption of different sugar-containing snacks and soft drinks. In Finland the most common sugar habit is the consumption of sugar-sweetened coffee, which is used daily by over half of all Finnish adolescents (Honkala 1984; Honkala *et al.* 1991). In most European countries approximately half of the children consume sweets and soft drinks on a regular basis (Fig. 6.4). The main difference between countries is whether oral health promotion to decrease the daily use of sugar products among children and adolescents is seen as an important priority. Children's use of different sugar products is related to socioeconomic background, but there is also a strong relationship between the sugar habits of children and those of their parents (Honkala *et al.* 1983). Use of sugar products is negatively correlated with children's school performance, school career, and positively with available pocket money (Honkala *et al.* 1982). In a recent study the amount of money spent on sweets per week had a clear association with caries experience (Dummer *et al.* 1990).

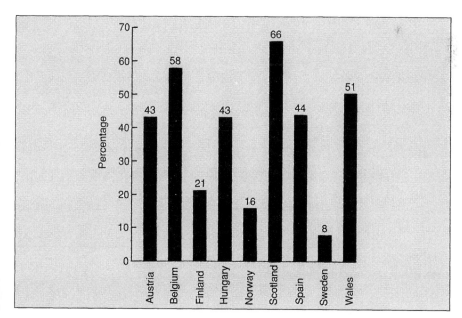

Fig. 6.4   Daily consumption of sweets among 77-year-olds in some European countries (Honkala *et al.* 1990).

There have been attempts to deny children all sugar products, but this would mean major changes in common behaviour and in the social norms of those societies where sweets are given as presents. There is also the danger of overestimating oral health issues among the priorities of life, and this kind of approach could be termed 'healthism' and in practice could result in 'victim blaming' (Ryan 1976). In the Nordic countries, therefore, the practical step for restricting sweets consumption has been to recommend a 'candy day' for children. This allows a compromise for parents and especially grandparents, who have found it very difficult to accept total prohibition, because giving sweets is one way to show love and concern for their grandchildren. It is much easier to modify their behaviour than to completely change it.

Sugar-using habits are adopted early in childhood (Rossow *et al.* 1990), and it has been shown that some preference for sweet taste exists during infancy (Beauchamp and Moran 1982) and is emphasized by a sugary diet or suppressed by a sugar-free diet. Sweetened comforters such as feeding bottles containing sugar-sweetened liquids, dipped dummies, and reservoir (dinky) feeders are dangerous to teeth (Health Education Council 1984), especially after the first six months when the primary teeth start to erupt. There is clearly a danger of 'nursing bottle caries', also referred to as 'baby bottle mouth' (Goepferd 1986). Dietary counselling for parents of preschool children is of great value in controlling caries in this vulnerable age group (Persson *et al.* 1985).

Murray (1987) has made some practical suggestions for restricting childrens' sugar consumption:

1. Give up sugar-containing boiled sweets that are packaged for frequent consumption.

2. Restrict confectionery consumption to meal times.

3. If sugar is used in coffee, substitute an artificial sweetener.

4. If fruit drinks and squashes are consumed, substitute sugar-free varieties.

5. If fizzy drinks are consumed frequently, suggest 'diet' versions.

6. Try to replace some sweet snacks by fruits, crisps, nuts, or cheese.

7. Try to limit sugar in both food and drinks to mealtimes only.

8. Never allow a sugar-containing drink to be consumed last thing at night.

Continuous use of fluorides

The preventive effect of water fluoridation on dental caries has been extensively documented (Murray and Rugg-Gunn 1982). Caries reductions in these studies have varied from 20 per cent to 80 per cent for deciduous teeth and from 20 per cent to 90 per cent for permanent teeth (Naylor and Murray

1983). Adjusting the fluoride level in public water supplies is the most cost-effective measure in preventive medicine (Davies 1974). Its effectiveness is based on the population strategy of comprehensive delivery of fluoride in the drinking water, a method that demands no effort from the recipients. Unfortunately, this measure has not met with universal acceptance and its implementation has been opposed in some countries. The same positive effect as provided by fluoride in the drinking water has in some cases been achieved by school fluoridation programmes (Jenny and Heifetz 1978). The cost of this public health measure has also been low (about US $1.50 per child annually) (Horowitz and Heifetz 1979) and it may be more acceptable to some people than fluoridation of the public water supply. Other possible ways to offer the benefit of systemic fluoride are fluoride tablets and drops and fluoridated milk and fruit juices. Regular consumption of fluoride tablets or drops requires an established daily habit, where the main responsibility is taken by the parents. This demands a high degree of health consciousness and concern by at least one parent, and compliance has been quite low (Honkala et al. 1988). If the tablets are given regularly at school the coverage has been better, but then it requires a time commitment from the teachers, which is often not forthcoming.

Topical fluoride also increases tooth resistance to caries. The most common topical application of fluoride is obtained during brushing with a fluoride toothpaste. Fluoride toothpastes have contributed considerably to the recent caries decline in the industrialized countries. Their effect is based more on the frequency of use than on their concentration (Naylor and Murray 1983).

Fluoride rinsing programmes have been based on either the population strategy, covering all schoolchildren, or the risk-group strategy, as a special programme for those with high risk of caries. When conducted in schools, however, it demands quite a lot of the school personnel and has been shown to be ineffective even when used in addition to comprehensive use of fluoride toothpaste (Klein et al. 1985; Haugejorden et al. 1990). Such rinsing programmes have commonly been implemented in the Nordic countries, but the coverage has been decreasing as the caries trend has declined (Honkala et al. 1991). Thus, general school rinsing may not be appropriate, but the risk group strategy targeting handicapped schools and schools in areas with high caries rates is probably cost-effective. Considerable efforts are still needed to promote fluoride programmes in every country among children in areas without adequate fluoride concentration in drinking water. There are considerable national differences in Europe in the use of different forms of fluorides by children (Table 6.3).

Concentrated fluoride solutions have to be used under supervision and fluoride varnishes must be applied by professionals, therefore in recent years their cost-effectiveness has been questioned (Klein et al. 1985). They may be used for high caries risk groups, but give little benefit when used in addition to the regular use of fluoride toothpaste.

Table 6.3 Use of different fluoride measures (given as percentages) among 11-year-olds in some European countries (Honkala *et al.* 1990)

Country	Toothpaste (daily)	Rinses		Tablets	
		Daily	Weekly	Daily	Weekly
Austria	52	13	16	4	3
Belgium	76	5	3	6	8
Finland	87	3	38	12	12
Hungary	38	11	7	3	3
Israel	58	16	8	2	3
Norway	93	12	22	34	11
Scotland	85	6	47	4	8
Spain	76	32	25	9	11
Sweden	87	4	45	1	2
Switzerland	–	23	9	6	6
Wales	80	11	12	2	7

Socialization

The way in which children learn and adopt behaviour is called socialization. It is the process whereby knowledge, values, attitudes, and routines are transmitted to children through social interaction. 'Primary socialization' is the term applied to the early influence of the home, parents, relatives, and close friends. The process of primary socialization operates via a system of reward and punishment and involves a modelling process. Parents reward or punish their children for developing desirable or undesirable attitudes and values, and children model their behaviours on parental example and internalize key values (Tones 1979). Adoption of consistent behavioural habits takes place at home and the parents, especially the mother, are the primary models for behaviour (Blinkhorn 1981). It has been shown that towards the end of the first year of life, most children are weaned and start to eat solid food. The child adapts to the family eating pattern, which also means that sugar-eating patterns are established at this age (Holm 1990). The move from families to the more formalized community-based networks takes place during the secondary socialization phase. Other agencies transmit norms; the school is probably the major secondary socializing agency. The mass media are also the purveyors of values and norms at a secondary level. Secondary socialization is characterized by greater formality and less emotional involvement with the person, and so the school typically teaches its pupils in a more formal and detached way than parents do (Tones 1979). Adolescence is the stage at which an individual develops an identity, and some kind of identity crisis may well be a necessary component of the developmental process (Petersen 1982). This crisis of identity may be accompanied by a decline in self-esteem and therefore requires special attention in behavioural programmes, of which health promotion programmes are one type. The other important aspect of adolescent development is that the media, especially television and music, have a powerful impact upon young people. Adolescents look to their society for what they should be and become, and they learn a great deal from television and radio (Petersen 1982). Where intervention attempts to change existing values, attitudes, and routines, the term 'resocialization' is often used. Health care professionals need to pay greater attention to those adolescents who have been called 'invulnerables'. These are the adolescents who by any standards could be 'losers' — delinquent, emotionally disturbed, or alienated — because of a history of parental loss, abuse, absence, neglect, extreme poverty, and often a series of early losses and separations (Green and Horton 1982). The ultimate goal of health for all demands special efforts for those at greatest health risk. Tones (1979) also defined 'anticipatory socialization' as a process of adopting the values, attitudes, and behaviours of social groups to which children would like to belong or whose attributes they admire. Such groups are called reference groups. One of the major functions of the school may be to provide some kind of anticipatory guidance. Children may adopt the norms of a valued peer group as a kind of entry qualification. Social norms consistently influence behaviour such as toothbrushing, dental visiting, and use of sugary foods (Traen and Rise 1990).

Programmes of oral health promotion for children

Whenever efforts are made to change behaviour through health promotion the key issues are programme planning, implementation, and evaluation. The general principles of developing programmes of oral health promotion can best be described by considering the concepts proposed by Sheiham (1990):

1. Integration: oral health education should be integrated with general health education into the activities of teachers, all health workers, community leaders, trade unionists, sports people and all members of the dental team. Oral hygiene education should be integrated with general health education dealing with body cleanliness, grooming and self-esteem (Blinkhorn et al. 1983). It has also been demonstrated that it is beneficial to involve the parents in health promotion programmes for children (Blinkhorn et al. 1981). This also means that teachers must take responsibility for teaching and resist attempts by eager and well meaning doctors and nurses to come into the school and teach about health and illness (Tones 1979). It is also much more cost-effective to support teachers to teach oral health education messages than to use external oral health personnel at school (Blinkhorn and Wight 1987).

2. Diverse educational approaches are needed because individuals have different needs and are at different stages of behavioural development. Individual instruction, group discussion, mass media, and community development methods can be used, but they need to be cumulative and

consistent. There is and can be no best method. In addition to educational methods, fiscal, legal, and organizational changes should also be used in these programmes (WHO 1984). Encouragement of modelling and reinforcement are important elements of behavioural change.

3. The earlier the intervention in the health education of a child, the more effective is the result. Primary and secondary socialization have a paramount influence in establishing the habits and therefore the parents, teachers, and peer groups are the 'significant others' whose role is important for children. Children working as teachers of their peers are also likely to involve teachers and the parents (Plamping *et al.* 1980).

4. More emphasis should be placed on the educational process and on the target groups than on the substantive content of the programme. Educational efforts should optimize salience, pertinence, credibility, habit formation, long-term change, and reinforcement.

5. Community, public, and staff participation in the planning process should increase the probability of success. Fostering of negotiation between the learner and the educator involves the participation of the children themselves in the education process.

6. Encourage self-efficacy: empowerment of the child means encouraging his or her self-esteem and making change more a matter of personal control. Therefore, the focus should be on the whole person, or on certain central characteristics of the person, such as self-esteem, or the sense of internal control over his or her own life, or the belief in personal responsibility for his or her own health (Jessor 1982).

7. Healthier choices — easier choices: the programme should include practical procedures for making the environment of children healthier at home and at schools. Appropriate school meals should be one goal for any health promotion programme, and efforts should be devoted to banning sweet snacks during the school day.

8. Dental anxiety prevents children from taking advantage of the health education message, and so fear-providing messages should be avoided.

9. Educational and behavioural outcomes — objectives should be clearly stated. The basic question asked should be 'Who is expected to achieve how much of what and by when?' These objectives are needed as a basis for evaluation.

10. The goals should, according to Myers (1987), be: appropriate, realistic, measureable, positive, important to the person, and time-related. Many disappointments can be avoided if the goals are clearly stated and are appropriate for the target group before the programme is implemented.

11. The evaluation of a programme is necessary for its continuation and for further development (see Chapter 7). A new programme can only be developed when there is knowledge about whether an existing programme is achieving its objectives.

In general, a programme of oral health promotion should emphasize lay competence, be supportive, and not 'blame the victim' (Sheiham 1990). This also means that these programmes should involve groups other than health professionals; to be effective they need to be multisectoral. In addition, they should be planned to fit into the everyday life of the children and be concerned with the situations and organizations in which the children live.

Craft (1984) summarized the experiences of the 'Natural Nashers' school-based oral health education programme, in which teachers' acceptance is gained by gradually introducing several critical factors:

1. Presenting a content that overlapped and complemented the biology syllabus. This was chosen as a convenient point of entry and at least ensured a whole-body context; the content included experimental activity, classroom reinforcement, and homework.

2. Using a design which did not significantly distort the teacher's perceived role.

3. Providing a wide variety of materials for teachers and individual pupils.

4. Providing classroom fieldworkers as a resource and back-up for teachers in the initial runs of the programme.

The other approach, used in the Life Skills Training (LST) programme (Botvin 1984), is designed to focus attention primarily on the major psycho-social factors for promoting health behaviour, which can be divided into the following components: cognitive, decision-making, anxiety-reduction, social skills training, and self-improvement. This approach is needed for individual-based interventions.

The programmes which have the most important effect at a population level are the national programmes. These national programmes should be planned well in advance so that oral health professionals can implement them locally, working together with other personnel. One example of a successful and comprehensive national programme is the Finnish programme of oral health promotion, which was introduced by the Public Health Act in 1972. The directives of this programme are described in Table 6.4.

In addition, oral health promotion programmes should try to involve other educational enterprises such as community leaders, public education, mass media, promote environmental change, and professional education (Sheiham 1984b).

Table 6.4   Directives to dentists from the National Board of Health of Finland. The main points of the letter of general instructions, 28 July 1972 (Honkala *et al.* 1991)

The emphasis should be put on preventive oral health care

Special attention should be focused on health behaviour
1. Dental dietary instructions should be part of general nutritional advice, where especially the frequency of consumption of sugar-containing foods should be reduced.
2. Oral hygiene instructions should include use of toothbrush, toothpaste, and toothpicks.
3. Increasing tooth resistance by fluorides should be recommended.

Oral instructions should include use of accepted oral health education material
1. Children under 17 years of age should be given a toothbrush.
2. A first package of fluoride tablets or fluoride rinse should be given in conjunction with dental health education.

Oral health education should be conducted in conjunction with all dental treatment given, and in nurseries and in schools

Activities in Mother and Child Health (MCH) clinics
1. Instruction should be focused towards pregnant mothers and the parents of 0–2-year-olds.
2. The pregnant mothers should be invited for oral health education sessions.
3. Annual treatment of children under school age should always include oral health education of the parents.

Activities in schools
1. School meals should be planned properly for dental health by avoiding unnecessary consumption of sugar.
2. Each school class should receive at least one oral health education lesson during every school term.
3. Supervised toothbrushing sessions should be organized 2–4 times a year.
4. Topical fluoride applications should be conducted.

Activities in dental clinics
1. Importance of home-care should be emphasized to all children.
2. Every child should brush his or her teeth under supervision before the dental treatment and rinse with fluoride solution.

Healthy environment for children and adolescents

Population strategy may be considered radical when its aim is to influence the underlying causes of diseases, however it is behaviourally important to create social norms based on healthy behaviour (Rose 1985). This kind of population approach in relation to implementing the British NACNE recommendations has been suggested to be divided into five different strategies (Sanderson 1984):

(1) education

(2) substitution

(3) pricing

(4) provision

(5) regulation

This kind of approach could also be called macro-level prevention and . should be considered in all oral health behaviours.

Macroprevention in oral hygiene

Education has been the most common method of promoting good oral hygiene and is an important method for improving knowledge and for changing attitudes and values, but it is quite inefficient for changing behaviour. However, when mass-media campaigns of health education are connected to other behavioural interventions, they seem to facilitate learning (Schou 1987).

Substitution could be used, for example, for developing toothbrushing practice in kindergarten, nursery schools, day-care or child-care centres, and in schools as an alternative or in addition to oral hygiene practices at home. Although brushing in the mornings and in the evenings would be quite appropriate, brushing exercises at school with their peers might be behaviourally crucial, especially for children who are not encouraged by their parents to brush their teeth at home. Cheaper prices for toothbrushes, toothpaste, and dental floss would encourage usage, but unfortunately, these products are often heavily taxed in some countries as they are considered as cosmetics rather than health items. Toothbrushes and toothpaste could also be distributed free to children, because this would be an investment in the oral health of future generations. Their provision could be seen as providing the appropriate equipment for good hygiene.

Macroprevention in sugar restriction

Education to help children control their use of sugar has been used much less than education to improve oral hygiene. Only one fifth of the children in Finland have had instruction in the use of sugar products (Honkala *et al.* 1991). Substitution has, of course, been common among diabetic children, but it could also be used much more effectively for other children. Many more xylitol-sweetened products are available and the use of xylitol in the most frequently used food products could be increased. The results are especially promising, where xylitol chewing gum has been added to existing caries-preventive measures (Isokangas *et al.* 1988). More professional pressure is also needed to require the pharmaceutical industry to rapidly and urgently substitute xylitol or other sweeteners for sucrose in medicines, especially in medication for children such as cough syrups.

Pricing could be a very effective means of decreasing consumption of products containing sugar and for increasing the use of xylitol products. The system of taxation could be modified according to the goals of healthy behaviour. A special disadvantage tax for sugar products would probably be as effective as it has been for tobacco. Such a provision would also mean, for example, healthier school meals.

Regulation could be used to prohibit the sale of cariogenic chewing gums, sweets, or soft drinks in schools, where they are sometimes sold by the school-children themselves. It would be quite helpful for parents if in supermarkets cariogenic sweets, chewing gums, and other snacks were not allowed near the cashiers or on the lowest shelves, where they are near at hand for small children. In general, dietary changes call for a food policy to limit the consumption of refined sugars (Sheiham 1984a). Food policy needs to be formulated, implemented, and evaluated.

Macroprevention and fluorides

Education has been used to facilitate the decision to start programmes of water fluoridation in communities, but oral health personnel have not been very successful in promoting the broad use of this cost-effective measure. The value for money argument has been used to promote water fluoridation, but even these price advantages have continuously failed to assure the public and the municipal decision makers of the safety and effectiveness of water fluoridation (Tuutti et al. 1985). Education has also been ineffective for increasing the use of fluoride tablets. Low pricing and free provision have also been used to increase the use of fluoride tablets and fluoride rinses. More effort is needed to increase worldwide coverage of water fluoridation schemes.

The targets for macroprevention measures have been stated by Sanderson (1984) as follows: producers, processors, manufacturers, intermediaries, distributors, caterers, government, professional pressure groups, consumers, and treaters. All these groups should be considered when population strategic planning takes place in the community.

Conclusion

A healthy environment means the policy of making healthy choices the easier choices (Tones 1990). Health education has much to contribute to health promotion by raising consciousness, providing skills, setting agendas, and faciliting healthy choices (Tones et al. 1990). These are really needed when oral health professionals are working for a new public health policy which could facilitate the improvement of global oral health. Oral health promotion activities need to be combined into a comprehensive preventive programme of oral health care, which also means reorientating restorative care (Elderton 1987) for children and adolescents. Oral health promotion demands that dentists should review their caries diagnostic skills in the light of changes in the pattern of dental disease. This has been successfully achieved in the New Zealand school dental service, where the number of caries-free children increased by 35 per cent within a few years by discouraging the use of a sharp probe and only restoring teeth with frank cavitation (Sheiham 1986b). The final task would then be to integrate an oral health programme into the general health programme and then into the everyday lives of all children.

References

Beauchamp, G. K. and Moran, M. (1982). Dietary experience and sweet taste preference in human infants. *Appetite Journal for Intake Research*, **3**, 139–52.

Blinkhorn, A. S. (1981). Dental preventive advice for pregnant and nursing mothers — sociological implications. *International Dental Journal*, **31**, 14–22.

Blinkhorn, A. S., Taylor, I., and Willcox, G.F. (1981). Report of a dental health education programme in Bedfordshire. *British Dental Journal*, **150**, 319–22.

Blinkhorn, A. S., Hastings, G. B., and Leather, D. S. (1983). Attitudes towards dental care among young people in Scotland. Implications for dental health education. *British Dental Journal*, **155**, 311–13.

Blinkhorn, A. S. and Wight, C. (1987). An assessment of two dental health education programmes for Scottish secondary school children. *Health Education Research*, **2**, 231–7.

Botvin, G. J. (1984). The life skills training model: a broad spectrum approach to the prevention of cigarette smoking. In *Health education and youth. A review of research and developments*, (ed. G. Campbell), pp. 205–22. Falmer Press, Basingstoke.

Craft, M. (1984). Natural Nashers: a programme of dental health education for adolescents in schools. *International Dental Journal*, **34**, 204–13.

Davies, G. N. (1974). *Cost and benefit of fluoride in the prevention of dental caries*. World Health Organization Offset Publications, Geneva.

Dummer, P. M. H., Oliver, S. J., Hicks, R., Kingdon, A., Kingdon, R., Addy, M., *et al.* (1990). Factors influencing the caries experience of a group of children at ages of 11–12 and 15–16 years: results from an ongoing epidemiological survey. *Journal of Dentistry*, **18**, 37–48.

Elderton, R. J. (1985). Six-monthly examinations for dental caries. *British Dental Journal*, **158**, 370–4.

Elderton, R. J. (1987). Preventively-oriented restorations and restorative procedures. In *Positive dental prevention. The prevention in childhood of dental disease in adult life*, (ed. R. J. Elderton), pp. 82–92. Heinemann Medical Books, London.

Frandsen, A. (1986). Mechanical oral hygiene practices. State-of-the-science review. In *Dental plaque control measures and oral hygiene practices*, (ed. H. Löe and D. V. Kleinman), pp. 93–116. IRL Press, Oxford.

Goepferd, S. J. (1986). Infant oral health: a rationale. *Journal of Dentistry for Children*, **53**, 257–60.

Green, L. W. and Horton, D. (1982). Adolescent health: issues and challenges. In *Promoting adolescent health. A dialog on research and practice*, (ed. T. J. Coates, A. C. Petersen and C. Perry), pp. 23–44. Academic Press, New York.

Haugejorden, O., Lervik, T., Birkeland, J. M., and Jorkjend, L. (1990). An 11-year follow-up study of dental caries after discontinuation of school-based fluoride programs. *Acta Odontologica Scandinavia*, **48**, 257–63.

Health Education Council (1984). *Dental health in infancy*. A report of a seminar organised by the Health Education Council (mimeo).

Holm, A. -K. (1990). Education and diet in the prevention of caries in the preschool child. *Journal of Dentistry*, **18**, 308–14.

Honkala, E. (1984). Dental health habits of Finnish adolescents. *Proceedings of the Finnish Dental Society*, **80**, Suppl. II.

Honkala, E., Eskola, A., Rimpelä, M., and Rajala, M. (1982). Consumption of sweet foods among adolescents in Finland. *Community Dentistry and Oral Epidemiology*, **10**, 103–10.

Honkala, E., Paronen, O., and Rimpelä, M. (1983). Familial aggregation of dental health habits in Finland. *Journal of Pedodontics*, **7**, 276–86.

Honkala, E., Nyyssönen, V., Knuuttila, M., and Markkanen, H. (1986). Effectiveness of children's habitual toothbrushing. *Journal of Clinical Periodontology*, **13**, 81–5.

Honkala, E., Kannas, L., Rimpelä, M., Wold, B., Aaro, L. E., and Gilles, P. (1988). Dental health habits in Austria, England, Finland and Norway. *International Dental Journal*, **38**, 131–8.

Honkala, E., Kannas, L., and Rise, J. (1990). Oral health habits of schoolchildren in 11 European countries. *International Dental Journal*, **40**, 211–17.

Honkala, E., Karvonen, S., Rimpelä, A., Rajala, M., Rimpelä M., and Prättälä, R. (1991). Oral health promotion among Finnish adolescents between 1977 and 1989. *Health Promotion International*, **6**, 21–30.

Horowitz, H. S. and Heifetz, S. B. (1979). Methods for assessing the cost-effectiveness of caries preventive agents and procedures. *International Dental Journal*, **29**, 106–17.

Hurrelmann, K. (1989). *Human development and health*. Springer-Verlag, Berlin.

Isokangas, P., Alanen, P., Tiekso, J., And Mäkinen, K. K. (1988). Xylitol chewing gum in caries prevention: a field study in children. *Journal of American Dental Association*, **117**, 315–20.

Jenny, J. and Heifetz, S. B. (1978). Prevention update. *Dental Hygiene*, **52**, 187–94.

Jessor, R. (1982). Critical issues in research on adolescent health promotion. In *Promoting adolescent health. A dialog on research and practice*, (ed. T. J. Coates, A. C. Petersen, and C. Perry), pp. 447–65. Academic Press, New York.

Klein, S. P., Bohannan, H. M., Bell, R. M., Disney, J. A., Foch, C. B., and Graves, R. C. (1985). The cost and effectiveness of school-based preventive dental care. *American Journal of Public Health*, **75**, 382–91.

Kolbe, L. J. (1984). Improving the health of children and youth: frameworks for behavioral research and development. In *Health education and youth. A review of research and development*, (ed. G. Campbell), pp. 33–59. The Falmer Press, London.

Lembariti, B. S. (1990). Tanzania — the development of an oral health care service. In *Evolution of dental care*, (ed. R. J. Elderton), pp. 60–3. Clinical Press Ltd, Bristol.

Löe, H. and Kleinman, D. V. (ed.) (1986). *Dental plaque control measures and oral hygiene practices*. IRL Press, Oxford.

McHale, M., McHale, J., and Streatfield, G. (1979). World of children. *Population Bulletin*, **33**, 6.

Milen, A., Tala, H., Hausen, H., and Heinonen, O. P. (1986). *Dental health status, habits and care of Finnish children and youths in 1981–82. A feasibility study of an information system*. Health Services Research by the National Board of Health in Finland, Helsinki.

Murray, J. J. (1987). Diet counselling and oral hygiene in caries control. In *Positive dental prevention*, (ed. R. J. Elderton), pp. 46–57. W. Heineman Medical Books, London.

Murray, J. J. and Rugg-Gunn, A. J. (1982). *Fluorides in caries prevention*, (2nd edn). Wright, Bristol.

Myers, G. (1987). *Mnemonic proposed at workshop on moving toward preventive dentistry in the Royal Navy*. 27–28 September, Portsmouth.

Naylor, M. N. and Murray, J. J. (1983). Fluorides and dental caries. In *The prevention of dental disease*, (ed. J. J. Murray), pp. 83–158. Oxford University Press, Oxford.

Persson, L. -Å., Holm, A. K., Arvidsson, S., and Samuelson, G. (1985). Infant feeding and dental caries — a longitudinal study of Swedish children. *Swedish Dental Journal*, **9**, 201–6.

Petersen, A. C. (1982). Developmental issues in adolescent health. In *Promoting adolescent health. A dialog on research and practice*, (ed. T. J. Coates, A. C. Petersen, and C. Perry), pp. 61–71. Academic Press, New York.

Plamping, D., Thorne, S., and Gelbier, S. (1980). Children as teachers of dental health education. *British Dental Journal*, **150**, 113–15.

Rose, G. (1985). Sick individuals and sick populations. *International Journal of Epidemiology*, **14**, 32–9.

Rossow, I., Kjaernes, U., and Holst, D. (1990). Pattern of sugar consumption in early childhood. *Community Dentistry and Oral Epidemiology*, **18**, 12–16.

Ryan, W. (1976). *Blaming the victim*. Vintage Books, New York.

Sanderson, M. E. (1984). Strategies for implementing NACNE recommendations. *Lancet*, Dec. 10, 1352–6.

Schou, L. (1987). Use of mass-media and active involvement in a national dental health campaign in Scotland. *Community Dentistry and Oral Epidemiology*, **15**, 14–18.

Sheiham, A. (1984a). Changing trends in dental caries. *International Journal of Epidemiology*, **13**, 142–7.

Sheiham, A. (1984b). An analysis of existing dental services in relation to periodontal care. In *Public health aspects of periodontal disease*, (ed. A. Frandsen), pp. 59–67. Quintessence Publ. Co. Inc., Aalborg.

Sheiham, A. (1986a). Response. In *Dental plaque control measures and oral hygiene practices*, (ed. H. Löe and D. V. Kleinman), pp. 117–19. IRL Press Ltd, Oxford.

Sheiham, A. (1986b). *The limitations of dentistry*. Joint Department of Community Dental Health and Dental Practice, Monograph Series, London.

Sheiham, A. (1990). *Public health approaches to the promotion of periodontal health*. Joint Department of Community Dental Health and Dental Practice, Monograph Series No. 3, London.

Tones, B. K. (1979). Socialisation, health career and the health education of the schoolchild. *Journal of the Institute for Health Education*, **17**, 23–8.

Tones, K. (1990). *The power to choose: health education and the new public health*. Health Education Unit, Leeds Polytechnic, Leeds.

Tones, K., Tilford, S., and Robinson, Y. (1990). *Health education. Effectiveness and efficiency*. Chapman and Hall, London.

Traen, B. and Rise, J. (1990). Dental health behaviours in a Norwegian population. *Community Dental Health*, **7**, 59–68.

Tuutti, H., Honkala, E., and Laurinkari, J. (1985). Acceptability of fluoride use in Finnish municipalities. *Scandinavian Journal of Social Medicine*, **13**, 109–12.

Ulich, D. (1987). *Krise und Entwicklung*. Psychologie Verlagsunion, München.

WHO (1984). *Health promotion. A discussion document on the concept and principles*. World Health Organization, Regional Office for Europe, Copenhagen.

6D

Oral health promotion in the workplace

LONE SCHOU

Introduction

It has long been recognized that using the dental surgery as the only way to promote oral health among children is insufficient. The regular or irregular visit to the dentist has only a minor influence on children's dental health and dental health behaviour. Therefore, most dental health education efforts have concentrated on reaching children where they spend most time — in the family, at schools, or in nurseries or playgroups. However, when it comes to adults, the situation is quite different. Most oral health promotion efforts are concentrated on trying to get people to visit a dentist regularly. For many reasons, the payment system being the major one, these activities at the dentist's office are mainly orientated towards treatment of oral diseases rather than prevention of diseases or promotion of oral health. It thus seems appropriate to try to get out of the dental office and reach people where they are. Most adults spend about half of their waking life in a place of work. Here they are often surrounded by peers with whom they largely share norms and values and by whom they are often influenced. The workplace thus appears to be an obvious target for health promotion efforts. In this chapter the many advantages of using the workplace as a setting for oral health promotion are illustrated by using existing literature on general health, as well as specific oral health programmes.

General health promotion programmes in the workplace

During the last decade an increasing number of general health promotion programmes have been organized in various workplace settings (Shain *et al.* 1987; Weinstein 1983; Yenney 1984*a*, 1984*b*; ODPHP 1986; Sloan *et al.* 1987). The majority of these programmes have concentrated on either broad concepts such as wellness, quality of life, or fitness, or they have focused on more specific topics such as hypertension, stress, weight control, smoking or alcohol use. A recent review of potentials and pitfalls of work site health promotion stated that work sites are potentially the single most accessible and efficient site for reaching adults for health education (Conrad 1987). Rather promising results have been achieved. For instance, a workplace smoking programme demonstrated an overall quit rate of 21 per cent over 20 months which is markedly higher than the expected population quite rate of 2 – 5 per cent per year (Sorensen *et al.* 1991). Another workplace health promotion programme showed a 47.5 per cent decline in hourly employee absenteeism over six years (Bertera 1990*a*).

Comprehensive workplace health promotion programmes can not only produce a reduced number of disability days but also provide a good return on investment. Bertera (1990*b*) thus showed a $2.05 return for every dollar invested in a comprehensive programme in a large, multilocation, diversified industrial company.

Dooner (1990) summarizes the many good reasons why action should be taken to improve workplace health and highlights the factors that make the workplace in Canada a good site for promoting health:

1. Canadians spend approximately 60 per cent of their waking hours at work.

2. A range of occupational hazards endanger worker health and safety.

3. Persistent workplace stress erodes individual and organizational self-efficacy, and can lead to illness, accidents, and unhealthy lifestyle practices.

4. Workplace policies, rules, and regulations can effect employee health.

5. The workplace provides opportunities to level the 'health playing-field' by addressing socioeconomic inequalities in employees' health status.

6. Short and long-term benefits can be derived from workplace health programmes, for example lower rates of absenteeism, reduced health care costs, and increased morale.

7. Most employees (69 per cent) consider the workplace to be an appropriate site for promoting good health (Canada's Health Promotion Survey).

8. Workplace health programmes tend to have higher participation rates than health programmes offered at other sites.

These reasons are obviously not specifically related to an oral health promotion programme. Only a limited number of programmes have reported an oral component or focused specifically on oral health. Using merely empirical data from actual dental programmes would thus be rather limited. Instead, and more appropriately, the potential benefits will be analysed from the point of view of the main involved parties: the management, the dental profession, and, not least, the employees (the patients).

The management perspective

When confronted with new suggestions the main concern of any management or organization is related to cost–benefit aspects.

Regarding cost, national differences in financing health care are of importance. Unlike European and Canadian organizations which function in an environment of nationalized health care, American organizations have much greater responsibilities for direct payment for health care costs. Consequently a major motivating factor for development of workplace health promotion programmes in the United States has been companies' interest in reducing their high health care cost (Sloan 1987; Bly *et al.* 1986).

However, apart from savings on direct health care costs (described in relation to dentistry by Spencer and Wright (1985)) the main argument for oral health promotion programmes (OHP programmes) from the employers' point of view lies in the broad consideration of increased productivity and reduced absenteeism.

If we want to persuade employers to adopt and implement healthy policies, data which relate oral health to productivity and absenteeism are needed. Although the dental profession in the past has provided numerous data on dental health, these might have been of more use to the profession than they have been for policy makers.

One of the few studies of dental health and public policy (Reisine 1985) concluded:

... traditional measures of oral health status — such as decayed, missing and filled teeth and the periodontal index — should be linked to measures of social outcome in order to place dental conditions within the broader context of health status in terms that are relevant to policy makers.

Measures of social function rather than traditional measures of oral health are far more relevant as health indicators, particularly when attempting to promote oral health through the workplace. Disability days or work loss due to dental problems are more effective arguments for decision and policy makers because of cost implications.

It has been estimated that up to 12 million working days may be lost in the United Kingdom through dental causes each year (Feaver 1988). In 1979, acute dental conditions in the United States as a whole resulted in 6.1 million days of work loss or 0.06 days per employed adult (Bailit *et al.* 1982). This estimate includes only work loss of four or more hours' duration and is, therefore, mainly a measure of 'serious' health problems — preventive or curative visits were not included. In this context Cohen (1985) stated 'Further examination of specific workplaces in local United States areas suggests that the national study had seriously underestimated the problem. Anywhere from 15–56 per cent of adults reported taking time off from work because of dental visits.' Thus, apart from the employees' possible benefits, it is evident that productivity could be increased simply by reducing the amount of work loss due to dental visits outside the workplace. In a state-of-the-art report on the relationship between dental diseases and work loss (Bailit *et al.* 1982), it was concluded that the primary factors associated with people taking time off from work to visit the dentists were their oral health status, the cost of work loss to them and their employers, and access to dental care.

The same report also indicated that the use of preventive services and good oral health were negatively associated with work loss. In other words, an effective preventive workplace programme has the potential, without including any treatment services, of reducing the amount of work loss.

This potential was utilized in the Johnson and Johnson dental programme. The programme separates 'well care' given at the corporate site from 'treatment' provided by private sector practitioners. Recognizing that the most common reason for not seeing a dentist has been identified as lack of perceived need, the approach was to divide the employees into two groups. A nucleus of employees, viewed as a core group of enthusiasts, registered for the programme believing they had need. It was assumed that the remainder would register later as a result of positive feedback from the initial users of the programme. These assumptions were correct. At the time of reporting approximately two-thirds of the employees and their families were registered (Meadow and Rosenthal 1983). Only patients who had been in the programme for at least one year were included in the evaluation. All health indicators showed statistically significant changes during the one-year period. Of those patients requiring dental treatment, 73 per cent received the needed dental care within the first year of the preventive programme. Dental insurance record data revealed that the programme participants obtained 35 per cent more dental care than the average for all Johnson and Johnson employees.

The separation of treatment and preventive services also overcomes another hesitation possibly arriving from employers. Hicks (1985) argues that companies which set up new schemes of health care are liable to run into considerable problems with a backlog of untreated morbidity and that the worker newly improved to base levels of dental health is all too likely to move on, taking his newly refurbished mouth to another employer who has not invested capital in the refurbishing. However, if the workplace dental programmes refer all treatment to general dental practice the employer's cost of treatment will not be an issue.

The dental profession's point of view

Utilization of dental services has recently attracted the attention of the dental profession in many countries.

Numerous reviews have identified variables related to utilization and also shown that a high proportion of the population is not utilizing the dental service (Gift 1985). Among the most common variables reported to be associated with dental utilization are age, sex, race, income, education, and region of the country. Although no other category of variables has been employed to the extent of demographics, it is seen that economic variables, personal and psychological background variables, and variables related to the structural characteristics of the delivery system are also associated with utilization of dental services. At present no conclusive evidence exists showing that the workplace as a setting for oral health promotion will increase utilization, but it seems clear there is a great potential. In particular, the reasons which people give for not going to a dentist lend themselves to optimism with regard to the workplace. Among the eight most mentioned reasons were: access problems, lack of knowledge about the system (such as not knowing a dentist), and problems related to work (such as losing wages). All these reasons could be overcome by having the dental service at the place of work.

Most existing delivery systems for adults have hitherto been restrained by the payment system and the physical environment in which dental services have been delivered. The fee-per-item payment system usually includes fees for fillings, extractions, and other treatments but rarely fees for preventive or health promotion activities. Dentists employed in industry are usually salaried and therefore do not rely upon fee-per-item.

Traditional dental offices have an operating chair taking up most of the room space. Industrial dentists have the possibility of creating a more stimulating place for individual or group preventive activities. Indeed, many periodontal epidemiological studies (Bellini and Gjermo 1973; Markkanen 1978; Lie *et al.* 1988), and in particular studies of the effect of oral hygiene instruction and preventive periodontic procedures, have been carried out in workplace settings (Lightner *et al.* 1968; Suomi *et al.* 1971; Lightner *et al.* 1971; Tribhawan *et al.* 1975; Tan and Saxton 1978; Tan 1979; Hetland *et al.* 1981).

Every developed country has, by now, some form of dental health service and therefore all dental programmes in workplace settings are offered either as an addition, or an alternative, to that existing service. Hence, it could be perceived by the dental profession as a competitive factor. Cohen (1985) reported, in relation to a major American project, that although the programme met initial resistance from the private sector, dentists accepted the programme because of the demand generated at the worksite and further stated 'acceptance by the profession is no longer an issue'.

Instead of obstructing, members of the dental profession should act as advocates for oral health promotion in the workplace as well as in other settings. Indeed, many enthusiastic members of the profession have done so, but health promotion is not just the responsibility of the health sector. It demands coordinated action by all concerned: by governments, by health and other social and economic sectors, by non-governmental and voluntary organizations, by local authorities, by industry, and by the media. If the dental profession want to be advocates, they will need to adopt a very different role from the one they are used to.

Employees' point of view

The immediate advantages from the employees' point of view are reduced
travel time and waiting time, easy access, and possible reduction in loss of
wages. People who do not normally visit a dentist regularly, might for these
reasons become regular attenders. There is a potential for reaching and motivating people who normally have a low dental health awareness and whose
behaviour would otherwise lead to oral problems rather than good oral
health.

A further reason for a dental occupational health service is the consideration that some workers are exposed to additional dental hazards by the
nature of their work in industry. It has been argued (Conrad 1987) that the
promulgators of health promotion with respect to 'wellness' are uninterested
in the traditional concerns of occupational health and safety and turn their
attention from the environment to the individual.

In one of the few existing overviews of dental care in industrial settings,
Ayer *et al.* (1987) concluded that programmes in the US were initially
concerned with work-related injuries, then shifted to more comprehensive
non-work-related treatment, and finally, in the 1970s, to some preventive
efforts. This development does not seem to have happened in other
countries. Most of the available literature related to the workplace, from the
Soviet Bloc countries, is still mainly concerned with the effect of the working
environment on dental health (Rode and Vrobosek 1972; Ilewicz *et al.*
1978; Fahmy 1978; Kurnatowska and Pawlicka 1979; Kimak 1979;
Remijn *et al.* 1982; Borysewicz-Lewicka and Kobylanska 1983). Also,
studies from Scandinavia are at present concerned with dentally related
health hazards. An example is the recent change in Danish legislative
regulations which allows economic compensation for dental diseases caused
by the working environment (Petersen 1987). This regulative change
occurred partly on the basis of dental research among confectionery
industry workers, which showed that they were at risk of work-related
dental hazards (Petersen 1983).

However, avoidance of dental hazards is preferable to economic compensation. At the workplace, special measures can easily be instituted for high
risk groups such as food tasters and confectionery workers (Feaver 1988).
Ideally, the prevention of occupational diseases should imply modification of
the working environment.

Finally, screening services can be provided which benefit people such as
denture wearers who normally would not seek a dental opinion. This would
also give them an opportunity to benefit from the early diagnosis of oral
pathological conditions or oral manifestations of systemic diseases.

Examples of oral health promotion programmes in the workplace

Some examples of workplace based programmes will be presented to give an indication on what types of programmes have been evaluated so far, and with what results. Table 6.5 shows a selection of different programmes from various countries.

A workplace project in the USA involved a total of six companies. Traditional dental health education as well as a mass media approach were used at weekly sessions over an eight-week period. Efforts were made to determine the needs of the blue-collar workers and to respond to them, rather than inflict on them a programme that might be inappropriate. Preliminary findings showed that 74 per cent of the participants found the programme extremely useful, particularly the dental screening examinations.

Company team members and the investigators reviewed employee survey comments, on-site employee responses, management needs, and baseline data to plan the second phase of the intervention strategy. Among the findings were: timing recommendations; problems with video players and cassettes; and posters, pamphlets, and brochures were too numerous and distributed to everybody rather than only the ones who were interested in a particular topic.

At the time of reporting no data on changes in dental diseases or self-care activities were available. However, the investigators recommend that combining mass screening examinations with the availability of company resource teams, as well as appropriate educational materials, may be the most effective plan (Ayer *et al.* 1984).

Several programmes have been reported from Sweden. The result of a programme including restorative as well as preventive care in a shipyard showed: improved standard of oral hygiene; reduced amount of calculus and overhanging restorations; arrested loss of previously progressive periodontal bone loss; decrease in the need for treatment; and decreased rate of tooth mortality. The author concluded that 'improved dental health can be achieved by a dental care programme with a preventive emphasis provided to individuals under routine care. The major part of the preventive care can be delivered by dental auxilaries.' (Soderholm 1979). In addition he stated 'One of the advantages of a dental clinic within an industrial estate is that individuals previously being sporadic dental visitors could be recruited to a maintenance programme with frequent recalls' and 'fee per item may be one of the factors impeding a preventive type of care'.

Dental health behaviour and attitudes towards dental health care were studied among 500 adults with and without dental services in the work-place (Rickardsson and Soderholm, 1986). In the group of unskilled workers who

Table 6.5 Examples of oral health promotion programmes in the workplace

Author (year), country	Workplace	Programme	Results	Conclusion
Ayer et al. (1984), USA	Blue-collar workers in six companies	Needs-orientated 8-weekly sessions and use of mass media	74% found the programme extremely useful	Recommendations of mass screening examinations combined with company resource teams and appropriate education materials
Soderholm (1979), Sweden	Shipyard employees	Restorative and preventive care	Improved oral hygiene, arrest of progressive bone loss, decreased need for treatment, decreased rate of tooth mortality	Improved dental health can be achieved with a dental care programme with preventive emphasis. The major part of the programme can be delivered by dental auxillaries.
Rickardsson and Soderholm (1986), Sweden	Unskilled workers	Dental health services with preventive perspective	Higher proportion of regular attenders. Employees' appreciation due to reduced travel time, being called automatically, and preventive perspective	With workplace programmes it is possible to reach groups of people who normally have no, or only sporadic, contact with the dental service. More cost-effective than general dental service provided in the same area
Lindeborg (1975) Sweden	Car industry	Information meetings distribution of material, film-showing exhibition. Employees actively involved in running the campaign	Improved oral health attitudes, oral hygiene and gingival health	Programme recommended in other companies
Hager and Krasse (1983), Sweden	Insurance company	18 of 507 employees trained as dental health educators, informing fellow	Employees positive and claiming to have reduced sucrose intake. Reduction in lactobacilli. Raised	This type of programme recommended for use in other health areas

		workers in groups on prevention	level of knowledge		
Hiraiwa et al. (1986), Japan	Department workers	Intra-oral brushing instruction	Improved oral hygiene and gingival health		The intra-oral brushing instruction recommended for dental public health programmes
Schou (1985), Schou & Monrad (1989), Denmark	Unskilled workers in factory	Monthly group discussions among peers over 6 months at the place of work in working hours. Active involvement of participants	Increased knowledge. More positive attitudes. Improved plaque and gingival health $3\frac{1}{2}$ years after termination of programme		Reinforcement, active involvement, use of peer groups, and programme being carried out at place of work in working hours are the determinants of success
Petersen (1989), Denmark	Chocolate workers	Active involvement, health education plus clinical prophylaxis	Improved behaviour and dental health		Reinforcement, active involvement, regular preventive visits important determinants
Masalin (1988), Finland	Sweet and bakery industry	Xylitol-containing products provided at workplace free of charge	86% reported daily use. Positive attitudes. Increased salivary flowrate and buffer capacity. Number of people at risk decreased		Other measures also needed. Use of xylitol not recommended as single activity but as part of an oral health promotion programme
Towner (1988), United Kingdom	Wide range of workplaces: food and pharmaceutical companies, tyre manufacturers, chain stores, general hospital	Co-work between occupational health dept, personnel dept, community dental service and employees. A flexible package allows four levels: an awareness campaign, screening, personal advice session, and behaviour change support system	Formative evaluation showing that the programme was acceptable and could be used in a wide range of workplaces		Possible to involve employees in planning and running campaign. Materials acceptable to the majority. Competition and incentives important. Organizations and companies willing to provide time and money. Campaign can be starting point for other health activities

had dental services at their place of work, 86 per cent were regular attenders whereas in a similar group without workplace dental services only 63 per cent were regular attenders. The patients' reasons for appreciating work-based dental services were: reduced travel time, being called at regular intervals, and that the service had a preventive perspective. It was concluded that with oral health programmes in the workplace it is possible to reach groups of people who normally have no or only sporadic contact with the service and also that it was possible to run it more cost-effectively than the general dental service provided in the same area.

Improved dental health attitudes, oral hygiene and gingival health were reported after an information campaign in a Swedish car-industry (Lindeborg 1975). The campaign included information meetings, distribution of leaflets, film-shows, and a dental health exhibition. A subsample of the employees were actively involved in the running of the campaign.

'Barefoot doctors' were used for dental health education in a Swedish insurance company (Hager and Krasse 1983). Eighteen of the 507 employees were trained as dental health educators. They then informed their fellow workers about prevention of caries and periodontal disease in groups of ten persons. Two information meetings were held. Eighty-nine per cent of the employees were positive about this educational programme. Twenty-two per cent said that they had reduced their intake of sucrose after the first meeting. Even more people reduced their sucrose intake later. Saliva secretion rate and buffer capasity were analysed; a significant reduction in the number of lactobacilli was found, confirming the change in sugar intake. The information raised the level of knowledge about dental health among the employees. It was suggested that this type of educational programme should be used in other health areas.

The effect of toothbrushing instruction among department workers was studied in a small Japanese survey (Hiraiwa et al. 1986). Among the subjects who followed the instructions, oral hygiene and gingival health was improved at the one-year follow-up. The intra-oral brushing instruction used in the survey was recommended for dental public health programmes.

A dental health education programme including discussions in peer groups among unskilled workers in a Danish company showed a long-term effect. Increased knowledge, more positive attitudes, and better oral health measured by levels of plaque and gingivitis was recorded three-and-a-half years after the termination of the programme. The reason for the long-term effect was the use of the principle of active involvement of the participants in the programme (Schou 1985).

Active participation was obtained by various means;

1. Teaching was carried out in pre-existing peer groups.

2. The participants' own goals and needs were included.

3. The traditional dentist–patient barriers were excluded.

4. The traditional dentist–patient roles were changed.

5. The sessions were repeated.

In a follow-up survey (Schou and Monrad 1989) a selection of the participants were interviewed. There was a strong agreement between the investigators' suggested active-involvement principle and the participants' own expressions of the reasons for the behavioural changes. The most important single factors stated three-and-a-half years after the termination of the programme were:

(1) the programme carried out in working hours at the place of work;

(2) peer-groups;

(3) the feeling that they had a voice in deciding the content of the programme.

Another Danish study among chocolate workers, which included clinical prophylaxis as well as health education based on active involvement, was evaluated after two years. The results showed improvements of dental health and reported dental health behaviour. It was concluded that the reinforcement strategy, the active involvement of participants and opinion leaders, as well as the regular preventive visits including fluoride applications, should be considered very important determinants (Petersen 1989).

A Finnish programme (Masalin 1988) provided xylitol-containing products in the sweet and bakery industry. The employees showed rather positive attitudes and as many as 86 per cent reported daily use. A clinical examination showed increased salivary flow rate and improved buffer capacity. Although the programme achieved its aim of decreasing the number of people at high risk, it was concluded that the use of xylitol should not be recommended as a single activity but as part of an oral health promotion programme.

In the UK a flexible oral health promotion programme for adults has been developed to be used in a wide range of workplaces (Towner 1988). The programme consists of a package which can be used at various levels depending on the company involved. The levels include: an awareness campaign, screening, personal advice session and a behavioural change support system. At the time of writing only formative evaluations have been reported. This showed that the programmes were acceptable to all involved parties in a wide range of UK workplaces. The author concludes that it is possible to involve employees in planning and running a campaign. Most organisations and companies were willing to provide time and money.

Theoretical considerations

It could be argued that many of these OHP programmes are missing a sound theoretical base. Indeed, most of the dental programmes could be described as 'trial and error' attempts rather than interventions built on principles from existing theories. Perhaps future dental programmes could benefit from 'borrowing' elements or principles from theories used in general health programmes. Sorensen *et al.* (1990) describes an intervention model (The Treatwell Program) for promoting healthy eating patterns in the work site. The key elements in the model which could most easily be adopted to dental programmes include:

(1) adaptation of an intervention model to the work site based on knowledge of the work site, its organization and norms, and the potential barriers to intervention that exist at the worksite (Orlandi 1986);

(2) worker and management participation at the earliest phases of planning and implemention to facilitate the programme to the work site and eventual incorporation of programmes into existing structures (Farquhar *et al.* 1984);

(3) work site 'ownership' in which the work site is involved in the planning process, sets priorities about intervention activities, and is part of the decision-making and implementation process (Carlaw *et al.* 1984);

(4) integrating multiple channels of influence to target individuals at different risk levels (Farquhar *et al.* 1984), at varying stages of readiness for change (Abrams *et al.* 1986), and occupying differing target market segments (Lefebre and Flora 1988);

(5) incorporating intervention efforts into existing social structures and places frequently used by the target audience, such as cafeterias (Lafebre and Flora 1988).

(6) emphasis on social support and peer group influences to promote behaviour change throughout all levels of intervention (Syme and Alcalay 1982);

(7) opinion leaders and early adopters of behaviour change serving as role models and initiators in the process of diffusion of health behaviour changes (Rogers 1983; Orlandi 1986);

(8) enhanced adult learning through motivation, shared responsibility, active participation, and experiential learning (Knowles 1978);

(9) environmental changes to increase the ease of behaviour change and support its maintenance (Glanz and Mullis 1988; Mayer *et al.* 1989).

These key elements were integrated in the theoretical model show in Fig. 6.5 which incorporates three overall components of the Treatwell Program: the organization and mobilization of employees to plan, promote, and implement interventions; the focus of the intervention programme on both individual behaviour change and change in environmental structures that

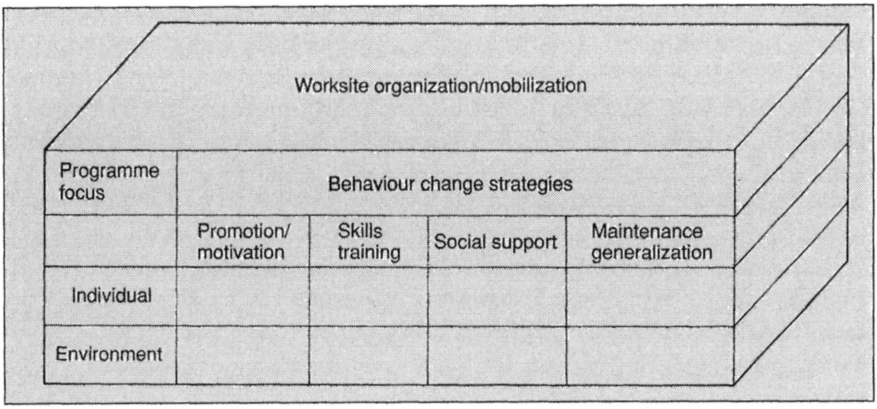

The figure shows a three-dimensional box model with the following labelled cells:

Worksite organization/mobilization			
Programme focus	Behaviour change strategies		
	Promotion/ motivation	Skills training	Social support	Maintenance generalization
Individual			
Environment			

Fig. 6.5   The theoretical model for the Treatwell programme (from Sorensen *et al.* 1990).

support healthy dietary behaviour; and the use of a variety of the behaviour change strategies.

The intervention model incorporated principles from theories of community organization (Bracht 1990), social learning (Bandura 1986), diffusion of innovations (Rogers 1983), and adult learning (Knowles 1978).

The Treatwell intervention model is but one example of how workplace programmes can be theoretically based. This particular model may not be ideal for dental programmes but at least it is hoped that it can inspire future dental researchers or initiators of programmes to go beyond the 'trial and error' attempts.

Conclusion

The workplace as a setting for oral health promotion is a novelty without history or tradition. Although many general health promotion programmes have been workplace based, only few include or focus specifically on oral health. It should be remembered in this context, that all health promotion activities are still in their infancy despite the increased attention and importance paid to them in both developed and developing countries around the world. Perhaps other areas of health or other settings for promotion have had higher priorities hitherto among policy makers, administrators, or the general public. Nevertheless, the present review of the literature points to numerous potential benefits. The main arguments from the employers' point of view are increased productivity and reduced absenteeism, reduced health care costs (mainly the USA), and perhaps a more satisfied workforce. The benefits to the dental profession are a possible increase in utilization and less restraint from payment structure and physical environment. The immediate benefit to the employees is easy access to the dental service. In addition, work-related dental hazards can be compensated for or prevented, and screening activities can be more easily organized. Although the literature is at present scattered and programmes may not be suitable at all types of workplaces it appears as if the workplace is a vastly underused area for oral health promotion for adults. In addition a 'spillover' effect to the home environment is possible. Several authors have claimed that 'money spent is an investment' and 'organizations can ill afford *not* to be involved'.

However, somebody needs to take the initiative and try and make workplace programmes part of future oral health policy. The dental profession is, to a certain extent, responsible for public oral health development. Perhaps we could take the advocacy role in this new area.

References

Abram, D. B., Elder, J. P., Carleton, R. A., Lasater, T. M., and Artz, L. M. (1986). Social learning principles for organizational health promotion: an integrated approach. In *Health and industry: a behavioral medicine perspective*, (ed. M. F. Cataldo and T. J. Coates), pp. 28–51. Wiley, New York.

Ayer, W. A., Seffrin, S., Davis, D., Deatrick, D., and Wirthman, G. (1984). *Dental health promotion in workplace settings. Progress report and final report to the American found for dental health*, pp. 1–174. American Dental Association, Chicago, Illinois.

Ayer, W. A., Seffrin, S., Wirthman, G., Deatrick, D., and Davis, D. (1987). Dental health promotion in the workplace. In *Health and industry. A behavioral medicine perspective*, (ed. M. F. Cataldo and T. J. Coates), pp. 255–69. Wiley, New York.

Bailit, H. L., Beazoglou, T., Hoffman, W., Reisine, S., and Strumwasser, I. (1982). *Work loss and dental disease*. Report to the Robert Wood Johnson Foundation. University of Connecticut Health Center.

Bandura, A. (1986). *Social foundations of thought and action: a social cognitive theory*. Prentice Hall, Englewood Cliffs, NJ.

Bellini, H. T. and Gjermo, P. (1973). Application of the periodontal treatment need system (PTNS) in a group of Norwegian industrial employees. *Community Dentistry and Oral Epidemiology*, **1**, 22–9.

Bertera, R. L. (1990a). Planning and implementing health promotion in the workplace: a care study of the Du Pont Company experience. *Health Education Quarterly*, **17**, 307–27.

Bertera, R. L. (1990b). The effects of workplace health promotion on absenteeism and employment costs in a large industrial population. *American Journal of Public Health*, **80**, 1101–5.

Bly, J. A., Jones, R. C., and Richardson, J. E. (1986). Impact of worksite health promotion on health care costs and utilization. *Journal of American Medical Association*, **256**, 3235–40.

Borysewicz-Lewicka, M. and Kobylanska, M. (1983). Periodontal disease, oral hygiene and fluoride content of dental deposits in aluminium workers. *Fluoride Quarterly Report*, **16**, 5–10.

Bracht, N. F. (ed.) (1990). *Organizing for community health promotion: a guide*. Sage Publications, Newbury Park.

Carlaw, R., Mittlemark, M., Bracht, N., and Luepker, R. (1984). Organization for a community cardiovascular health program: experiences from the Minnesota Heart Health Program. *Health Education Quarterly*, **11**, 243–52.

Cohen, L. K. (1985). Market and community responses to changing demands from the workplace. In *Dentistry and the workplace: proceedings of a conference, Melbourne Victoria*, (ed. J. Spencer and C. Wright), Suppl. *Community Health Study*, **IX 1**, pp. 18s–24s.

Conrad, P. (1987). Wellness in the work place: potentials and pitfalls of work-site health promotion. *Millbank Quarterly*, **65**, 225–75.

Dooner, B. (1990). Achieving a healthier workplace. Organisational action for individual health. *Health Promotion*, Winter 1990/1991, 2–6.

Fahmy, M. S. (1978). Oral and dental affections in mercury-exposed workers. *Community Dentistry and Oral Epidemiology*, **6**, 161–65.

Farquhar, J. W., Fortmann, S. P., Massoby, N., *et al.* (1984). The Stanford Five City Project: an overview. In *Behavior health: a handbook of health enhancement and disease prevention*, (ed. J. D. Matrazzo, S. M. Weiss, J. A. Herd, and N. E. Miller), pp. 1154–65. Wiley, New York.

Feaver, G. P. (1988). Occupational dentistry: A review of 100 years of dental care in the workplace. *Journal of Social and Occupational Medicine*, **38**, 41–3.

Gift, H. C. (1985). Utilization of professionel dental services. In *Social Sciences and Dentistry. A critical bibliography*, Vol. II, (ed L. K. Cohen and P. S. Bryant), pp. 202–66. Quintessence Publishing Company Ltd, London.

Glanz, K. and Mullis, R. M. (1988). Environmental interventions to promote healthy eating: a review of models, programs and evidence. *Health Education Quarterly*, **15**, 395–415.

Hager, B. and Krasse, B (1983). Dental health education by 'barefoot doctors', *Community Dentistry and Oral Epidemiology*, **11**, 333–6

Hetland, L., Midtun, N., and Kristoffersen, T. (1981). Effect of oral hygiene instructions given by paraprofessional personnel. *Community Dentistry and Oral Epidemiology*, **10**, 8–14.

Hicks, N. (1985), Unions, employers and health services. In *Dentistry and the workplace: proceedings of a conference*, (ed. J. Spencer and C. Wright) Supplement to *Community Health Studies*, IX, **1**, pp. 5s–10s.

Hiraiwa, H., Tsurumi, M., Morita, M., Sakata, M., Kishimoto, E., and Watanabe, T. (1986). The effect of tooth brushing instruction on department workers. *Nippon Shishubyo Gakkai Kaishi*, **28**, 670–80.

Ilewicz, L., Waszkiewicz-Golos, H., Szczucka, Z., Mniszek, M., Klimkiewicz, K., Zubek, G., *et al.* (1978). The condition of parodontium and oral mucosa in workers of the casting division of the mining machinery factory in Zabrze. *Czasopismo Stomatologiczne*, **31**, 1125–30.

Kimak, A. (1979). The effect of working environment on the condition of the parodontium in workers from a glass plant. *Czasopismo Stomatologiczne*, **32**, 113–16.

Knowles, M. (1978). *The adult learner: a neglected species*. Gulf Publishing Company, Houston.

Kurnatowska, A. and Pawlicka, H. (1979). Incidence of dental caries and parodontal disease in workers of the optima candy factory. *Czasopismo Stomatologiczne*, **32**, 757–62.

Lefebre, R. C. and Flora, J. A. (1988). Social marketing and public health intervention. *Health Education Quarterly*, **15**, 299–315.

Lie, T., Due, N. -A., Abrahamsen, B., and Boe, O. E. (1988). Periodontal health in a group of industrial employees. *Community Dentistry and Oral Epidemiology*, **16**, 42–6.

Lightner, L. M., O'Leary, T. J., and Jividen, G. J. (1968). Preventive periodontic treatment procedures: results after one year. *Journal of American Dental Association*, **76**, 1043–46.

Lightner, L. M., O'Leary, T. J., Drake, R. B., Crump, P. P., and Allen, M. F. (1971), Preventive periodontic treatment procedures: results over 46 months. *Journal of Periodontology*, **42**, 555–61.

Lindeborg, P. (1975). Effekten av tandhalsoupplysning vid en svensk industri. *Tandlakartidningen*, **67**, 745–53.

Markkanen, H. (1978). Periodontal treatment need in a Finnish industrial population. *Community Dentistry and Oral Epidemiology*, **6**, 240–4.

Masalin, K. (1988). Finnish examples of oral health promotion in the workplace. In *Oral health promotion in the workplace*, (ed L. Schou). pp. 32–44. Scottish Health Education Group, Edinburgh.

Mayer, J. A., Dubbert, P. M., and Elder, J. P. (1989). Promoting nutrition at the point of choice: a review. *Health Education Quarterly*, **16**, 31–43.

Meadow, D. and Rosenthal, M. (1983). A corporation-based computerized preventive dentistry program. *Journal of American Dental Association*, **106**, 467–70.

(Office of Disease Prevention and Health Promotion, U. S. Public Health Service, Department of health and Human Services) (1986). Worksite health promotion: a bibliography of selected resources. ODPHP, Washington.

Orlandi, M. A. (1986). The diffusion and adoption of worksite health promotion innovations: an analysis of barriers. *Preventive Medicine*, **15**, 522–36.

Petersen, P. E. (1983). Dental health among workers at a Danish chocolate factory. *Community Dentistry and Oral Epidemiology*, **11**, 337–41.

Petersen, P. E. (1987). Erhvervssygdomme og loven om arbejdsskade-forsikring. *Tandlagebladet*, **91**, 91–4.

Petersen, P. E. (1989). Evaluation af a dental preventive program for Danish chocolate workers. *Community Dentistry and Oral Epidemiology*, **17**, 53–9.

Reisine, S. (1985), Dental health and public policy: The social impact of dental disease. *American Journal of Public Health*, **75**, 27–30.

Remijn, B., Koster, P., Houthuijs, D., Boleij, J., Willems, H., Brunekreef, B., *et al.* (1982). Zinc chloride, zinc oxide, hydrochloric acid exposure and dental erosion in a zinc galvanizing plant in the Netherlands. *Annals of Occupational Hygiene*, **25**, 299–307.

Rickardsson, B. and Soderholm, G. (1986). Tandvardsvanor och attityder till tandvard hos anstallda med och utan foretagstandvard. *Socialmedicinsk tidskrift*, **3**, 112–116.

Rode, M. and Vrbosek, J. (1972). Influence of the working milieu on the changes of soft and hard tissues in the mouth cavity of the workers in factory 'Saturnus'. *Zobozdravstveni Vestnik*, **27**, 167–176.

Rogers, E. M. (1983). *Diffusion of innovations*, 3rd edn. The Free Press. New York.

Schou, L. (1985). Active-involvement principle in dental health education. *Community Dentistry and Oral Epidemiology*, **13**, 128–32.

Schou, L. and Monrad, A. (1989). A follow-up study of dental patient education in the workplace: participants' opinions. *Patient Education and Counselling*, **14**, 45–51.

Shain, M., Suurvali, H., and Boutilier, M. (1987). *Healthier workers. Health promotion and employee assistance programs.* Lexington Books, Toronto.

Sloan, R. P. (1987). Workplace health promotion: the North American experience. In *Health promotion in the workplace,* (ed. H. Matheson), pp. 8–13, Scottish Health Education Group, Edinburgh.

Sloan, R. P. Gruman, J. C., and Allegrante, J. P. (1987). *Investing in employee health. A guide to effective health promotion in the workplace.* Jossey-Bass Publishers, San Francisco.

Soderholm, G. (1979). Effect of a dental care program on dental health conditions. A study of employees of a Swedish shipyard. Thesis, pp. 1–94. Department of Periodontology, University of Lund, Malmo Sweden.

Sorensen, G., Hunt, M. K., Morris, D. H., Donnelly, G., Freeman, L., Ratcliffe, B. J., *et al.* (1990). Promoting healthy eating patterns in the worksite: the Treatwell intervention model. *Health Education Research,* **5**, 505–15.

Sorensen, G., Rigotti, N., Rosen, a., Pinney, J., and Prible, R. (1991). Effects of a worksite non-smoking policy: evidence for increased cessation. *Americal Journal of Public Health,* **81**, 202–4.

Spencer, J. and Wright, J. (1985). Dentistry and the workplace. Proceedings of a conference, Supplement to *Community Health Studies* IX **1**, pp. 1s–38s.

Suomi, J. D., Greene, J. C., Vermillion, J. R., Doyle, J., Chang, J. J., and Leatherwood, E. C. (1971). The effect of controlled oral hygiene procedures on the progression of periodontal disease in adults: Results after third and final year. *Journal of Periodontology,* **42**, 152–160

Syme, S. L. and Alcalay, R. (1982). Control of cigarette smoking from a social perspective. In *Annual review of public health* (ed. L. Breslow, J. E. Fielding, and L. B. Lavel, pp. 179–99. Annual Reviews Palo Alto, **3**.

Tan, H. H. and Saxton, C. A. (1978). Effect of a single dental health care instruction and prophylaxis on gingivitis. *Community Dentistry and Oral Epidemiology,* **6**, 172–5.

Tan, H. H. (1979). Effect of dental health care instruction and prophylaxis on knowledge, attitude and behavior in Dutch military personnel. *Community Dentistry and Oral Epidemiology,* **7**, 252–8.

Towner, E. (1988). 'Brush up your smile'. A UK workplace dental health education programme. In *Oral health promotion in the workplace,* (ed. L Schou), pp.61–72. Scottish Health Education Group, Edinburgh.

Tribhawan, N. C., Nanda, R. S., and Kapoor, K. K. (1975). Dental prophylaxis procedures in control of periodontal disease in Lucknow (Rural) India. *Journal of Periodontology,* **46**, 498–503.

Weinstein, M. S. (1983). *Health promotion and lifestyle change in the workplace.* World Health Organization, Copenhagen, Denmark.

Yenney, S. L. (1984a). *Health promotion and business coalitions: current activities and prospects for the future.* Office of Disease Prevention and Health Promotion, Department of Health and Human Services, Washington.

Yenney, S. L. (1984b). *Small businesses and health promotion: the prospects look good.* Office of Disease Prevention and Health Promotion. U. S. Department of Health and Human Services, Washington.

6E

Oral health promotion in old age

H. Asuman Kiyak

Introduction

As the number of older adults increases in the world's population, and as many of these older people retain their natural teeth, oral health promotion becomes more important for maintaining their quality of life. In this chapter we will examine why oral health is an important concern for the older population and their care providers as well as for the health professionals who must treat them when oral conditions become unmanageable at home, and the methods and benefits of health promotion to maintain the older person's well-being. Throughout this chapter we will use a *systems perspective* to discuss the interaction of multiple individual and social systems in creating the need for and influencing the success of health promotion efforts. Age-related changes in the older person's organ systems interact with the individual's expectations about health and disease in old age; these changes in turn interact with society's willingness and ability to provide oral health services for older adults. These interactions influence health beliefs, behaviours and subsequently the oral health status of older adults.

An important objective of oral health promotion, as of any health promotion effort, is the enhancement of *quality of life*, defined here as the individual's feelings of being free of pain, experiencing healthy function in physical, social, and psychological domains, and maintaining a positive self-concept. Improvements in oral health status can influence some of these areas by reducing or even eliminating oral–facial pain, improving mastication, and thereby enhancing the quality of food ingested, digestion, communication (more specifically smiling and speaking), confidence in social situations, and of course freedom from disease. The importance of attractiveness as a motive for oral health maintenance in all ages is discussed by Gift in Chapter 3 of this volume and in an earlier book (Gift 1986). There is little research on the role of attractiveness in motivating older adults, but clinical evidence and preliminary data from a cross-cultural survey by the author suggests that, in most cultures, attractiveness is equivalent to or more important than mastication or freedom from pain as a reason for seeking dental services and maintaining one's oral health. Self-esteem has been found to be negatively correlated with poor oral health in non-institutionalized elderly (Berkey *et al.* 1985), although it is difficult to determine from such a correlational approach whether poor oral health lowers self-esteem or whether depression and its less severe manifestations result in poor self-maintenance and inattention to health in general. Some evidence for the former argument comes from studies by the author and colleagues in which self-esteem improved significantly following a successful oral health promotion effort in both institutionalized and non-institutionalized elderly (Kiyak and Mulligan 1987). These studies will be discussed in the last section of this chapter. Thus, we need to consider both motivational *contributors to* health as well as motivational *consequences of* health (McClelland 1989). This is because motivational contributors influence future disease states, whereas motivational consequences play a role in people's ability to recuperate from past diseases and their vulnerability for future diseases. Self-esteem, attractiveness, improved mastication and choice of diet, communication, and social acceptability can serve both as motivational contributors *and* consequences for oral health promotion efforts aimed at older adults.

In the next section of this chapter we will examine demographic patterns that make it imperative for developed countries to become more concerned about oral health promotion for older adults, as well as normal and pathological changes in physiological and cognitive functions with ageing that highlight the need to use a systems perspective in developing oral health promotion efforts with older persons. A further reason for examining age-related changes in physiological functions is to illustrate the value of reducing the impact and even the extent of decline through health promotion programmes aimed at improving exercise and nutrition.

Changing patterns of ageing

The demographic imperative of geriatric dental care

Perhaps the single most important reason for the increased interest in ageing is demographics. In 1900, people over 65 accounted for approximately four per cent of the population in the United States. By 1990, one in nine Americans, or 12.6 per cent, was 65 or older (US Bureau of the Census 1991). Growth patterns are even more dramatic in European countries. For example, in 1985 15 per cent of the population of Germany and the United Kingdom was age 65 or older. The median age of Europe is 40, compared with 32 in the United States (Rauch 1988). While high fertility and mortality rates in less developed regions of the world have kept the median age at about 20, these countries are expected to show an even greater *rate* of growth in their oldest population, from a current level of less than five per cent to 17 per cent by 2075. Indeed, by the year 2025, only 28 per cent of the world's elderly are expected to reside in industrialized nations, while 72 per cent will live in developing countries (United Nations Secretariat 1989).

As birth rates in industrialized countries fall below population replacement levels and the proportion of people living beyond age 75 increases, these countries will experience a growing demand on their social and health services for older persons. In the area of dental care the demands may be compounded by three factors: the increased number of people retaining most of their natural dentition in old age, as will be discussed in the third section of this chapter; changes in preventive dentistry attitudes from one of seeking dental care only for emergencies when the current cohort of elderly were children and young adults to the current emphasis on regular preventive visits; and changes in patterns of utilization of dental services, with a reduction in use in countries where dental care is an out-of-pocket expense, when the older person's financial resources diminish, and among those who cannot make the trip to a dental office. To the extent that older people in developing countries can be encouraged to maintain their personal oral hygiene and to seek preventive dental services, one can expect the use of more costly services for acute dental problems to decline.

Physiological ageing and medical conditions in the elderly

When asked to describe the physical aspects of ageing, most people think only of the visible signs such as greying hair, balding, wrinkled skin, and a slower walk or shuffling gait. Numerous other changes occur in all organ systems with ageing. Both the appearance and function of organ systems change with *senescence* or biological ageing. This is defined as the normal process of deterioration in all living organisms, resulting in a slowing down of many systems but not necessarily disease or death. A useful analogy of the ageing process is with a machine that gradually accumulates damage to its parts, some more than others, and eventually loses capacities in some functions that are accommodated by substituting functions and activities. For example, older people may alter their physical and social environment to reduce the demands placed on their remaining functional capacity. They may choose health care providers within walking distance rather than attempting to manipulate the local transportation system.

Such adaptive mechanisms may protect the older person's level of physical and social equilibrium but may also make it difficult to engage an older person in any form of health promotion effort that places demands on their learning and behavioural skills. Perhaps the most obvious change with ageing is in body composition, where the proportion of body weight contributed by water decreases by about six per cent; lean body mass is replaced by fat (in many older people it can double), and both extracellular and intracellular water is lost. There is a loss of elasticity and flexibility in muscles and decreased mass of bone, although recent studies of general health promotion with older adults have shown significant improvements in strength and bone mass following a regular programme of weight-bearing exercise.

Both *renal* and *bladder functions* decrease with ageing. Of all the organ systems, the kidneys show the greatest deterioration with ageing. There is a decrease in volume and weight, with a corresponding reduction in the total number of glomeruli by 30 per cent from age 30 to 65. This results in a significant reduction of renal blood flow (as much as 50 per cent), and impairs the older person's ability to metabolize many medications. These drugs remain active longer in the kidneys and may become more potent for older patients. Thus, the adage 'start low and go slow' is a crucial one for physicians and dentists prescribing medications for older persons. Sodium and acids are also not excreted efficiently by the ageing kidneys, contributing to problems with hyponatraemia and dehydration for older persons (Rockstein and Sussman 1979). Urinary function also decreases with age, due in general to a reduced capacity of the bladder and loss of efficiency in the muscles that control the bladder. As a result, urinary incontinence is common in the elderly, with at least 15 to 30 per cent of community dwelling older adults and at least half of those in nursing homes suffering from difficulties with bladder control. The problem may be aggravated by a stroke, dementia, or other diseases associated with the nervous system.

Changes in the *gastrointestinal system* are also observed in normal ageing. In particular, there is decreased contraction of the muscles of the oesophagus, slower opening of the sphincter into the stomach, and less secretion of digestive juices in the stomach, resulting often in atrophic gastritis; less efficient operation of the small and large intestines, and structural changes in the colon that often result in chronic constipation in many older persons.

The *normal* age-related declines in the structure and function of organ systems do not necessarily result in disease or death. Chronic disease represents the extreme of normal ageing. As Fig. 6.6 illustrates, chronic diseases begin in the middle years, with the incidence of these conditions increasing in old age. Thus, the pattern of diseases does not change but the proportion of people with each condition increases from age 45 to 65. In the US, more than 80 per cent of persons aged 65 and over have at least one chronic condition, with multiple conditions being common (National Center for Health Statistics 1987). The most frequently reported chronic conditions are *arthritis, hypertension, hearing impairment,* and *heart disease.* All of these, as well as others such as orthopaedic problems and cataracts, result in limitations in older persons' activities of daily living (ADLs). For example, an individual with arthritis and heart disease may have difficulty with mobility, self-care, and household maintenance. For this reason, oral hygiene may

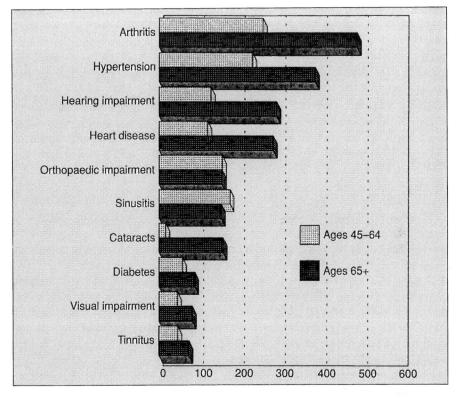

Fig. 6.6 Morbidity from the top ten chronic conditions, 1989 — rates per 1000 people (National Center for Health Statistics 1989).

suffer and regular dental visits may become burdensome for an older person with these chronic conditions.

The accumulation of long-term, degenerative diseases together with a declining immune system may also mean that an acute condition such as the flu may be devastating for an older person. With reduced resistance to disease, the older person may experience what has been described as a 'cascade of disasters', whereby a seemingly innocuous cold or flu virus can result in bronchitis, pneumonia, weight loss, dehydration, weakness, hospitalization, and its sequelae. It is not unusual for an older person to become institutionalized after a severe bout of the flu, or to remain bedridden for months following a case of pneumonia. It is therefore important to recognize that the boundary between health and disease is more blurred in elders than in the young.

Cognitive ageing

Cognitive functioning is comprised of three elements: learning, memory, and intelligence. The question of whether or not normal ageing results in decline or stability in these functions has long been explored in gerontology. It appears that ageing has no impact on our storage capacity for learning and retaining new information, but the problem may be due to inefficient mechanisms to store newly learned material and to retrieve information that has been stored in secondary or long-term memory. Time constraints are particularly detrimental to older learners. Psychomotor and sensory systems slow with ageing, resulting in *longer time to encode new information.* Yet, when given more time, more repetition of the new material, and presentation of it in multiple modes (for example the written word, illustrations, or an oral presentation), older learners do as well as younger persons. Educational level and verbal ability also can impair an older person's learning ability. Given that the current cohort of elders has less than a high school education, it is doubly important to assist them in the learning process. Pacing the information at a rate that is comfortable for older learners, giving them opportunities to practise this new knowledge (for example demonstrating flossing and brushing techniques, then asking *them* to perform this task immediately under the guidance of a health educator), can help older people to learn and retain this material longer.

Older persons learn more if the material to be learned is high in meaning and personal significance (Fozard 1980). Therefore it is imperative for the health promotion programme to emphasize the value of new health information and techniques for the older person's own quality of life; perhaps most important is the need to de-emphasize knowledge that is foreign to the individual's daily habits and to gradually introduce these behaviours. These include flossing for an older person who has never before flossed, and performing oral cancer self-exams for one who has never done so in the past *and* is at high risk for this disease.

Because of difficulties in the retrieval of information from secondary memory, it is useful to provide cues to aid this recall process: older people do worse in tests of recall than in those of recognition (Inman and Parkinson 1983). That is, asking an older person to write down all their medical conditions and medications may be risky, resulting in *errors of omission.* Instead, a recognition technique that lists the most common illnesses and types of medications, followed by a probing interview, is most likely to elicit correct responses. As with the process of learning new information, older people can recall old information if they are given more time and multiple cues to aid their recollection of stored material. These normal, age-related changes in learning and memory must be considered if health promotion efforts with older people are to be successful.

Why be concerned about older people's oral health?

Oral disease patterns in older people

As more and more people live beyond the age of 65, more of them are also retaining their teeth. In the 1985–6 NIDR National Survey of US Adults

(NIDR 1987), the age group under 29 had an average of 26.5 teeth, those aged 65–69 had 18.1, and those over the age of 80 had an average of 15.1 teeth remaining! This is an astounding number, especially for the oldest group, and raises the question of what the condition of these teeth might be. In this section we will examine further the results of US surveys that provide some indication of older people's oral health status. Note, however, that cross-national differences may exist and are not covered in this review. For example, the 1985–6 NIDR survey (NIDR 1987) also revealed that 41 per cent of people 65 and older were edentulous, compared to 45.5 per cent in 1971. The only cross-national comparisons available are for the 1971 survey, when 82.6 per cent of elderly were edentulous in the Netherlands and 74 per cent in the United Kingdom. Unless significant gains have been made in recent cohorts of elderly, one would expect continued high rates of edentulousness in elderly in many other countries.

Dental attitudes of practitioners and the public have undergone significant changes in the past 30 years in the United States, where the emphasis is now on saving teeth at any cost, rather than extracting decayed teeth. This is reflected in the differences between elderly cohorts separated by just 15 years; in the 1985 survey (NIDR 1987) 32 per cent of the 65–69-year-olds were edentulous, compared with 49 per cent of those aged 80 or older. This represents a 50 per cent decline in tooth mortality within just one generation! Regional surveys such as the Iowa study of elderly show even greater differences; 29 per cent of the 65–69-year-olds were edentulous, compared with 54 per cent of those 80 and older (Hunt et al. 1985).

This suggests that oral health promotion efforts with older people will become more relevant with the increase in the population trying to retain whatever remaining teeth they have. As recently as 1977 it was difficult to find people over the age of 75 interested in oral health promotion; many argued that they had nothing to promote, since they had already lost all their natural teeth anyway. While it is also valuable to work with older adults to maintain their oral health after they have begun to use dentures, those with some teeth remaining are more motivated to keep the teeth they have. It is important to teach older persons also that ageing per se does not place their teeth at greater risk for extraction; in the Iowa survey less than two per cent of teeth were extracted from these older persons over an 18-month period (Hunt et al. 1988).

It has been observed that the teeth that do survive in many older people do so with some 'battle scars'. In the NIDR (1987) survey, mean decayed and filled surfaces (DFS) for coronal caries peaked at 29 for those aged 40 to 50, compared with a mean DFS of 20 for the 65–69 age group and 17 for those aged 80 and older. This apparent decline in coronal caries with age may be associated with the fact that many teeth lost previously in this population were lost to caries. Conversely, DFS for root caries increased with age; 67 per cent of men and 61 per cent of women had one or more lesions, many of which were unrestored.

It is important to emphasize with older persons the need for a daily oral hygiene routine and regular visits to a dentist or hygienist to maintain the teeth they already have, and to treat a carious lesion early, whether it is at the root or the coronal surface, in order to prevent tooth loss. One major goal of oral health promotion with older audiences is to prevent complacency, or the attitude that people as old as 80 who have retained some of their natural teeth are somehow blessed or lucky, and that they need not continue to maintain their oral health. It is also important to emphasize that many of the systemic chronic diseases from which they suffer and the medications they use for these conditions may impair their oral health. For example, despite the prevalence of diabetes, especially in African American and Hispanic elderly, few people with this condition realize that their oral soft tissues may be at greater risk for disease and, as a result, do not devote special attention to their periodontal health. Many of the medications used by older people, especially several classes of antihypertensives and antidepressants, place them at risk for xerostomia and subsequently for the development of root caries. Unfortunately this problem is compounded by the lack of awareness of these risks among many physicians whose primary objective is to counter the effects of the systemic disease, with less concern about side-effects such as reduced salivary flow and increased rates of caries. In a recent health promotion study by this author, a 73-year-old woman with severe hypertension had complained of having a dry mouth to her physician several weeks after starting a course of hydrochlorothiazide. The physician recommended sucking on hard candies, which the woman proceeded to do during the health promotion classes! She was surprised to learn that the sugar in those candies was aggravating her already high risk for developing root caries.

The NIDR (1987) survey has also revealed that periodontal health in older people is worse than in the young, although active disease is less common. For example, 34 per cent of the over-65 age group in the NIDR survey had one or more sites with 6 mm or more of attachment loss; the mean attachment loss on buccal and mesial surfaces was 3.5 mm in the oldest group, compared with 1.5 mm in the under-29 age group. Pocket depth was also greater in older people; 22 per cent had one or more sites with a pocket depth greater than 4 mm, compared with less than 10 per cent of the under-29 age group. This survey found an almost linear increase in pocket depth with increasing age beyond 30, although even in the oldest group pocket depths of 6 mm or more were rare. A third indicator of periodontal health, gingival bleeding (defined here as a site that bleeds after gentle probing of the sulcus), was similar in frequency in both the younger and older persons examined; approximately 47 per cent of the youngest and oldest had one or more sites that bled. Nevertheless, twice as many elders had affected sites as did the younger sample. These indicators of periodontal health suggest that older persons are more likely to have had a history of periodontal destruction, but active disease is relatively rare.

Oral cancers are less common in North America and western Europe, where the frequency has been estimated to be two to five per cent (Smith 1979).

However, in Asia, Southeast Asia, and the Middle East, they account for as much as 50 per cent of all cancers. However, in all these regions, the prevalence appears to increase with age; malignant neoplasms of the lip and the floor of the mouth as much as doubled in frequency after the age of 65 compared to the age of 45. These conditions may become less prevalent as the incidence of smoking and alcohol consumption declines in adult populations. Nevertheless, it will continue to be a problem for current cohorts of elderly, making it necessary to include material on prevention and self-exams for oral cancer in any oral health promotion effort aimed at older adults. This information must be emphasized with some high risk populations even more than in the general populations of elderly.

Oral health attitudes of current and future elderly

The previous sections of this chapter have provided a *rationale* for oral health promotion for the elderly. That is, given the growing numbers of older people who will continue to live for a long time but with some deterioration in their physiological and cognitive functions, with multiple chronic conditions, and having retained more teeth than in previous generations, it is important to raise the level of oral health and functional capacity in older people. The challenge is made more difficult by the fact that the current cohort of elderly grew up in an era before preventive dentistry was widely practised. The value of fluoride, especially of adding fluoride to the community water supply, was not accepted until the 1940s. Routine dental check-ups and prophylaxes were rare for this population until the 1950s. As a result, many experienced early and unnecessary caries, periodontal disease, and tooth loss, accompanied by an attitude that dental disease and tooth loss are inevitable consequences of ageing. Not surprisingly, these early dental experiences have shaped older people's current values and attitudes about oral health. These attitudes subsequently affect their current dental care behaviours, including the decision to seek dental care.

Evans (1984) cites four dental 'myths' embraced by older people that are detrimental to their oral health. These include: ageing is naturally associated with tooth loss; dental care is expensive; dental treatment requires lengthy visits; and dentists and dental care delivery systems are all the same. Such attitudes may prevent the older person from seeking dental care and, worse yet, prevent their participation in any type of oral health promotion effort. Indeed, the primary barrier faced by anyone attempting to develop a health promotion effort for any age group is the attitudinal one by potential recipients of such a programme. To the extent that an individual believes that there is nothing to be done about their health and that what treatment there is will be too costly and long-term, they will be less likely to participate. In the area of geriatric health promotion, it is often those elders with the most entrenched distrust of the health care system who have the greatest health needs! This is compounded in dentistry by the historical factors described above, with a lack of a preventive approach to dental care in their childhood resulting in poor oral health conditions currently. For these reasons, it is important to first overcome attitudinal barriers, and later to deal with knowledge and behaviour changes specific to dentistry. For example, in their survey of Iowa adults, Ettinger and Beck (1982) found that the oldest group (aged over 75) was more likely to agree with such statements as: 'I don't have dental problems'; 'There is no sense in seeking dental care'; and 'Problems with my teeth and gums don't affect my lifestyle'. Compared with the young-old (aged 65–74), the old-old (aged 75 and over) were more accepting toward dentures. It is therefore imperative for health educators to first explore the dental values and attitudes of older audiences, evoking from them such beliefs as those above, before working with them to overcome these attitudes through an educational and behavioural intervention. It may even be necessary to offer a different approach for different cohorts of elderly; for example, young-old participants in oral health promotion efforts may already be convinced that natural teeth are superior to dentures and will be ready to accept new information about improving their oral health. In contrast, a group that does not even believe that it is necessary to seek preventive dental services is not ready to accept information about how to find a dentist. As with any educational programme, oral health promotion efforts must first determine the *readiness* of their target audience for the material to be taught.

What is the goal of oral health promotion with older adults?

Changing dental attitudes among older people

Before describing the components of a successful oral health promotion effort, it is first important to determine the criteria for success. As with any age group, oral health promotion for elders should have as its primary goal the *enhancement and improvement of oral functions* such as mastication, diges-tion, and speech, as well as the *improvement of appearance and psychological well-being* such as the enjoyment of eating and communication, and enhanced self-confidence. All of these outcomes relate to an important aspect of well-being, *quality of life*. While dentistry has only recently begun to examine its role in maintaining quality of life, medicine has long asserted that treatment outcomes should enhance the individual's quality of life, as expressed in the ability to perform activities of daily living, to live indepen-dently and with a minimum of pain and discomfort, and to maintain psy-chological well-being. Because ageing is often accompanied by physiological and cognitive changes, as well as systemic diseases and social losses that can impair one's quality of life, it is particularly important to address this issue of enhancing quality of life in older people. It may be that improved oral function and appearance can significantly alter the older person's overall quality of life, as will be demonstrated below with examples of research in this area.

In the previous section we emphasized the importance of addressing older people's oral health attitudes and level of dental awareness before undertaking an effort to change behaviour. In this section we will review the need to consider primary, secondary, and tertiary prevention with older adults. *Primary prevention* is needed for diseases that they have not yet experienced, most commonly oral cancers for this population. As with most other cancers, behavioural changes such as smoking cessation efforts and reducing heavy alcohol consumption are examples of primary prevention. Other behaviours must be learned, such as proper techniques of oral self-exams and the need to seek regular check-ups by a dentist who will also perform an oral cancer screening.

Secondary prevention is most likely the approach to be used for the majority of aged persons, since some tooth loss and periodontal destruction has already occurred in many elderly, as we have noted earlier. Secondary prevention may include attempts at changing knowledge *and* attitudes related to oral health. Such dysfunctional attitudes as those described above (for example 'tooth loss is inevitable with ageing', 'dental care is expensive', and 'problems with teeth and gums don't affect the older person's lifestyle') must be overcome in order to prevent further disease and tooth loss. Attempts to elicit the older person's belief system about oral health and *explanatory models* of disease (such as 'What is the cause of the person's disease?' and 'Who is responsible for treating the disease?') will prove useful in the long run if health promotion efforts are to be successful in changing older people's health status and behaviours.

Other secondary prevention techniques are the use of chlorhexidine by older people who have a history of periodontal disease, professionally applied fluoride or a fluoride rinse to be used at home, and regular check-ups at a place that is convenient for the older person (for example in a senior citizens' centre, nursing home, or meal site rather than in a dentist's office).

Tertiary prevention is most often aimed at those who have lost all their teeth and must cope with the day-to-day problems of dentures. A programme that combines some of the educational and attitudinal goals described above for secondary prevention is probably most beneficial for this population. In some cases, cognitive and behavioural retraining may be necessary to assist the individual who is having unusual difficulties adjusting to dentures, or whose dentures cannot be adjusted for an ideal fit because of structural changes in the ageing mouth. It may also be helpful to direct such a patient to other alternatives such as implants, if cost considerations are not unrealistic. At the very least, tertiary prevention should help the older person to prevent discomfort and maximize whatever oral functions remain.

Successful methods of oral health promotion

The preceding discussion highlights the need for a multidimensional approach to oral health promotion, with a strong educational component as well as clinical interventions to provide chemotherapeutic and prophylactic procedures that can improve function. It is surprising that older people have been neglected as targets of oral health educational programmes. As noted above, information regarding appropriate dental behaviours may never have been learned by some elderly. Other types of information, such as correct methods of oral hygiene, use of fluorides, and prevention of periodontal disease, have changed or expanded over the years, so that elderly persons who received dental health information in their youth may hold on to outdated information (for example, many elderly people believe that brushing vertically against the gums and using a hard toothbrush are correct brushing techniques). This is compounded by the lack of regular dental care, making it difficult for older people to learn about new developments in dentistry.

The few reports of preventive dental education for the elderly have shown successful results. A preventive program in Denmark that combined frequent prophylaxes with oral health education was found to result in significant reduction of gingivitis (Gron 1981). Scores on the gingival index, attachment loss, and pocket depth improved within one year of this programme. Gron notes that a frequent prophylaxis without education was *not* found to be effective with elderly patients. In another Scandinavian study, Ambjornsen and Rise (1985) compared the effects of a verbal information programme with one that combined this method with a demonstration of denture cleaning methods. The information and demonstration were repeated 14 days later. Both groups experienced short-term improvements in oral hygiene and in caring for dentures, but only the latter group showed improvements in oral hygiene six months later. This study highlights the need to combine active learning with a strictly educational approach. Social reinforcement by the health educator and peers provides the third important component of a successful approach to health promotion efforts with older people.

The author has conducted research on improving oral health in older people over the past 14 years. The premise of these studies has been that older persons can still benefit from oral health promotion and can change their behaviour, even if the goal is secondary or tertiary prevention. Both dental and psychological outcomes have been measured, including plaque scores and gingival bleeding, frequency of oral home care behaviours, oral health knowledge, perceived control, morale, and self-esteem. It has been hypothesized that improved oral health can enhance psychological well-being and quality of life among older people. That is, the realization that one can improve one's own oral health and can see changes in a short period should result in improved morale and a greater sense of control over one's life. Furthermore, if one develops an improved perception of oral health, this perception should generalize to other aspects of health. Thus, the individual who comes to evaluate his or her general health status in a more positive manner will also develop a better sense of self-worth. These variables — perceived oral health, general physical health, morale, and self-esteem — have been measured before and after the experimental interventions in four of the six studies.

These studies have been conducted with cognitively intact elderly in an intermediate care nursing home (Kiyak 1980), in senior citizens' centres serving ethnic elderly (Price and Kiyak 1981), among depressed elderly in a nursing home (Kiyak and Mulligan 1987), as a demonstration project throughout the state of Washington (Kiyak and Grayston 1989), in a study comparing oral health promotion alone or integrated with a general health promotion effort (Kiyak and Grayston 1991), and most recently with high risk elderly (Kiyak 1991). In this section we will describe briefly the methods and results of these studies, their objectives, and some findings. Finally, the implications of these studies for future research in oral health promotion with elderly will be examined.

Self-monitoring has been defined as a behaviour management technique in which the individual keeps a daily or weekly record of his or her behaviours that are to be changed. Self-monitoring techniques have been applied successfully in programmes of weight loss, exercise, stress reduction, and, in gerontology, in programmes to discontinue repetitive behaviours among institutionalized elderly (Sachs 1975).

In the case of our oral health studies, we have predetermined the behaviours to be improved by all participants. As Fig. 6.7 illustrates, each participant is given a weekly chart on which he or she records daily the frequency of brushing natural teeth or dentures, rinsing the mouth, and soaking dentures. Flossing is not recorded because this has not been emphasized in previous studies. Each participant is asked to post this weekly chart on a wall by the sink at home where daily oral hygiene is performed. Group members are asked to bring their chart to the first of the two sessions held each week. At that time, individual charts are reviewed with the group as well as individually. Participants who have recorded more than one brushing and mouth rinsing per day are given verbal reinforcement by the group leader, and other group members are encouraged to praise that person. Initially this intervention strategy began with tangible rewards (such as books, magazines, and knitting supplies) to participants who successfully completed their charts each week. However, it soon became clear that most older persons responded more favourably to the verbal reinforcement, and were uncomfortable about receiving prizes.

The use of social reinforcement as a reward for successfully completing their dental charts is consistent with Ajzen and Fishbein's (1980) theory of reasoned action. According to this model, behaviour change takes place because people hold specific beliefs about the consequences of that behaviour and about other

Week _____
Home care for: _____
Put an 'X' every time you do any of the following things.

Days	Brushed teeth	Cleaned mouth
Monday		
Tuesday		
Wednesday		
Thursday		
Friday		
Saturday		
Sunday		

Fig. 6.7   Self-monitoring chart for subjects with natural teeth.

people's approval or disapproval if that behaviour is performed (subjective norms). These two sets of beliefs lead to intentions which result in actual behaviour. Thus, in the case of a group learning situation, members of the group provide each other with reinforcement for performing health behaviours that have been described as beneficial or desirable (a social norm that endorses increased attention to and performance of preventive behaviours). Each member of the group receives information about the benefits of preventive behaviours, as well as social approval for performing these activities. One would expect a change in behaviour if the individual's beliefs are consistent, or become consistent, with group norms over the course of the oral health promotion effort, according to Ajzen and Fishbein's model.

The usual procedure has been to first perform a thorough oral exam on volunteer subjects, recording plaque, decayed, missing, and filled surfaces (DMFS), and treatment needs. Those needing treatment for acute dental problems are generally seen on site by a project dentist. A hygienist performs a baseline prophylaxis on all participants. They are then interviewed by a trained interviewer. Subjects in the nursing home study (Kiyak 1980) were asked questions about their dental history, current oral health status, perceived oral and physical health, morale (Lawton 1975), and self-esteem using Coopersmith's (1967) measure revised for the elderly. Locus of control, using Rotter's (1966) measure of generalized locus of control, was used as a covariate, as were cognitive status and manual dexterity. The Mini-Mental Status Exam (Folstein *et al.* 1975) was used to screen for cognitive disorders. In addition, a test of hand function (Jebsen *et al.* 1969) was used to assess manual dexterity and to determine if problems with manual and finger dexterity might affect oral self-care. Although some variation was found on this test, problems were not serious enough to affect tooth or denture brushing, or to require the use of assistive devices for brushes. Differences in manual dexterity did not influence oral hygiene and psychological outcomes in the experimental groups. Subjects were assigned to a self-monitoring condition, an oral health promotion group with no self-monitoring, a placebo group, and a control group with no interventions. After a six-week intervention, all subjects were re-examined by the dental hygienist and reinterviewed by the research assistant. Both of these project staff members were kept blind to the group assignment of participants. Six weeks later, and again six months after that, another follow-up was conducted with all participants. The greatest improvements were found in the self-monitoring condition; the least in the health education-only group. Most significant was the finding that self-monitoring groups continued to show lower plaque scores, higher frequency of home care behaviours, and higher morale scores six months after the intervention than before the programme began; the education-only groups had reverted to their preintervention levels on all variables.

In the second study (Price and Kiyak 1981), focusing on Japanese–American or Caucasian elderly in the community, the tests of cognitive functioning and manual dexterity were discontinued. Three of the four conditions tested in the nursing home were also tested in the senior citizens' centre; the placebo group was not included. In addition to a preintervention assessment, subjects were tested immediately after the intervention. The self-monitoring group again showed the greatest improvement in oral health (measured by plaque scores), and in self-reported oral and general health. Those in the oral health education group without self-monitoring did not differ from the control condition in their plaque scores following the intervention. While ethnic differences were observed in the degree of improvement in plaque scores and oral health knowledge (with Japanese–American elders showing greater gains), both ethnic groups who used self-monitoring techniques reported significantly higher levels of general and oral health immediately after and six weeks after the intervention. These gains were also significantly greater than for the education-only conditions.

Because of the dramatic effects of these oral health interventions on psychological well-being, a third study was undertaken among nursing home residents who were mildly depressed or at risk for depression (Kiyak and

Mulligan 1987). The sense of worthlessness, loss of autonomy, and loss of health which are associated with depression may be aggravated in the nursing home environment where the individual often forfeits control over his or her lifespace and activities. Self-care in oral health, bathing, and dressing may be replaced with dependence on others. This is more likely to occur among depressed patients because the apathy and social withdrawal that accompanies depression may be interpreted by staff as an inability or unwillingness to do things for oneself. Research by Langer and Rodin (1976) and by Rodin and Langer (1977) has shown that elderly nursing home residents who are given control over their environment experience increased self-worth.

In this third study (Kiyak and Mulligan 1987), we hypothesized that oral self-care should increase the depressed person's perception of autonomy and self-worth. This, coupled with self-monitoring in a group setting, was expected to reduce depressive symptoms and to improve self-esteem. These hypotheses grew out of the results of the two studies described above.

Residents without serious cognitive impairments and who were ambulatory (independently or with a wheelchair) were first screened by the director of nursing, who did an initial assessment for depression, then referred them to the project psychologist for further evaluation. Those who were currently on antidepressant medication and whose clinical picture of depression was severe or non-existent (using the Community Epidemiological Studies of Depression (CESD) scale) were eliminated from the sample. However, because apathy and lack of self-care are hallmarks of depression, it was difficult to encourage people who fit our research criteria to participate in the study! Thus, instead of the anticipated 60 subjects, the project was able to recruit just 36 depressed elders from two nursing homes. These people were assigned to one of three groups: a self-monitoring oral health educational group or an education-only group that each met once a week for six weeks, or a control group that was examined and interviewed only at baseline and at the termination of the project. Because of attrition due to death or refusal to be re-examined, only 26 people were available at the second follow-up.

Despite the high attrition rate, the two intervention groups experienced declines in plaque levels, resulting in an overall effect for time ($F = 4.5$; $df = 2$, 23; $p < 0.02$). The self-monitoring group experienced the greatest decline from their pre-intervention levels of plaque ($\bar{x} = 67$ per cent of surfaces covered by plaque) to the immediate post-intervention assessment ($\bar{x} = 58$ per cent of all surfaces), and even at the six-week post-intervention assessment ($\bar{x} = 60$ per cent), but these differences were nonsignificant.

Self-reported health status also changed for the two intervention groups, but remained stable for the control group, resulting in an overall group × time interaction. These results support the value of an oral health screening programme combined with group discussion in improving the oral health status and overall sense of well-being among depressed elders. It was surprising to find, however, that the self-monitoring groups did not experience far greater increases in their hygiene status and perceived oral health than did group discussions alone. This was the first study in which results from self-monitoring were *not* significantly better than education alone, and may be attributed to small sample sizes.

Contrary to the hypothesis that enhanced oral health and a sense of increased control over one's health would effect improvements in morale and levels of depression in this population, no significant changes were found for the two intervention groups. However, the self-monitoring group did report *slightly higher morale* at the immediate post-intervention interview than they did initially. The finding of no significant change in the self-reported Beck depression scale is, to some extent, a function of a restricted range of scores (means of 2.4–5.7 on a 24-point scale), suggesting very low depression scores! This in turn may reflect a reluctance on the part of these older people to admit that they were depressed. This is supported by the finding that, during the clinical interview, these persons had been rated by the project psychologist as moderately depressed.

A clinical assessment of participants in the two intervention groups revealed increasing socialization and group communication among members of the group during the six-week interventions. Self-reports of morale showed some improvement in psychological well-being among the group that focused on oral health. Nevertheless, these effects were slight and had little impact on pre-existing depression.

In the fourth health promotion study conducted by the research team (Kiyak and Grayston 1989), funding was obtained from the US Administration on Aging to test the feasibility of the self-monitoring approach on a large-scale basis. Because this was *not* an experimental intervention but a demonstration project, no control groups were utilized. The programme consisted of six one-hour sessions held twice each week at 36 senior citizens' centres throughout the state of Washington. Baseline interviews and oral exams were conducted on 400 elders ranging in age from 60 to 97 ($\bar{x}$ age = 73.4). Classes were conducted jointly by a health educator and hygienist; the topics covered were typical of our other health programmes and are listed in Table 6.6. Participants reflected the national pattern of oral health status in persons over 65; 40.2 per cent wore complete dentures while the remainder had only natural teeth or a combination of natural teeth and prostheses.

In order to test the effects of attending all six sessions versus some of the sessions, we compared post-intervention plaque scores of those who attended all six vs. fewer than six sessions. The former group had significantly lower plaque scores at *all* measurement periods, including at baseline, indicating greater motivation and acceptance of the newly acquired information. Note that these analyses were made only of those who returned for both follow-up assessments (only 55 per cent of the original sample). Had we been able to include in the comparison those who dropped out altogether, the differences

Table 6.6   Representative topics for a six-week programme

Week 1
Discussion of participants' beliefs regarding oral health and disease
Highlight need for regular dental care, finding a dentist
Establish individual goals for behaviour change
Introduce self-monitoring charts

Week 2
Techniques for home care of natural teeth and dentures
Need for regular visits to dentist
Participants demonstrate their brushing techniques
Review self-monitoring charts
Audiovisual materials: slide-tape 'Teeth for life', handouts

Week 3
Demonstration of correct techniques and tools for brushing teeth and dentures
Importance of removing partial and complete dentures daily
Review self-monitoring charts

Week 4
Effects of nutrition on oral health, maintaining good nutrition in old age
Use food models to demonstrate and practise balanced, low sugar diet
Suggestions for relieving dry mouth
Review self-monitoring charts
Audiovisual materials: side-tape 'Nutrition and oral health', handouts.

Week 5
Osteoporosis and effects on the oral structures, denture mobility
New developments in denture construction
Review self-monitoring charts
Audiovisual materials: videotape 'Calcium is not just for kids', handout on osteoporosis

Week 6
Oral diseases (with an emphasis on oral cancer) in the later years
Demonstration and practise of self-exams for oral cancer and other disease
Review self-monitoring charts
Audiovisual materials: slide-tape 'Oral health in the later years', brochures on cancer

between regular and irregular attendees would have been even more dramatic.

These findings point to the importance of informing potential participants in oral health promotion programmes of the need to attend *all* sessions *or* trying to recruit only those who are motivated enough to complete the programme. Given the difficulty of achieving either goal — the former for ethical reasons, the latter because it would result in a positively biased sample — it may be more reasonable to condense all the oral health information into a maximum of three sessions, each lasting two hours. The current study we are conducting with elderly at high risk for caries and periodontal disease has eliminated much of the material covered in previous health promotion efforts, thereby resulting in a single two-hour session. This latest programme will be described in the final section.

The demonstration project described above resulted in significant improvements in the elders' oral health status and behaviours. Plaque levels were lower by 20–30 per cent in those with natural or dentures, both at the immediate and at the three-month post-intervention assessments. The finding of continued improvement at three months attests to the benefits of a self-monitoring approach, as we found in the first two projects. There was a corresponding increase in self-reported brushing frequency, from 52 per cent brushing more than once a day at baseline to 68 per cent and 66 per cent doing so immediately and three months later, respectively. Similarly, a significant increase was observed in the number performing regular oral self-exams, from none at baseline to 34 per cent at three months post-intervention. Perceived oral health also improved during this period, probably reflecting the greater sense of control and self-efficacy these elders experienced through their involvement in the programme. Indeed, the finding that plaque scores were inversely correlated with perceived oral health at all assessments supports this conclusion.

The same project attempted to provide oral health promotion for institutionalized elders by conducting free oral screenings of 1063 residents of 31 nursing homes and offering workshops for nurse aides and nurses working in these facilities. We found that the greatest problem faced by these frail elders was poor oral hygiene (72 per cent of dentate residents), followed by periodontal symptoms (43 per cent) and root caries (36 per cent) in dentate residents, while poorly fitting dentures were the greatest problem for edentulous elders (46 per cent) (Kiyak *et al.* 1992). The greatest advantage of a health promotion effort for dependent elders, as in this case, is the opportunity to provide an exam and prophylaxis, as well as educating their daily caregivers. Unfortunately, we have found it extremely difficult to recruit nurse aides into oral health educational programmes, whether these are offered as a one-time workshop as in this demonstration project, or as a series of group educational sessions, as provided in a subsequent study by Lingenbrink and Kiyak (1991), where we had difficulty recruiting and retaining participants in the study, even when they were reimbursed for their time. Perhaps most disturbing is the finding that many nurse aides who are responsible for the daily oral hygiene of institutionalized elders have very poor oral hygiene habits themselves and are often less knowledgeable about oral health than the elders themselves.

In a recently completed study (Kiyak and Grayston 1991), self-monitoring was again utilized. However, in order to test whether elderly persons would be more likely to participate in the programme if told that the health topics would be broader than oral health alone, volunteers at senior citizens' centres were randomly assigned to groups that *focused* on oral health with *some* general health topics or groups that *integrated* oral health into broader topics such as cancer, arthritis, nutrition, and drugs. While this strategy did not appear to increase the numbers of volunteers, both focused and integrated groups that used self-monitoring techniques showed consistently higher scores post-intervention than did non-self-monitoring groups. That is, regardless of the degree to which oral health was emphasized in the course, elders who used self-monitoring charts to track their oral hygiene and dietary patterns showed lower plaque scores and less gingival bleeding post-intervention than did those *not* monitoring their behaviour. Oral health attitudes and the perceived importance of oral and systemic health also improved in the self-monitoring groups, as did self-efficacy, or the conviction among these elders that they could control their health by the behaviours they performed. Given that these are important attributions for improving health status (Kiyak 1992), these findings provide even stronger evidence for the value of self-monitoring in any health promotion effort.

The latest in our series of oral health promotion studies has recently begun, with a focus on low income persons over the age of 60 who qualify as patients in the local health department clinics but who have used these services only on an emergency basis (Kiyak 1991). Because of the poorer oral health status of many minority elders in the US, this project aims to enroll at least 25 per cent minority elders (African Americans, Asian Americans, and Hispanics). Already we have seen dramatic differences in periodontal status and caries history between the Caucasian and minority samples. These participants will be followed for two years as they participate in one of four oral health promotion groups or a control group. Each experimental group adds a new intervention, ranging from: education alone; education *and* chlorhexidine; education *and* chlorhexidine *and* semiannual fluoride varnish applications; and education *and* chlorhexidine *and* semiannual fluoride varnish applications *and* a semiannual prophylaxis. All education interventions consist of a single two-hour session for small groups of participants, held at the health department semiannually. The focus of these sessions is on maintaining natural teeth (all participants in this study must have at least six teeth) and conducting self-exams to detect soft tissue lesions.

Is there hope for older adults? Some dos and don'ts

A broad perspective is necessary when developing and successfully completing an oral health promotion programme for older adults, because the boundary between health and disease is quite blurred in ageing, as illustrated by the 'cascade of disasters' phenomenon. For example, it is important to limit educational sessions to two hours or less if group discussion is involved, and to one hour or less if these sessions consist of lectures only.

A long-term intervention effort, such as many of the six studies conducted by the author, has the advantage of reiterating and reinforcing new information (which is valuable in light of normal age-related changes in learning and memory), and in terms of testing for long-term retention of newly acquired skills.

Attrition due to a loss of interest and conflicting social needs also is a problem in longitudinal programmes with the elderly. One of the most liberating aspects of ageing is the realization that one need not conform to societal expectations and demands! Even those elderly who in their working years kept rigid standards of commitment to a job or activity, no longer feel the necessity to fulfil such obligations in their retirement years. This is true for those in both long-term care settings and community settings. Indeed, senior citizens' activity centres may at first seem like an ideal place to recruit large numbers of active elderly, but in fact these settings offer numerous social opportunities as well. For this reason, elderly senior citizens' centre attendees who enroll in a health promotion programme may initially be committed, but a long-term programme has the potential of conflicting with other social activities at the centre.

It is also important to consider the content and methods of presentation. In our earlier research the sessions were described as oral health education that would be appropriate for both edentulous *and* dentate elderly. While this may have appealed to a small proportion of elders in that setting who were concerned about their oral health (thereby producing a ceiling effect for improvement in some cases), many older people with even greater needs did not participate. The addition of other topics such as cancer education, blood pressure and dietary needs increased the number of volunteers somewhat above our previous numbers, but it appeared that the best recruitment tool was a methodological, not a content approach! That is, potential volunteers were told that the programme would offer *free* dental exams (and emergency treatment if necessary), *free* blood pressure and cholesterol screenings, and *free* educational materials developed specifically for elders. In addition, a small stipend for each follow-up visit appeared to enhance both the recruitment *and* the retention rates. Indeed, retention in studies without a stipend has been as low as 50 per cent, whereas in studies with a stipend the rate has been as high as 75 per cent (most drop-outs in these latter studies have been attributable to death and disability). Thus, it is important to recognize the value systems of one's audience in any health promotion effort, especially when working with older adults.

Another important methodological approach is to repeat information presented in previous sessions. This argues for a multi-session programme, which in many cases is superior to a one-time-only educational effort. This may also limit the number of topics covered, but it is based on sound cognitive retraining principles for the elderly, that is the need to reiterate new information and allow a longer time for older people to learn and actively practise the new material, and to present the information in multiple modes (for example written handouts, oral presentation, demonstration, and individual practice in the group). If it is necessary to limit the educational programme to a single session, the material should *not* be condensed but instead reduced to just one or two topics.

Group educational sessions also offer the instructor time to query elderly participants about their current oral health problems, how they cope with these, and how they maintain their oral health. The example presented earlier of the older woman who was told to suck on hard candy by her physician in response to her complaints about her dry mouth is illustrative here. During the initial discussion with the group about medications that may cause a dry mouth, they were asked to share their experiences in this area and how they had coped with such problems. It was in this context that the older woman described her doctor's recommendation about hard candy, permitting the instructor to explain the problems with sucrose in an oral environment low in saliva. If specific situations such as this that require behavioural change arise during a health promotion session, it behoves the educator to follow up with the participant experiencing these difficulties, perhaps even providing alternatives such as artificially sweetened candy or, in severe cases, saliva substitutes in this situation. It may even require contacting the primary physician to discuss alternative medications for an older person who is experiencing anticholinergic side-effects from one or more medications prescribed by that physician.

Even with these special considerations in planning appropriate oral health promotion efforts for older people, it is impossible to eliminate totally potential problems that may arise. As stated earlier, volunteer participants often have better oral health and higher socioeconomic status than non-participants. This creates a situation of 'preaching to the converted', that is those people who have a history of relatively good dental care and are motivated to maintain their oral health by participating in a planned intervention. In some ways this is an ideal population, since they already have a reasonable level of health that is to be promoted, rather than focusing on secondary or tertiary prevention. On the other hand, from an ethical perspective, health professionals have an obligation to provide some health promotion opportunities for elders with the worst oral health. This may require the cooperation of administrators of long-term care facilities and senior service programmes to encourage *all* elderly in their settings to obtain a free health screening, including a thorough oral assessment and treatment or referral of acute conditions. Financial incentives such as a token remuneration (US$5 or US$10) can also attract the less motivated elderly. Nevertheless, it is also important to be realistic and to recognize the fact that no incentive will be sufficient to encourage those who have no interest in maintaining or improving their oral health, or those who see no association between their oral conditions and quality of life.

Finally, it is critical to involve other professionals in any oral health promotion effort. The tacit and active support of facility administrators was described above. In long-term care settings, the director of nursing services and charge nurses must be committed to the programme and believe in its efficacy. This will increase the chances of greater cooperation on the part of nurse aides responsible for bringing elders to a health promotion programme and, in the long run, ensure that behavioural changes made during the life of that programme will continue. Social service directors in such settings must also be involved in establishing a programme consistent with the social and physical needs of the population, ensuring that the programme will not conflict with other activities and encouraging elderly residents to enroll in and continue with the programme. Such involvement is also more likely to result in social services staff continuing or re-establishing the health promotion effort even after the dental providers are no longer present. Directors of community-based social services for older people (for example hot lunch programmes and senior citizens' centres) are similarly crucial for the success of oral health promotion efforts in these settings. Visiting nurses or other health educators who visit these sites regularly should also be made aware of and, if possible, become involved in conducting oral health promotion programmes both for cooperation and collaboration, and to avoid conflict with other health promotion efforts. Because of the growing awareness of health promotion for older adults, it is not unusual to find several disjointed programmes in many senior citizens' centres today — a nutritionist conducting a programme on fat-free diets, a nurse teaching hypertension awareness, and an aerobics instructor teaching low impact aerobics! The inclusion of an oral health promotion effort in such settings will be unsuccessful unless it can become integrated with all or some of these other programmes.

Conclusions

This chapter has attempted to provide a background on the processes of ageing, both normal and pathological, and how these age-related changes in physical and cognitive functions can influence the design and outcomes of an oral health promotion programme. The increased number of people living to the age of 65 and beyond and, more importantly, the number retaining their natural teeth (albeit with extensive histories of decay and periodontal disease), make it imperative for dental professionals and health educators to develop age-appropriate oral health promotion programmes for this population. This includes the development of educational materials (slide/tape-programmes, videotapes, and brochures) directed specifically at elders.

The type of audience one can expect in an oral health promotion effort has been described in terms of changing oral epidemiologic patterns *and* in the context of who volunteers to participate in programmes to change oral health or any health behaviour. The rigidity of many older persons in terms of their refusal to adapt new knowledge and behaviours into their oral health belief systems must be acknowledged and addressed through an active learning approach that includes behaviour modelling by the older person's peers. New information must be presented within the context of the elder's belief system and relative to their specific needs. For example, in our current study, an individualized behaviour change plan is developed for each participant by a hygienist who determines the elder's current oral health routines and makes recommendations for improving or changing these behaviours.

The author's research in this area has been described as an illustration of successful and unsuccessful methods. The impact of these programmes on oral health status, knowledge, and behaviours, as well as on psychological outcomes such as perceived health, morale, self-esteem, and self-efficacy, have been discussed. It is hoped that these studies will serve as examples of what can be done with diverse populations of elderly, as well as limitations of oral health promotion efforts with older people.

References

Ajzen, I. and Fishbein, M. (1980). *Understanding attitudes and predicting social behavior.* Prentice-Hall, Englewood Cliffs, NJ.

Ambjornsen, E. and Rise, J. (1985). The effect of verbal information and demonstration on denture hygiene in elderly people. *Acta Odontol, Scand.*, **43**, 19–24.

Berkey, D. B., Call, R. L., and Loupe, M. J. (1985). Oral health perceptions and self-esteem in non-institutionalized older adults. *Gerodontics*, **1**, 213–16.

Coopersmith, S. (1967). *Antecedents of self-esteem.* Freeman, San Francisco.

Ettinger, R. L. and Beck, J. D. (1982). The new elderly: what can the dental profession expect? *Spec. Care Dent.*, **2**, 62–9.

Evans, R. W. (1984). The aging dental patient: myth and reality. *Gerodontology*, **3**, 271–2.

Folstein, M. F., Folstein, S. E., and McHugh, P. R. (1975). Mini-mental state: a practical method for grading the cognitive status of patients. *Journal of Psychiatric Research*, **12**, 189–98.

Fozard, J. L. (1980). The time for remembering. In *Aging in the 1980s: psychological issues*, (ed. L. W. Poon), pp. 273–290. American Psychological Association, Washington DC.

Gift, H. C. (1986). Current utilization patterns of oral hygiene practices. In *Dental plaque control measures and oral hygiene practice*, (ed. H. Loe and D. V. Kleinman), pp. 39–71. IRL Press, Oxford.

Gron, P. (1981). Preventive dental health program for the elderly: rationale and primary findings. *Spec. Care Dent.*, **1**, 129–32.

Hunt, R. L., Beck, J., Hand, J., and Kohout, F. (1985). Edentulism and oral health problems among elderly rural Iowans: the Iowa 65+ rural health study. *Amer. J. Publ. Health*, **75**, 1178–81.

Hunt R. L., Hand, J., Kohout, F., and Beck, J. (1988). Incidence of tooth loss among elderly Iowans. *Amer. J. Publ. Health*, **78**, 1330–2.

Inman, V. W. and Parkinson, S. R. (1983). Differences in Brown–Peterson recall as a function of age and retention interval. *Journal of Gerontology*, **38**, 58–64.

Jebsen, R. H., Taylor, N., Trieschmann, R. B., Trotter, M. J., and Howard, L. A. (1969). An objective and standardized test of hand function. *Archives of Physical Medicine and Rehabilitation*, **50**, 311–19.

Kiyak, H. A. (1980). Clinical test: preventive dentistry for the elderly. Final report submitted to NIDR (Grant No. R23-DE05235). University of Washington, Seattle.

Kiyak, H. A. (1991). *Evaluation of cost-effective preventive regimens for high risk older adults.* NIDR Contract No. NO1-DE125686. University of Washington, Seattle.

Kiyak, H. A. (1992). *Self-efficacy as a predictor of oral health improvements. Journal of Dental Research*, **71**, 750.

Kiyak, H. A. and Grayston, N. (1989). A successful oral health promotion effort for independent elderly. *The Gerontologist*, **29**, 140.

Kiyak, H. A. and Grayston, N. (1991). Does health promotion improve health practices? *The Gerontologist*, **31**, 85.

Kiyak, H. A., Grayston, N., and Crinean, C. (1992). Oral health problems and needs of nursing home residents. *Comm. Dent. Oral Epidem.* In press.

Kiyak, H. A. and Mulligan, K. (1987). Studies of the relationship between oral health and psychological well-being. *Gerodontics*, **3**, 109–12.

Langer, E. and Rodin, J. (1976). Effects of choice and enhanced personal responsibility for the aged. *Journal of Personality and Social Psychology*, **33**, 191–8.

Lawton, M. P. (1975). The Philadelphia Geriatric Center Morale Scale: a revision. *Journal of Gerontology*, **30**, 85–9.

Lingenbrink, P. and Kiyak, H. A. (1991). Oral health promotion for nurse aides in nursing homes. *J. Dent. Res.*, **70**, 1799.

McClelland, D. C. (1989). Motivational factors in health and disease. *Amer. Psychol.*, **44**, 675–83.

National Center for Health Statistics (1987). *Current estimates from the national health survey: US 1986* (National Health Survey). Vital and Health Statistics, Series 10, No. 164, DHHS Publication No. 82-1569, US Government Printing Office, Washington, DC.

National Center for Health Statistics (1990). *Current estimates from the national health survey: US 1989*. Vital and Health Statistics, Series 10, No. 176, DHHS Publication No. 88–1872, US Government Printing Office, Washington, DC.

NIDR (National Institute for Dental Research) (1987). *Oral health of US adults: 1985–1986*. US Government Printing Office, Washington, DC.

Price, S. C. and Kiyak, H. A. (1981). A behavioral approach to improving oral health among the elderly. *Spec. Care Dent.*, **1**, 267–74.

Rauch, J. (1988). Economic report: growing old. *National Journal*, December 31, 3234–44.

Rockstein, M. and Sussman, M. (1979). *Biology of aging*. Wadsworth, Belmont, CA.

Rodin, J. and Langer, E. J. (1977). Long-term effects of a control-relevant intervention with institutionalized aged. *Journal of Personality and Social Psychology*, **35**, 897–903.

Rotter, J. B. (1966). Generalized expectancies for internal versus external control of reinforcement. *Psych. Monographs*, **80**, 1–28.

Sachs, D. A. (1975). Behavioral techniques in a residential nursing home facility. *Journal of Behavioral Therapy and Experimental Psychiatry*, **6**, 123–7.

Smith, E. (1979). Epidemiology of oral and pharyngeal cancers in the United States: review of recent literature. *Journal of the National Cancer Institute*, **63**, 1189–8.

United Nations Secretariat (1989). *World population prospects, 1988*. Population Studies #106. Department of International Economic and Social Affairs. United Nations, N. Y.

US Bureau of the Census (1991). 1980 and 1990 censuses of the population. *General Population Characteristics* PC80-1-B1, Table 45. Bureau of the Census, Washington, DC.

6F

Oral health promotion in developing countries

MURRAY DICKSON

Recent textbooks on public health or epidemiology frighten me by showing how much public health has lost its original link to social justice, social change, and social reform, and how it has opted for behavioural victim-blaming instead.

Dr Halfdan Mahler (1988)

Many people associate oral health promotion with health talks and posters, but to others it is more encompassing, as in the words of the World Health Organization: 'health promotion is the process of enabling people to increase control over, and to improve, their health' (Epp 1986). In the application of health promotion to oral health, one must come to consider an expanded sphere of determinants that influence oral disease in order to develop interventions that are effective, acceptable, and sustainable.

To that end, several themes weave through this chapter: the multideterminant nature of oral disease, the capacity of oral health promotion to be enabling for both communities and dental workers, the desire for sustainability, and the fact that these apply to situations existing in both industrialized and third world countries.

Imagine... You are a 25-year-old woman with three children and a husband away in the city in search of work. You are totally preoccupied trying to cope with daily events that seem overwhelming. You feel frustrated and angry about your own life situation as even dental workers berate you saying that you must 'do better', for both yourself and your children. If only your children were able to go to school and you had a chance to make something of yourself, maybe then you would be able to work on your family's oral health.

As it is now, the dental system delivers neither general improvements in the quality of life nor ideas as to its relationship with dentistry. The scenario of the mother and her children is all too common and is not limited to developing countries. The fact is that a majority of people worldwide are struggling just to survive and are not deserving of our chastisement. We must recognize that people's realities are not always of their making and that they often have limited opportunities to adopt new health behaviours. For many people, health is simply surviving without major debilitating disease. At best, health is having enough land, food, and water, educating one's children, living in peace, and safe-guarding values like caring, sharing, belonging, and being able to look forward to a better tomorrow.

Unfortunately, dental workers often see themselves and their services as the solution to people's oral problems and the means for achieving oral health. This thinking has even influenced their public who come to believe that their own oral health is really the responsibility of dental workers. Dental training contributes to this dependency by preparing dental workers to treat and to prevent sickness rather than enable people to achieve their own oral health. Our professional solutions often ignore the complexity of the human condition and the importance of self-care and empowerment. Professional training tends to nurture a certain arrogance in which knowledge and skills are seen as the prerogative of professionals, giving us a certain superiority. Poor people, whether they live in cities or rural areas, are perceived as uninformed and backward, having only themselves to blame for both their poverty and their poor oral health. Inevitably, dental services tend to ignore vulnerable, poor populations. Urban-based dental professionals and government officials do not see poor people and do not know their realities or their real needs. Worse, as Chambers (1983) astutely points out, professionals do not know that they do not know!

There are exceptions. Some professionals consciously choose to work with neglected populations; they challenge the status quo, and are redefining public health dentistry and the kind of dental personnel needed to practise it. We can learn from them and benefit.

Promoting oral health is a phrase which means different things to different people. The result is a spectrum of views which spans 'services' for people to 'development' of people through programmes of oral health promotion that have as their basis human and societal well-being. The service approach is the conventional one and predominates. It sees oral health as something to be delivered to people by professionals. Thus, the primary participants are seen as being either 'providers' or 'beneficiaries' and oral health a variation on clinical dentistry. While providers direct information *at* people and prescribe prevention to people as a form of care, beneficiaries soon learn *to* see themselves as recipients of helpful procedures. The service approach sets up the typical paradox between treatment and prevention. Despite prominence being given to disease prevention and oral health promotion, national expenditures continue to go towards more facilities, equipment, local anaesthetic, and restorative materials rather than to public health. Further, most resources are expended on the elite who are able to pay and who demand ever more sophisticated services.

Meanwhile, the greater population remains voiceless and welcomes almost any dental service, whether it is appropriate or not. There then occurs a kind of dental iatrogenesis in which additional dental problems arise as a result of the care that exists to prevent and treat them.

In many African countries dental workers insist on saving more teeth through root canal treatments. They have requested, even demanded, proper equipment, instruments, and filling materials, and more clinical training. But, it is all too much for the meagre budgets of most Ministries of Health. Besides, more clinical care would take dental workers away from programmes considered to be an equal priority.

Yet, root canal treatments continue, often to the immediate satisfaction of patient and clinician. However, seldom seen or appreciated by them is the asymptomatic root resorption that occurs and then the chronic osteomyelitis which is more often seen and treated by doctor and nurse colleagues at the hospital.

This kind of situation is of concern to many countries and explains why a 'development' view of oral health promotion is increasingly being seen by them as a means for addressing the unhealthy and unacceptable state of dental dependency that currently exists. The development view situates oral health within the context of overall well-being of people in their communities. Well-being is not restricted to biology and behaviours; rather, it extends to the political and social structures that permit — or do not permit — people to have control over their lives and, in turn, over their oral health. The result is a shift from caring for people to working with people. This emphasis moves the worker–patient relationship to a more informed partnership between a supportive professional and an involved community.

Oral health promotion focuses on working with people to remove barriers to health, barriers that are seen to be very much a part of people's social and physical environments (Grossman 1990). It is this multideterminant, empowerment view of oral health promotion that is emerging in developing countries. It contests the current practice of promoting only personal life-style changes and advocates for healthy public policy and overall community development.

The intent is to create a supportive living and working context that nurtures an increasing sense of personal control and participatory competence (Lord and McKillop Farlow 1990). The challenge that follows is to prepare oral health workers with relevant skills and attitudes, and to support them for roles in that process.

Realities

Certain fallacies continue to afflict oral health promotion in developing societies.

The **fallacy of global affliction** views the situation of oral disease in developing countries as endemic with rates of caries that are escalating, and rates of periodontal disease that remain high and destructive.

Developing countries are often described as if their populations are one coherent group. Indeed, there are similarities in disease patterns and standards of living; however, the variations are many and great, and these demand individual and unique oral health approaches.

While there is a decline in caries experience in children and adolescents living in highly industrialized countries, observed levels of caries in developing countries vary, but generally remain low to very low (Leclercq *et al.* 1987; Barmes 1989). A particular problem is that unadjusted averages do not indicate who is seriously affected and, as a result, programmes often do not focus on individuals and groups who are most at risk.

Meanwhile, data suggest that periodontal diseases may not be a greater problem in developing countries and that severe stages of periodontal destruction may not be as common as previously thought. More epidemiologists tend to agree with local clinicians who have long stated that periodontal disease is not the major cause of tooth loss (Pilot 1988).

The **fallacy of single causes** highlights the interrelationship of oral structures with micro-organisms and substrates. This leads logically to the development of single interventions which aim at interfering with that relationship, in particular by altering the behaviour of people.

People's reality, however, varies and their social, economic, and physical contexts present unique limitations such that the efficacy of an intervention that is broadly seen to be universal may be less so in some situations. Limitations may be, for example, a lack of water, children attending school in shifts, or culturally bound understandings of oral disease such that tooth pain equates with punishment for past wrongdoings. Alternative means of understanding, explaining, and practising oral hygiene have been developed; they simply await proper recognition for the positive and popular results that they might provide (Enwonwu 1988).

The **fallacy of scarce resources** underlines the constant and critical shortage of dental equipment and materials which becomes the rationale for explaining why initiative is low and why outreach programmes are not occurring.

Not sufficiently acknowledged are local dental workers and their public who are, themselves, resources. They are reservoirs of ideas for explaining and promoting acceptable and beneficial practices. For example, just as a mother knows to clean and plait her daughter's hair, so she can help to clean her mouth (Figs 6.8 and 6.9).

In this case a traditional practice is used as the basis for a new skill, teeth cleaning. Knowing local practices, ones that are helpful, and being able to teach in non-formal ways, make a dental worker relevant and appreciated. Local cleaning materials like a chewing stick are not discouraged. In fact, they are used deliberately, for it is important to be clear about the intent: the first step in achieving a cleaner mouth is the development and acceptance of a cleaning habit (Dickson 1983).

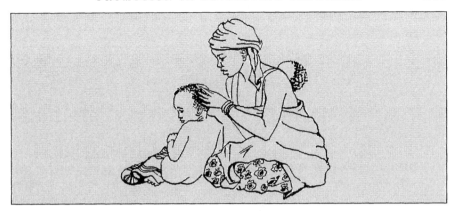

Fig. 6.8 Hair grooming

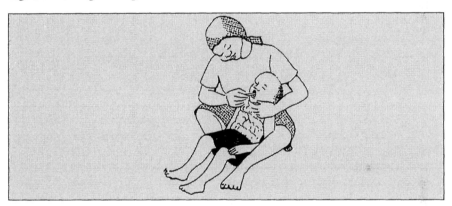

Fig. 6.9 Teeth cleaning

Scarce resources often pose a dilemma for the oral health worker. At one level, the job description and training of the worker may not reflect the realities and needs of the people in the community. At another level, the worker's efforts contribute to a system which continues to increase expenditure on clinical interventions that often waste scarce resources and make no real impression on overall oral health.

Risk factors

Oral epidemiological research has long documented that oral health status is jeopardized by self-imposed risks. 'If only people would practise better oral hygiene, consume less sugar, eat more locally grown foods, buy toothpaste containing fluoride, be more interested in their children's teeth, go to the clinic earlier for care ...'

The effect is to create the impression that oral health is primarily dependent upon individual lifestyle choices and that these are best addressed by transferring knowledge and providing scientifically based biological and behavioural interventions (Labonte and Penfold 1981). Seldom considered or addressed as risk factors are such things as physical and emotional poverty, feelings of helplessness, vulnerability, isolation, poor self-esteem, and diminished self-confidence. Yet, recent research suggests that these amount to being confounders of the more conventional risk factors (Wallerstein and Bernstein 1988). Taken together, they present a web of risk factors (Fig. 6.10) that explain an underlying susceptibility to oral disease.

By describing oral health only in individual terms, the social context in which personal choices are made remains hidden. Dental personnel must learn to include problems that lie outside individual control and must participate with colleagues on actions which aim to improve individual and group literacy, self-esteem, dignity, leadership, power, and control.

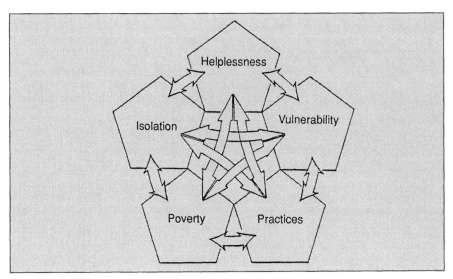

Fig. 6.10   The web of risk factors (adapted from Chambers 1983).

Shifting the focus

A problem with the behavioural approach to improving oral health is that the amount of control that people have over their own health is overestimated. In fact, health is determined by much more than behaviour. Health is, for instance, equally influenced by the environment in terms of resources and supports available. A classic example of this involves people's expectations which are often the product of advertising; the result is that throughout the world there are populations who feel there is no point in brushing when they have no toothpaste.

Equally important is the need to realize that health is more than simply the absence of disease.

Mothers at a maternal and child health clinic in rural Africa are being given a dental health talk. A poster is shown. It has two children: one is happy and the other sad. The sad child is obviously thin and her mouth shows swollen gums and black caries. In between the children is a toothbrush. The caption below reads *Cleaning your child's teeth makes a healthy and happy mouth.*

Presenting the solution to children's mouth problems as simply being better teeth cleaning may seem logical but it is neither appropriate nor acceptable in a poor society. By being insensitive to the child's social circumstances, mothers and children are unfairly held accountable for economic and social inequities that affect both nutrition and hygiene in their society. Many mothers *do* have children who are sad and have bleeding gums, just as in the poster. This is not because mothers are uncaring or are unwilling to act, but because that is what happens when a child is thin and debilitated. Illness is part of the familiar pattern of life.

Oh love, oh my love,
tell me
are we poor because we do not
have riches
or
is it that we don't have riches
because we are poor ?
                    Translated from an old Columbian folk song

By restricting our social analysis, we fail to recognize how poverty and oral health are linked in a vicious cycle. Poor people are poor because they are underemployed, because they have insufficient skills to compete in the work force, because they are raising children while their partners are away seeking work, and because they are often sick and not able to work. The subculture of poverty contributes to poor education, and that leads to inadequate understanding of how the body works, how sickness occurs, what are the early warning signs, and how certain principles of nutrition and personal hygiene can make a difference.

Mothers who are poor deliver babies with low birth-weights and these children are later seen with linear hypoplasia, a condition that makes their teeth vulnerable. Incipient dental problems go unattended and worsen steadily over time until the afflicted person finally arrives at the clinic with a life-threatening complication.

Poor people feel distanced socially from the better off and well-informed professionals who purport to serve their needs. It is said that we, the dental professionals, 'just don't speak their language'. Communication becomes directive and is limited to a simple dialogue around procedures. Many poor people are functionally illiterate and that seriously limits their comprehension of post-operative instructions and health education messages. Since they are continuously unemployed and unacknowledged, their self-esteem may suffer and their view of their own poverty and resulting poor oral health becomes rationalized as punishments for personal inadequacy.

What, then, is meant by poverty? It is not so much a matter of limited possessions, for the income and possessions of an unemployed North American would be like a king's ransom to a member of a farming community in central Africa. Poverty is a more subtle and significant affair; it means limited power. The majority of people living in developing countries are poor, and poor people have no meaningful control over many events in their lives. Is oral health any different? To what extent do people really control their own oral health?

Oral health promotion as community development

The dominant aspiration of our times is development — of individuals, groups, communities, and society as a whole. To this end, Jenkins and Bryant (1979) describe development in human terms like belonging, caring, counting for something, sharing, becoming... being on the way.

Development becomes a reality for a person only when it has become a reality for all; when the whole of an individual and all individuals have benefited. The aim is human promotion. To meet immediate needs, such as the sickness of oral disease, is undoubtedly a useful action. But, such measures only relieve need temporarily; sickness will return. Community development means increasing awareness of problems and possibilities, channelling energy into self-care and mutual help experiences, and using these experiences to crystallize a new consciousness — in both professionals and the public — and then keeping it going through organization.

Community development is the backbone of community health promotion (Labonte 1987). The intent is to integrate traditional 'top–down' approaches with newer 'bottom–up' approaches. In this way, 'top–down' people receive the guidance they need for their work to be relevant and effective, and 'bottom–up' people are adequately supported with information, training, and finances. It is a process that acknowledges local people as resources to build upon. The aim of community development is to openly and supportively create community self-reliance which might then help ensure that oral health promotion programmes reach the greater population and are sustained.

A community development approach to oral health moves us beyond focusing on individual behaviours to social actions that provide and create conditions for improved health. In this, the critical contribution is the active involvement of local people in confronting issues that they know more intimately than anyone else. As George Kent (1981) is fond of asking, 'Why should local people be the beneficiaries but not the producers of their own development?'

Strengthening community capacity and action is emphasized in the Ottawa Charter that emerged from the 1986 international conference on health promotion.

Health promotion works through concrete and effective community action in setting priorities, making decisions, planning strategies, and implementing them to achieve better health. At the heart of this process is the empowerment of communities, their ownership and control of their own destinies.

In the context of their communities, people develop and become empowered when they decide and act for themselves on issues that are theirs to live with over the long term. Thus, mothers choose to breast feed instead of bottle feed not because they have been told to do it, but because they arrive at their own understanding of the situation and decide for themselves that breast feeding is in their baby's best interest.

A caring and skilled community dental worker can be instrumental in helping local people identify issues and realize their own capacities for confronting issues and affecting overall community health and development. For instance, showing a drawing of a local child with caries, and using a popular education method called 'But Why?' (Werner and Bower 1982), a dentist helped members of an Indian Tribal Council in Canada analyse their own dental state of affairs.

What do you see?
  A child with caries.
What else?
  I see a sad face.
But why?
  Probably the child is hungry.
But why?
  Maybe it has something to do with that baby bottle.
But why?
  Perhaps it is the sugar that we add to tea.
But why?
  Sweet tea quietens a baby.

At this point, discussion occurred about sugar, baby bottles, teeth, and comforting a young child who is upset. The analysis then continued on to such overriding health concerns as equity, justice, and self-reliance.

Okay, let's talk about sugar. On this day the mother had no sugar in her house.
Why?
  The mother was not given any money.
But why?
  There was no more money. Her husband has no work.
But why?
  He has only grade 4 education and so is not able to work for the Company.

But why?
  There is no point returning to school. What is taught does not relate to what is important to us.
But why?
  Because decisions are made by outsiders.
But why?
  Because we are not involved.
But why?
  Because we never tried.
But why?
  Yeh... Why not ! Then, our children could learn our traditions and want to stay 'on the land'.

AMEN ! !

Helping people to analyse their own problems is a key, initial step to gaining control over their lives. It is part of an overall strategy for oral health that begs to be legitimized.

Supportive strategies

Drawing on the Ottawa Charter framework, five key strategies are identified which can be built into a model for improving oral health promotion (Fig. 6.11).

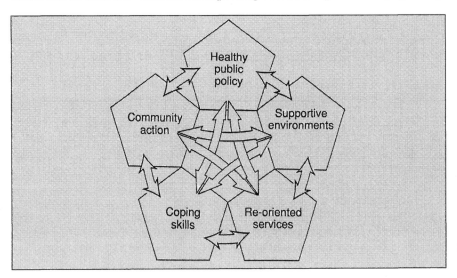

Fig. 6.11   Strategies for oral health promotion.

Building healthy public policy

Policy is a consensus on ideas that form the basis for coordinated actions which, in turn, ensure that services are provided equitably and healthy environments are maintained. Governments are ultimately responsible for the health of populations through conditions they permit or create. Oral health promotion policies that are the profession's and community's to recommend and the government's to legislate include:

(1) a national food policy which controls the production of processed, sugar-added foods (Sheiham and Plamping 1988) and supports the growth and distribution of traditional foods;

(2) a national policy on baby bottles, restricting their purchase to women who present a prescription attesting to the fact that they are not able to breast feed;

(3) a national policy on water or salt fluoridation and on fluorides in toothpaste (Sheiham and Plamping 1988);

(4) a national dental policy, compelling dental workers to spend half of each day working in such outreach programmes as school health, maternal and child health, and literacy.

Creating supportive environments

The aim is to contribute to the improvement of environments which support health. Areas of attention for oral health workers to act upon include:

(1) encouraging trade stores that are near schools to stock, promote and display non-sugared foods.

(2) periodically sampling sources of drinking water and requesting that they be analysed for contaminants and natural occurring fluoride;

(3) fostering supportive attitudes towards breast feeding;

(4) participating in community programmes which are aimed at improving the lives of women, young children, and adolescents.

Strengthening community action

It is important to involve more people in situational analyses, programme planning, and action. Dental workers can:

(1) join with community activists in networks and coalitions and work together on community issues of common concern;

(2) support school gardens as a means for both encouraging cooperative action and growing and eating healthy food;

(3) become members of teams engaged in literacy and maternal child health programmes;

(4) organize a dental planning committee, fill half of the positions with lay members, and allow the committee to make meaningful dental decisions.

Developing coping skills

The intent is to increase people's abilities for controlling oral disease and for improving oral health. Critical is the strengthening of self-confidence such that people feel an element of control over the options that are being presented and, therefore, over their own oral health. To that end, dental workers can help people to:

(1) differentiate between traditional beliefs and practices that are good and worth keeping and those that are harmful and need to be changed;

(2) be role models to family members and neighbours in terms of food that is grown, purchased, and eaten, and practices of oral hygiene;

(3) examine at home the mouths of younger children, recognize developing problems, and know where and when to get help;

(4) choose toothpastes that contain fluoride and sources of drinking water having optimum amounts of fluoride.

Reorientating dental services

The desire is twofold: to nurture a more holistic practice of dentistry and oral health promotion, recognizing the importance of people's emotional, cultural, and social well-being; and to challenge the professional status quo such that strategies of care include restructuring established delivery systems (Hobdell and Sheiham 1981: Sheiham and Plamping 1988).

Movement in this regard is possible when dental officials accept for themselves the principles of primary health care and prepare dental workers, through training and support in the field, to:

(1) reach out to groups that are disadvantaged by taking their services to people and not require people to always come to them;

(2) deliberately solicit public opinion about their work in order to be accountable to the people they serve;

(3) focus on prevention instead of only cure, promote practices of self-care, and prepare others to become nonformal teachers for oral health;

(4) create systems and technologies that are not dependent on the capital city or other countries for maintenance;

(5) function not in isolation but in association with other community health and development workers and their programmes.

Participatory research

The usual arguments for research remain valid, especially so in societies where populations are particularly at risk and where material resources are expensive and scarce. Thus, it remains important to know through research that education is well targeted, that preventive agents like sealants and fluoride are being used in cost-effective ways, and that oral health is improving as a result.

A problem, however, is that present approaches to oral health research focus heavily on quantifying data, while minimizing the contextual influences on this data. They also tend to demand the skills of an external 'expert'. The effect is to separate people from their own problem identification, analysis, and resolutions by handing that process over to others. Instead of being enlightening and liberating, research is often one more example of people's issues being in another's control (Dickson 1992).

Participatory research is different. It offers an alternate paradigm for viewing and conducting research with the explicit intent of not only describing reality but changing it — and who better than community members to observe and measure their own realities in democratic interaction with researchers? The role of the researcher becomes one of joining a community group and working in solidarity with members to understand and overcome specific issues of concern (Society for Participatory Research in Asia 1982).

Using participatory research, there can be a greater likelihood of posing the kinds of questions that affect health over the longer term and of developing manageable tools for conducting qualitative research into social pathologies like disunity, poor participation, poor integration of primary care services, worker apathy, and system abuse, all of which continue to plague dental care and so equally need to be understood in order to be addressed.

Can local people with a minimum of education actually conduct research? The answer is, yes — if it is directed at a question that is of concern to people and if the process for answering the question is theirs to decide upon. The role of the oral health worker is to learn to assist and guide community members in their own research process.

A participatory approach to oral health research generates benefits at two levels. First, it helps to ensure that a variety of dental questions are asked which provide an analysis of the most neglected sectors of society. Second, participatory research builds skills and self-confidence of those involved, dental worker and lay colleagues alike. It therefore promotes human development, essential if oral health promotion is to move from rhetoric to action, and from short term to long term.

The challenge

Where sustainable development may be the public health issue for the 1990s, promoting oral health through community development must become the priority strategy of dental public health everywhere. It is important to remember that probably no idea has had greater impact on our thinking about health and sustainability in this decade as the realization that ordinary people acting for themselves can do more to maintain personal and community health than scores of workers can do for them (Grossman 1990).

A serious problem is the fact that dental systems seldom nurture participation. When it is mentioned, there is a wide gap between the language and the reality of participation: often, organizations that espouse advocacy and participation, in reality continue to do things *for* people. Worse, participants may still want to be taken care of, thus extending dependency.

Clearly, an empowerment paradigm differs significantly from traditional approaches which are steeped in a dependency on scarce experts and, seemingly, specialized knowledge. Workers who practise oral health promotion need to think about participation and empowerment in broad terms. This includes learning from other areas of endeavour, including those of social sciences, adult education, and participatory research. We need to critically listen to people we say we serve and support. We must pay attention to the qualitative process of interventions and not just focus on their outcomes.

Moreover, we must recognize that adopting a community development perspective will call for significant changes in the structure and philosophy of both oral health promotion and of dental service systems. Moving from rhetoric to action will mean new roles for dental workers and for their organizations. Instead of simply transferring information and skills to those in need, they will be advocates for change both in terms of the meaning of community dentistry and the nature of training for its practice. If we direct ourselves at increasing such things as people's self-esteem, literacy, and leadership, we will be working to increase their strength. Interestingly, by so doing our own dental programmes may become markedly changed, even diminished, and yet oral health improve. What has been achieved is the growth of health and community but not necessarily the programme! The fundamental difference is in approach; instead of starting with disease and finding ways to attack and control it, one focuses on health and then finds ways to improve health whilst attacking disease.

A challenge now being faced head-on by dental structures in many developing countries is welcoming what others say that they need from dentistry and then being willing to change to work with people for oral health instead of trying to provide it for them. Clearly, a related challenge that awaits, one which is now being taken up by indigenous dental educators in countries like Mozambique, is preparing dental workers to have the consciousness and facilitative skills for working with people in the community development movement.

References

Barmes, D. (1989). International perspectives for the first quarter of the twenty-first century. *Swedish Dental Journal*, **13**, 1–6.

Chambers, R. (1983). *Rural development: putting the last first.* Longman Group Limited, Essex.

Dickson, M. (1983). *Where there is no dentist.* Hesperian Foundation, California.

Dickson, M. (1993). Community based research in dentistry. In *Proceedings: international (Berlin) workshop on improving oral health services for deprived communities.* German Foundation for International Development. In press.

Enwonwu, C.O. (1988). Societal expectations for oral health: response of the dental care system in Africa. *Journal of Public Health Dentistry*, **48**, 84–93.

Epp, J. (1986). *Achieving health for all: a framework for health promotion.* Health and Welfare, Canada.

Grossman, J. (1990). Health education: the leading edge of maternal and child health. In *Health care of women and children in developing countries*, (ed. H.M. Wallace and K. Giri), pp. 56–67. Third Party Publishing Company, California.

Hobdell, M. and Sheiham, A. (1981). Barriers to the promotion of dental health in developing countries. *Social Science and Medicine*, **15A**, 817–23.

Jenkins, D. and Bryant, J.H. (1979). *Moral issues and health care — the continuing debate.* In *Contact* special series No. 2. Christine Medical Commission, Geneva.

Kent, G. (1981). Community-based development planning. *Third World Planning Review*, **3**, 313–26.

Labonte, R. (1987). Community health promotion strategies. *Health Promotion*, **26**, 5–11.

Labonte, R. and Penfold, S. (1981). Canadian perspectives in health promotion: a critique. *Health Education*, **19**, 4–8.

Leclercq, M.H., Barmes, D.E., and Infirri, J.S. (1987). Oral health: global trends and projections. *World Health Statistics Quarterly*, **40**, 116–128.

Lord, J. and McKillop Farlow, D. (1990). A study of personal empowerment: implications of health promotion. *Health Promotion*, **29**, 2–8.

Mahler, H. (1988). *Keynote address.* At opening session of the Second International Conference on Health Promotion. Adelaide, Australia.

Pilot, T. (1988). Trends in oral health: global perspective. *New Zealand Dental Journal*, **84**, 40–5.

Sheiham, A. and Plamping, D. (1988). Strategies for improving oral health and reforming oral health care systems. *African Dental Journal*, **2**, 2–7.

Society for Participatory Research in Asia (1982). In *Participatory research: an introduction*, available from: International Council for Adult Education, Toronto, Canada.

Wallerstein, N. and Bernstein, E. (1988). Empowerment education: Freire's ideas adapted to health education. *Health Education Quarterly*, **15**, 379–94.

Werner, D. and Bower, B. (1982). Looking at how human relations affect health. In *Helping health workers learn*, Chapter 26, pp. 1–38. Hesperian Foundation, California.

7

Evaluation and planning of oral health promotion programmes

ANTHONY S. BLINKHORN

Introduction

Oral health promotion has as its central theme the improvement and maintenance of the oral health of the general population. This, together with the necessity of updating the knowledge of all health and allied professionals about relevant aspects of preventive dentistry, constitutes the main everyday activities of those involved in oral health promotion and education.

In all dental health care systems health promotion is a minor budgetary item, but by the very nature of its public profile it is open to more scrutiny than many other branches of dentistry. Indeed, health promotion as a whole attracts more criticism than money, and investigations into its potential value are the source of much debate.

The development of health education and promotion as a scientific and valued tool in the armamentarium to improve health has been gaining momentum in the last twenty-five years. Politicians and health care planners have grudgingly realized that in both the Third World and in industrialized societies the majority of ill health is attributable to human behaviour. The AIDS epidemic was the catalyst which provided the final recognition that lifestyle modification and promoting health was an essential part of any health service.

Although now accepted as a useful tool, health promotion has to be implemented in such a way that careful scrutiny of the use of resources as well as the attainment of stated objectives is a planned part of any programme. This means that evaluation and planning cannot just centre on effectiveness, but consideration must be given to efficiency. This may be defined, for the purposes of this chapter, as 'the realistic use of scarce resources to promote an improvement in health' (Dignan 1986). Evaluation and design are not as straightforward as one might expect, therefore the chapter will consider the subjects in nine sections. Eight will concentrate on the scientific basis and practical aspects of evaluation and the last topic will highlight some issues which will be of value to those involved in the practical planning of oral health promotion programmes.

What is evaluation?

Evaluation may be defined as an investigation into the performance of a programme in terms of its success or failure to achieve stated aims. Such a definition is highly specific and can be used to design an intervention which will certainly look appealing to those who demand more scientific rigour in the field of health promotion. There is, however, a broader view of evaluation which defines it as (Green 1977):

the comparison of an object of interest against a standard acceptability.

This definition implies that not only the outcome of a programme should be monitored but also how it is used — 'process evaluation'. Thus, all those involved in oral health promotion should try to split evaluation into a number of component parts, as this aids understanding of the different skills and scientific techniques which will be required. Table 7.1 gives examples of the different types of evaluation that will be required when planning and implementing a new oral health promotion programme.

Table 7.1 shows that there are two broad types of evaluation. Formative or process evaluation centres on the factors involved in the implementation of the programme, plus monitoring and improving the day-to-day running of the campaign. Summative evaluation, on the other hand, concentrates on collecting information once the programme has finished, and as such is detached from the problems encountered in the day-to-day running of a campaign. The aim of summative evaluation is not to influence the outcome of a project but to record success or failure in terms of stated aims and objectives.

Table 7.1   Types of evaluation which make up a typical assessment programme

Formative or process evaluation	Summative evaluation
Pilot assessment: including concept testing	Impact of programme: are target group aware of campaign?
Monitoring process: how is the programme used and what problems are encountered?	Qualitative and quantitative investigations: monitor attainment of stated objectives
	Costings: is intervention economically justifiable?
	Temporal: assess fade of programme over time

Medical commentators (Warner *et al.* 1988; Lancet 1988) have noted that evaluation information is only readily available to support health promotion in broad economic terms in two areas, namely smoking cessation and the control of hypertension. Such comments suggest that in the past investigators have concentrated on the success or failure of the education component, and evaluation as a whole has been confined within rather narrow limits. Hence, this chapter will take the broader definition of evaluation alluded to earlier (Green 1977) as the basis for further discussion.

Why evaluate?

The main reason for evaluating a programme is to assess what has happened as a result of expending human and economic resources in a particular way. However, the evaluation results can be considered from a number of different viewpoints (Rossi *et al.* 1979). For example, a health service manager may see a well publicized campaign as an indicator of the productivity of the health promotion unit, while a dentist in general practice may view advertisements promoting dental visits with some scepticism and concern when no new patients are forthcoming.

Despite these superficial differences, there are several key points which must be considered if the question 'Why evaluate?' is answered in a scientific manner. These are now described.

Should the programme be continued in its present form?

Medical and dental knowledge changes. Is the programme offering information that will actually improve health? For example, the Health Education Authority in England and Wales arranges for a panel of experts to review the scientific literature related to preventive dentistry and then publishes their deliberations in the form of a report entitled *The scientific basis of dental health education* (Levine 1989). This enables programme planners to check that the advice they are offering will benefit the client population, especially as the review is updated on a regular basis.

To determine that the programme is having the desired effect

If there is no evaluation, it is impossible to determine whether the programme is having either a positive or negative effect. This information is necessary as it can be used to modify or improve the programme.

Use of resources

Once a programme has been implemented it should be possible to record costs and then assess the benefits from the expenditure of resources. A programme may be highly effective but too expensive. Monitoring cost will enable investigators to adopt a realistic approach to health promotion programmes (Ledwith 1986).

Can procedures be improved?

Although the programme may be meeting the stated objectives, the evaluation may highlight the fact that a simpler approach might be as effective. This evaluation may encourage innovation.

Ethical considerations

By its very nature, health promotion is trying to alter people's attitudes or behaviour. It is essential to know whether the intervention is working to the benefit of the target population. Trying to change behaviour may involve creating feelings of anxiety and susceptibility (Downie et al. 1990). Is it ethically justifiable not to evaluate such a programme?

Scientific respectability

Many in the medical and dental professions are sceptical of the value of health promotion, so it is important to evaluate programmes in a scientific manner and present the results in the appropriate journals for consideration by the dental profession as a whole.

Defining what should be evaluated

Many health professionals claim that evaluation is a useful and important part of health promotion, but in practice there is concern and unease about what will be investigated. This stems in part from the fact that much of the training for health professionals is devoted to rote learning and little emphasis is given to the skills required for original scientific research.

The key issue is to define the aims and objectives of a programme in a succinct manner. However, many researchers tend to confuse aims with objectives, which has resulted in programmes being planned in such a way as to render scientific evaluation impossible.

Aims are 'planned for effects of an activity' and are usually expressed in general terms.

Objectives are more clearly stated as specific goals. Several objectives can be formulated to meet an overall aim.

Abramson (1984) emphasizes that objectives should be realistic, and formulated in operational terms which can be applied in practice. It is essential to state the objectives of a health promotion project in writing so that they can be assessed in terms of the following questions:

1. Are they clearly expressed?

2. Do they meet the requirements of the study population?

3. Are they expressed in such a way that measurements of success or failure are possible?

4. Do they fit within the budgetary constraints of the overall programme?

If these four questions can be answered positively then an evaluation exercise has a sound foundation.

Evaluation and measurement

Once the investigator has a clear idea of the aims and objectives of a health promotion programme it is possible to design a study to monitor whether these have been accomplished. In order to undertake evaluation there must be some way of measuring attainment of objectives. Indeed, the major factor limiting evaluation is the precision of the measuring instruments. Health promotion by its very nature is concerned with increasing knowledge, raising awareness, modifying behaviour, and changing attitudes; such concepts cannot be measured by a micrometer or ruler and it is up to the researcher to use well developed tests utilized by social scientists or formulate reproducible techniques specifically for the study.

Any measuring instrument be it laboratory or population based must be both reliable and valid (Marsh 1982). Reliability is concerned with consistency. Will the measuring device give the same answer when used on different occasions? If not, the research results would have to be treated with caution. However, the concept of reliability is based on the belief that some errors occur whenever measurements are made. Absolute accuracy exists only in theory. The task for an investigator is to choose measurement techniques that have acceptable levels of error.

Validity has two components, namely internal and external. Internal validity refers to the appropriateness of the methodology — does it measure what it intended to measure? At the end of the programme, can an investigator claim that the intervention has actually produced the results obtained? Internal validity also has another parameter, namely time. The extent to which measurement is valid for present conditions is termed concurrent validity, while the way in which a measurement will predict future developments is referred to as predictive validity.

External validity refers to generalizations that can be made to a broader reference population beyond the target group under investigation. If a study is too specific, the results cannot be applied on a wider basis.

Most programme evaluations are based on samples, as it is not feasible to collect information from every participant nor to monitor every part of a health promotion programme. Thus sampling will have an all pervasive influence on the success of the measurements (Tones *et al.* 1990). Also, an evaluation study not only collects information from a sample of participants but may also select representatives from programme staff, teachers, health professionals, and other groups involved in the dissemination of information.

Problems of measurement in the evaluation of health promotion

Health promotion programmes are designed to influence target populations through specifically planned interventions (**process**). These may have immediate effects (**impact**) as well as more long term influences (**outcomes**). For example, a programme to promote dental visiting could involve mass media as a way of promulgating the campaign's goals (process). An individual hearing the advice could be made aware that a dental visit was beneficial (impact) and might well arrange an appointment in the future (outcome). Clearly, evaluation could assess just one or all three components of a programme. Many investigators tend to concentrate on impact and rarely include data on the campaign activities (process) or the longer term effects (outcomes). Such omissions mean that in some campaigns the evaluation component is lightweight and superficial.

The perennial problem for behavioural scientists of 'how to measure human behaviour' is a spectre that haunts many involved in health promotion when items such as process, impact, and outcome are considered. Although a clear statement of the objectives of a health promotion exercise is crucial, there is still the problem of trying to record potential behavioural change through such proxy measures as knowledge and attitude changes. Sufficient knowledge and a positive attitudinal change are prerequisites to alterations in behaviour but the jump from high knowledge/positive attitudes to behaviour change is not straightforward. All too often, behaviour change does not occur despite increases in knowledge and changes in attitudes (Baric 1990). Therefore it is sensible wherever possible to devise some way of measuring behaviour change directly if the objectives of the programme are expressed in terms of altering behaviour.

The study population

The planning phase of an evaluation programme is detailed in Table 7.2. The formulation of objectives has already been discussed so the next problem is to consider the selection of the study population and the variables to be measured. Schou in her chapter on *Oral health promotion in the work place* (Chapter 6D) highlights the importance of having sufficient knowledge about a target group before implementing a health promotion exercise. She cites as an example the 'Treatwell Programme' devised by Sorensen *et al.* (1990) which sought to base a health promotional activity on a sound theoretical framework. Orlandi (1986) for example, suggests that knowledge of an

Table 7.2 Planning phase of an evaluation study

Aims described and specific objectives formulated		
Study design		
Population to be included	a) sample defined	
	b) size of sample	
Variables to be measured	a) agreed	
	b) scales of assessment chosen	
Method of data collection assessed and refined		
Data processing		

organization and the norms of a particular group, together with an assessment of potential barriers to health promotion are prerequisites to efficient planning and study group selection.

Investigators will usually have selected a study population because of their interest in solving a particular health problem. However, some researchers plan health campaigns without considering the appropriateness and practicality of their interventions. The appropriateness of a population under study refers to its suitability for the attainment of the objectives of the campaign. For example, a programme to reduce caries among 12-year-old children in a middle-class area in the south of England would be of questionable value as caries rates are so low (Todd and Dodd 1985) that further improvements would be difficult to achieve.

When considering the suitability of a population, it is wise to consider whether the way a sample is selected may affect validity and hence the practicality of making generalizations from the findings. Examples of ways in which the sample may be prejudiced are:

1. Volunteers. People who volunteer to enter a study may differ in many respects from those who refuse to participate. The results from a study based on a volunteer population will not necessarily apply to the population at large. One way around the volunteer problem is to allocate them to active and control groups and then at least a comparative study is available, but generalization will still be a problem. Another approach is to compare the effects of a health promotion programme on active and control groups but to try to record some information on people who did not agree to participate in the active group.

2. Hospital or clinic patients. People receiving dental care are clearly not representative of the general population or of all people suffering from oral diseases.

The problems of prejudicing the way in which a population is chosen can be reduced by having clear, well stated objectives and not generalizing results from a clearly specific group to the general population.

There are always practical difficulties when working with human beings. Laboratory-based scientists can 'pop back' in the evening to recheck a result or run a series of different studies within the same environment. No such luxury for the researcher evaluating a health education programme!

In order to make the research a little easier, it makes sense to ensure that the chosen population is accessible and that obtaining the required information and long-term follow up are possible. One of the tribulations for the health educator is that certain accessible populations are being 'over-researched' by a variety of scientists from different university and health board departments. Schools in particular are becoming resistant to the entreaties of researchers. Only well designed and relevant projects stand a chance of being accepted by education authorities. It is interesting to note that some clinicians have accepted that little is known about the value of a good many treatment regimes when assessed in terms of patient satisfaction and an improvement in the quality of life. This concern has led to a greater interest in medical audit, whereby both treatment planning and outcome are being scrutinized in more detail. Those working in health promotion have been in the forefront of this type of research.

In the majority of studies it is usually possible only to investigate part or a 'sample' of the total population involved in a campaign. The need to take a sample is usually necessary in order to optimize resources and it also allows more detailed information to be collected because the number of individuals to be studied is restricted.

There is usually no difficulty in applying the results obtained from investigating a sample to the main study group, provided that certain precautions have been taken. These are:

1. The sample should be representative of the total population under investigation.

2. The sample should be sufficiently large in order to keep sample variation to a minimum.

3. There must be adequate coverage of the sample in order to avoid bias. Non-respondents are a serious problem which can reduce coverage and lead to bias.

Researchers should make great efforts to sample correctly and avoid selecting the easy option, as this can lead to serious flaws in the research design. For example, interviewing people stopped at random in an out-of-town shopping centre is fairly straightforward but it will undoubtedly exclude people at work and those who are unable to afford transport to a site on the periphery of a conurbation.

There are two different techniques which may be employed by a researcher to aid in the selection of a sample in a scientific manner and can be encompassed by the terms probability and non-probability sampling.

A probability sample is one in which each person in a selected population has an equal chance of being included. This involves preparing a sampling frame, a list of all the people from whom the sample is to be selected, which is no easy task given that people move and lists are invariably out of date. Once the frame has been delineated and the sample size agreed, it is possible to draw a random sample. The size of the sample in relation to the total population in the sampling frame is referred to as the sampling fraction (Mausner and Kramer 1985). It is usually expressed as 1 in 'N'.

Other probability sampling methods include cluster sampling, stratified sampling, and two- or multistage sampling.

Cluster sampling selects groups or clusters of individuals at random rather than individual subjects. It is a convenient technique but care has to be taken to avoid selecting clusters containing similar people, as it then may be unwise to make generalizations about the general population forming the initial sampling frame. A way of overcoming this difficulty is to select a considerable number of small clusters rather than a few large clusters.

The stratified sampling technique, as its name implies, involves grouping individuals according to a category considered important for the research, such as age, school type, initial Decayed, Missing, and Filled Teeth (DMFT) scores, and dental knowledge. This procedure reduces sample variation with respect to the particular topics used in the stratifying process.

In two-stage sampling, the population is divided into a set of primary sampling units and a sample of these is then selected at random. The primary unit could be classes of schoolchildren or households. The multistage version is similar except that there can be a number of stages in the sampling technique. It is a useful method of arriving at a manageable sample if a large-scale survey is planned.

Probability sampling relies on the availability of a sampling frame. However, it may not be possible to devise a frame for certain groups, such as drug users. If one wanted to evaluate the value of a campaign directed at intravenous drug addicts discouraging the habit of sharing needles, a major difficulty would be finding the at-risk population, thus a non-probability sampling technique would have to be employed. The only way to gather information would be to ask social workers to suggest clients who might participate in a research project. Clearly, such a study could be biased but provided the results were treated with caution and the sampling problems discussed, some potentially useful information may well be collected.

Another type of non-probability sampling technique is the quota system, which is used a great deal by market research companies and those investigating the impact of mass media health promotion programmes. An interviewer is given a set of quota of specific types of people to question, and will endeavour to fill the set quota. It is not a truly random selection as the sampling frame is unknown, but it is commonly used to measure the impact of media-based programmes. The quotas can be predetermined so that they reflect specific characteristics of a population under study. For example, an interviewer would be given set targets of men and women in certain age bands. Although a popular technique, the results obtained must be viewed with some caution.

The most important aspect of any type of sampling procedure is to set up the selection rules in advance and thereby avoid the choice of subjects being based on ease of access or convenience.

Collecting the data

The type of data collection system used to monitor the value of a health promotion programme depends on the stated aims. Most programmes will be orientated to changing knowledge, altering attitudes, and modifying behaviour. However, in some instances, changes in environmental conditions or public policies may be investigated. The importance of policy and the implications for oral health promotion are discussed in Chapter 4.

Recording changes in knowledge before and after an intervention, preferably involving the use of a control group, is a popular and well proven way of evaluating a programme which seeks to improve people's information about a particular health risk. This can be undertaken in two ways — quantitatively or qualitatively. Qualitative research needs little introduction as it is based on the use of questionnaires or formally structured interviews to gain data. Questionnaires require considerable work and expertise to ensure that the data collected gives useful information. Davies and Ware (1982) suggested that greater reliability could be obtained by asking batteries of questions to investigate a topic rather than relying on a single question. In order to guard against subjects agreeing or disagreeing with statements regardless of their content, equal numbers of positive and negative statements about a particular health issue should be included in any battery of questions (Winkler *et al.* 1982). There is also a danger that respondents will give socially desirable answers to a question rather than reveal their true feelings. One way to overcome this is to try and keep questions neutral and thereby reduce socially acceptable responses. Quantitative research is also characterized by the requirement to select correspondents on a statistically representative basis.

Qualitative research, on the other hand, utilizes informal discussions with individuals, small group discussions, or the actual observation of groups or individuals (Blinkhorn *et al.* 1989). Qualitative research also allows the investigator to use complicated interviewing techniques concentrating on imagery, feelings, and motivation, areas where questionnaire-based methods may be criticized for lacking depth and subtlety. Research findings based on discussion do have some problems which must be considered when undertaking an investigation. The major one is 'response set biases', whereby people being interviewed often give socially desirable answers, or are defensive if they feel emotionally threatened. These difficulties are compounded in group discussions if one person is allowed to dominate the conversation. These problems can only be overcome by using well trained interviewers or group leaders (Blinkhorn *et al.* 1983).

Although the two techniques of quantitative and qualitative research are quire different, they are both useful research tools provided that the objectives of the health promotion programme are clearly stated, so that the collected data are not used to assess whether success has been achieved for objectives that were not included in the initial intervention.

Another way of collecting data is termed the ethnographic approach (Nettleton 1986) which relies heavily on participant observation. Although useful for problem definition work, it has only limited value in any evaluation research programme, being too small in scale, open to bias, and ethically questionable.

Apart from the decision to use qualitative or quantitative data collection techniques, it is also important to consider whether attitudinal changes will be recorded. Attitudes are central to health promotion since they tie together people's feelings and beliefs which are important determinants of health-related behaviour. Attitudes have several dimensions. Ajzen and Fishbein (1977) identified four specific elements:

(1) action element — what behaviour is required;

(2) target element — where should the behaviour be directed;

(3) context element — where is the behaviour to be undertaken;

(4) time element — when should the behaviour be undertaken.

They have suggested that the apparent lack of correlation between attitudes and behaviour may be due to the fact that measurements of the two do not take account of the four elements of an attitude. Thus, a measuring instrument for attitudes will be more complex than some earlier researchers had believed.

As attitudes have several dimensions, the measuring instrument will have to identify not only what attitudes are held but also determine how firmly they are held. The commonest way of measuring attitudes is to use 'attitude scales', which quantify attitudes in terms of a range of positive or negative values on an ordinal scale.[1]

The two principal attitude scales were devised by Likert (1932) and Thurstone (1928). The Likert scale is a five-point scale balanced around a neutral point (Table 7.3). An attitude score is then computed by summing the respondent's answer to different statements. The Thurstone scale is more complex and its construction is time consuming as it is based on an eleven-point rating scale indicating the positive or negative feelings towards the attitude object. The topics to be rated in the scale are selected from a large pool of items suggested and scored by a large number of judges, such that the whole continuum of an attitude is measured. While it was considered as a

---

[1] An ordinal scale is composed of categories, such as social class. The categories are distinct but have no inherent numerical distance between them.

Table 7.3   Likert attitude scale — example

Visiting a dentist every six months is important in maintaining my appearance.
The scale would run from:

+2 Strongly agree
+1 Moderately agree
 0 Neutral/don't know
−1 Moderately disagree
−2 Strongly disagree

There would be a series of statements such as the one shown to assess an
individual's assessment of the value of dental visiting. A summation of the
answers would indicate whether there was a positive or negative attitude to
dental visiting.

good way of measuring attitudes on an interval scale in the early years of its
use, the premise that attitudes can be measured in such a way is now thought
to be somewhat dubious, hence it is rarely used.

Another scale commonly used is the 'semantic differential technique' which
consists of a series of bipolar ratings (Osgood *et al.* 1957). The subject's
attitude is calculated by summing the total score from a series of ratings about
the attitude in question. Table 7.4 shows an example of the rating system.

Table 7.4   Semantic differential scale — bipolar rating system which
describes a person's attitude to the topic under investigation

Good	+3	+2	+1	0	−1	−2	−3	Bad
Pleasant	+3	+2	+1	0	−1	−2	−3	Unpleasant

The collection of data before and after a programme is necessary to monitor
attitude change which may well be a precursor to an alteration in health
behaviour. Recording changes in behaviour can be difficult, hence the need
for questionnaires and interviews, which are an attempt to record changes
'second-hand'. Observation is the obvious way of overcoming the problem of
'reported information' but it is time-consuming and not really practical other
than on a small numbers of subjects. However, changes in dental health
behaviour can be monitored by examining the oral soft and hard tissues
which respond in a relatively short time to changes in the oral environment.
This is particularly so when considering programmes aimed at improving oral
hygiene. There are a number of valid indices for recording changes in plaque
deposits and gingival bleeding (Blinkhorn and Mackie 1992).

Caries increment rates over a two-year period could be used to assess the
effectiveness of a preventive programme and sugar consumption rates are
reflected in the numbers of *Streptococcus mutans* and lactobacilli present in the
oral cavity (Blinkhorn and Geddes 1987).

Thus, data collection for recording the value of a programme can be based on:

(1) changes in knowledge and attitudes which may infer an alteration in behaviour;

(2) observation whereby changes in behaviour can be monitored directly, but this is difficult to organize other than in a small-scale project;

(3) changes in oral health, feasible and accurate way of assessing whether health-promoting habits have been adopted.

Evaluation and experimental methodology

Scientific experiments require close attention to standardization of procedures, precision, and careful matching of controls. However, the evaluation of health promotion programmes poses more difficulties in applying a rigourous scientific approach because allowances have to be made when working with communities. Evaluation may be impossible to implement if the scientific demands are too stringent. This being so, it is still essential to avoid the dangers of allowing poor scientific method just because working with 'human beings' can be difficult to organize. Every effort should be made to adopt experimental methods which will reveal useful and valid results (Campbell and Stanley 1963).

One such methodology adopted in health promotion is the comparative study, in which one group receives a programme and another does not. The two groups need not be identical in every other respect, but every effort should be made to match them as closely as possible. For example, a new dental health education initiative could be randomly allocated to half the schools in a region, the remainder acting as controls. Great care would be necessary to ensure that the programme was not offered only to schools interested and willing to undertake dental health promotion. True random allocation is necessary to avoid bias, although some stratification of schools in terms of the social background of the catchment area would be advisable.

The experimental design could be further improved by ensuring that the knowledge, attitudes, and oral health status of the control and experimental groups are measured before the health promotion programme, thereby ensuring that both groups are comparable. However, baseline testing can be a problem as it may encourage the control group to change their behaviour, or to take a greater interest in a particular health problem. Potential contamination of the control group by baseline testing can be monitored by increasing the complexity of the experimental design to include four groups, as is shown in Table 7.5. By comparing groups 2 and 4 in Table 7.5, it is possible to assess the influence of baseline testing. Groups 1 and 2, when compared, assess the value of the programme, with a further check on baseline testing available through a comparison of groups 2 and 3.

Table 7.5   Four-group design to monitor the effect of baseline testing

Group	Pretest	Programme	Post-test
1	Yes	Yes	Yes
2	Yes	No	Yes
3	No	Yes	Yes
4	No	No	Yes

Groups 2 and 4 compared to assess potential influence of baseline testing.
Groups 1 and 2 compared to assess value of programme.
Groups 2 and 3 compared to assess influence of baseline testing when programme is implemented.

Implementing and evaluating health promotion programmes is never as straightforward as laboratory work because the researcher has to rely on so many other agencies for cooperation. Schools may not agree to four groups being studied, employers want as little disruption as possible, and general dental practitioners will not want their patients to be kept waiting. Thus experimental methods may suffer, especially when the active group is self-selected. For example, some schools are innovative and want to try new programmes while others have so many problems that oral health is given a low priority. Clearly, a successful programme run in an enthusiastic school setting may well not translate to a more 'hostile' environment!

The problems of finding control groups has lead many researchers to utilize a design which uses the group involved in a programme as its own control. Measurements are made before and after the intervention and any changes noted. Although useful the results have to be treated with caution as outside influences may have affected the success or failure of the programme. For example, a programme in schools to promote dental visiting may appear successful, but the results could be attributable to a news item on television, or newspaper articles outwith the control of the researchers. If there is no control group it is impossible to assess the importance of these external factors.

Evaluation costs money and time, which may well reduce the funds available for the 'intervention' and this can jeopardize the research. Many health professionals want all the money spent on the programme because 'it must be better than doing nothing'. It is essential to counter such views by reminding people that without adequate evaluation health promotion will be seen as an easy option and not be taken seriously (Baric 1980). It is vital to convince dental professionals that the time has come to give oral health promotion more status and resources. However, that status will have to be earned through hard scientific endeavour rather than rushing from place to place saying 'Look at me, working hard at promoting health, I must be a valuable asset'. Frenzied activity is no substitute for science!

Common problems associated with the planning of health promotion programmes

Compliance with health orientated messages is highly variable and can depend on a number of factors, such as where advice is received, group support, personal relevance, intellectual development, and a particular dentist's communication skills. These topics are discussed in other chapters of the book as they are of sociological and psychological significance. In this section three topics which are related specifically to the practical aspects of planning oral health promotion programmes will be discussed:

(1) communication problems;

(2) use of mass media;

(3) appropriate use of leaflets and posters.

These topics are important and any planning exercise should not ignore these basic issues. It is rather galling and expensive for an evaluation project to report that fundamental problems such as communication difficulties, use of mass media, or leaflet design had not been considered at an early stage in the development of a programme.

Communication problems

Many dentists complain that while health promotion offers a positive route to good oral health, in practice patients do not seem to change their behaviour (Jacob and Plamping 1989). The answer to this problem is complex, but two overriding factors are of key importance. First, patients bring with them the values and norms of their own community and if oral health is given a low priority the messages given by the dental team may well be diluted or forgotten (Davis 1968). Second, dentists are trained to be clinicians. Intervention to treat disease is their main *raision d'être* and as such is given high status and priority. Health promotion is not so highly regarded and may well be viewed as an option to be discarded. Recent research by Croucher (1989) has noted that there is an 'information gap' between patients and their dentists. General dental practitioners consistently overestimate the amount of time and effort they give to educating their patients (see Croucher, Chapter 6B). It has also been noted by Wanless *et al.* (1990) that verbal interaction between dentists and patients is often minimal. People may want information but are somewhat constrained in questioning a health professional. The main point that dentists do not grasp is that empathy is important; failures in communication will occur if a practitioner is too formal and 'talks at', rather than 'with' the patient (Kreiberg and Treiman 1962).

Those involved in planning health promotion programmes which rely on members of the dental team offering advice to individuals or groups of people must ensure that adequate time and resources are devoted to staff training. For many, the art of communication is not an inate skill and has to be taught and reinforced on a regular basis.

One way to improve the success of surgery-based health education is to consider the application of behaviour modification techniques (Downer and Blinkhorn 1985). This involves the patient actively participating in the learning process and gradually working up to the required changes in behaviour through a process of self-discovery guided by the dentist, rather than being told what to do. Such an approach is time-consuming, but it could be made a practical alternative by using ancillaries and involving groups of patients with similar problems rather than focusing all the effort on to one individual.

However, the crux of the problem remains that for many dental practitioners, health education is a vague reminder to brush the teeth and avoid too much sugar! To be successful, information must be understandable, relevant, non-authoritarian, and most importantly, given with conviction (Becker and Maiman 1980).

The key points (Blinkhorn 1981) to remember when offering advice to either a single patient or a group of people are:

1. Only offer information which is appropriate to your particular patient or target audience.

2. Be realistic in the number of topics you cover in a given time. Attention begins to fade after 10–15 minutes and is prone to the problem of interference if too many new facts are given. They become jumbled and none is retained.

3. Make the information relevant to your patient or audience. If giving a presentation to a group of expectant mothers try to avoid phrases such as '95 per cent of expectant women in the USA'. Bring a more personal touch by saying 'the majority of women in this room'.

4. Practical demonstrations which involve the patient or audience help to increase interest. Such demonstrations do not have to be particularly complicated. Sucking a fluoride tablet or brushing the teeth in a set pattern are of interest to a non-dental audience. Abstract theories or concepts are difficult to understand.

Visual aids such as models, posters, photographs and slides can be useful but their value may be compromised if the objectives of the health promotion are not clearly stated.

Use of mass media

Mass media has an enticing aura which seems to suggest instant success for any health message given enough careful planning and money.

Mass media is defined as those institutions involved in the communication of ideas, information, entertainment, and persuasion to large-scale audiences. They include newspapers, radio, books, magazines, advertising on public transport, billboards, and television. Exposure to media products has become part of daily life for the majority of developed societies, occupying a considerable proportion of leisure time. Watching television is the principal leisure activity of most children and adults. The media, especially television, radio, and newspapers, are the major source of social knowledge, ideas, and beliefs. However, on careful examination there are certain problems in using mass media to achieve health education goals (Albert 1981).

The mass media cannot convey the complex messages which are often part of health promotion. For example, the interrelationship between diet and caries is outwardly quite simple, but trying to explain why sugar intake between meals is more harmful to teeth than sugar taken after a meal is not suited to being condensed as a media message. Trying to teach motor skills such as effective plaque removal is also not really the province of media interventions.

Trying to change behaviour in areas where social norms are actively against the media message are also unsuccessful. Dental visiting, for example, depends on many factors, one of the more important being the norms on visiting held by a particular community. Media campaigns urging people to visit a dentist have not been particularly successful in such an adverse social environment, where oral health care is given a low priority (Schou and Blinkhorn 1990).

Television will deliver a simple message which may alert the population to a particular health risk. There is, however, only a fleeting contact with the recipient and as audiences vary, one group may comprehend the message while others will not, so 'segmentation' is a key issue for all those involved in the mass media. If the watching, listening, or reading group can be identified then it is possible to design specific messages with the appropriate level of complexity or simplicity.

In general terms mass media will not in itself bring about a lasting behaviour change. Media-based campaigns must either involve locally based health care workers in a programme so that they can promote and reinforce on a more personal level within a specific community, or they must attempt to actively involve participants (Schou 1987).

Appropriate use of leaflets and posters

Patients frequently do not follow professional advice given in the form of posters and leaflets. This may be due in part to the fact that leaflets, in particular, are not successful unless backed up by the personal support of a member of the health care team. Posters have to achieve their impact without any interpersonal support, and it seems that many designers use overly complex messages, such that potential viewers ignore them or become confused.

Another reason why posters and leaflets may be of little value in enhancing campaign messages is the failure of designers to consider the suitability of educative material for a particular target group. This factor underlines the importance of pretesting during the planning phase of programme development. Therefore, before dispensing any health education literature, it should be assessed in terms of an ease-of-reading checklist, which is one way of matching the target group to the educative material (Blinkhorn *et al.* 1984). A simple checklist of points to consider when designing leaflets and posters are presented, namely:

1. Ease of reading. A number of tests are available which express readability in terms of a 'reading age'. This is a measure of an individual's reading development and is not directly related to chronological age. A simple readability test (Gunning 1952) is shown in Table 7.6. Most popular newspapers and magazines present their text in a format suitable for readers with a reading age of 12–13 years. Therefore, oral health promotion programmes which use literature with a higher reading age will be aiming for those people with a greater degree of reading development, and as such the potential target market will be somewhat more circumscribed than for simpler literature which would have more widespread appeal. The dental message is further complicated by jargon which may well be incomprehensible to a lay person, so every attempt should be made to substitute words in common usage for dental terms.

   It is important to note that reading ease measures are no substitute for pretesting a sample of the actual target group; they are, however, a useful guide (Gagne 1970). The layout of written material can also effect readability: too many changes of typeface, frequent use of italics, and diagrams dotted about in a random fashion will cause confusion.

Table 7.6   Description of how to compute the Fog Readability Index

1   Randomly select samples of 100 words

2   Determine the average sentence length: number of words divided by the number of sentences

3   Determine the percentage of 'hard' words by counting the number of words of three or more syllables.

4   Obtain the Fog Index by adding these two factors and multiplying by 0.4

5   Add 5 to the answer to give reading age.

   Example: Average sentence length = 10 words
                    Percentage of hard words = 15 per cent
                    Fog Index 0.4(10 + 15)   = 10.0
                    Reading age   = 10.0 + 5
                                                        = 15 years

2. Range. Learning new facts takes time, so a simple approach should be adopted. If too many new facts are given at one time they become jumbled and none is retained. This is termed interferance.

3. Interest. All health education programmes have to compete with a multitude of other media presentations, therefore the subject must be presented in such a way as to stimulate the interest of the particular target group. The messages should also be socially sensitive. For example, Player and Leathar (1981) stressed the importance of pretesting material to determine target group reactions rather than assuming that the health professionals know best.

The final aspect of posters and leaflets that must be considered is the need to convince fellow health professionals to use them. Too often, well designed and tested materials gather dust in office drawers or on waiting room tables because no-one was responsible for galvanizing the oral health care team into action, a fact which once again highlights the importance of pretesting to gauge not only 'consumer' acceptability but also 'user' reaction.

Conclusions

Dental disease is largely under the control of the individual and therefore oral health promotion/education is fundamental to its control. However, it is unwise to rely on programmes which have not been carefully evaluated and undergone adequate pretesting to ensure that the basic concept and delivery system are appropriate for both the proposed target group and the user group. Evaluation requires researchers to state their aims and objectives in a clear and precise manner so that measurement of success or failure is possible. It is also necessary to monitor how a programme is used rather than concentrating solely on outcome measures. Health promotion is not an exact science but every effort should be taken to ensure that the measuring instruments used to record human knowledge and behaviour are both reliable and valid. Thus research design must be carefully addressed and in particular random sampling should be used whenever possible. Both qualitative and quantitative information gathering systems provide useful data, provided the researcher is well trained and only investigates topics related to the stated aims of a health promotion project.

Compliance with health promotion programmes is often quite poor, so every effort should be made to take account of social factors affecting a message as well as ensuring that the design of any material used is relevant to the proposed target group.

This chapter has discussed the evaluation and design of health promotion programmes at a straightforward practical level, but it is important to bear in mind that governmental or commercial policies can greatly reduce the effectiveness of a programme. Thus all health promotion includes a political as well as a health dimension.

References

Abramson, J. H. (1984). *Survey methods in community medicine*, (3rd ed). Churchill Livingstone, Edinburgh.

Ajzen, I. and Fishbein, M. (1977). Attitude–behaviour relations: a theoretical analysis and review of empirical research. *Psychological Bulletin*, **84**, 888–918.

Albert, W. H. (1981). General models of persuasive influence for health education. In, *Health education and the media*, (ed. D. S. Leather, G. B. Hastings, and J. K. Davies, pp. 169–85. Pergamon Press, London.

Baric, L. (1980). Evaluation: obstacles and potentialities. *International Journal of Health Education*, **23**, 142–9.

Baric, L. (1990). *Health promotion and health education; module 1*, pp. 119–41. Barns Publications, Hale Barns, UK.

Becker, M. H. and Maiman, L. A. (1980). Strategies for enhancing patient compliance. *Journal of Community Health*, **6**, 113–35.

Blinkhorn, A. S. (1981). Dental health education In *Dental public health*, (2nd edn), (ed. G. L. Slack and B. A. Burt), pp. 270–86. John Wright, Bristol.

Blinkhorn, A. S. and Geddes, D. A. M. (1987). Assessment of caries risk and the potential for preventive management. In *Positive Dental Prevention*, (ed. R. J. Elderton), pp. 20–8. William Heinemann Medical Books, London.

Blinkhorn, A. S. and Mackie, I. C. (1992). *Practical treatment planning in paediatric dentistry*. Quintessence, London.

Blinkhorn, A. S., Hastings, G. B., and Leather, D. S. (1983). Attitudes towards dental care among young people: implications for dental health education. *British Dental Journal*, **155**, 311–13.

Blinkhorn, A. S., Fox, B., and Holloway, P. J. (1984). *Notes on dental health education*. Health Education Authority, London.

Blinkhorn, A. S., Leathar, D. S., and Kay, E. J. (1989). An assessment of the value of quantitative and qualitative data collection techniques. *Community Dental Health*, **6**, 147–51.

Campbell, D. T. and Stanley, J. C. (1963). *Experimental and quasi-experimental designs for research*. Rand University, Chicago.

Croucher, R. (1989). *The performance gap: patients' views about dental care and the prevention of periodontal disease*. Research Report No 23. Health Eduction Authority, London.

Davies, A. R. and Ware, J. E. Jr (1982). *Development of a dental satisfaction questionaire for the Health Insurance Experiment*. The Rand Corporation, Santa Monica.

Davis, M. S. (1968). Variations in patients' compliance with doctors advice: an empirical analysis of patterns of communication. *American Journal of Public Health*, **58**, 274–88.

Dignan, M. B. (1986). *Measurement and evaluation of health education*. Charles C. Thomas, Springfield Illinois.

Downer, A. C. and Blinkhorn, A. S. (1985). The use of behaviour modification techniques as an aid to improving adolescents' oral hygiene. *British Dental Journal*, **158**, 455–6.

Downie, R. S., Fyfe, C., and Tannahill, A. (1990). *Health promotion, models, and values*, pp. 73–4. Oxford University Press, Oxford UK.

Gagne, R. M. (1970). *The conditions of learning*, (2nd edn). Holt, Rinehart and Winston, London.

Green, L. W. (1977). Evaluation and measurement: some dilemmas for health education. *American Journal of Public Health*, **67**, 155–61.

Gunning, R. (1952). *The technique of clear writing*. McGraw and Hill, New York.

Jacob, M. C. and Plamping, D. (1989). *The practice of primary dental care*, pp. 29–36. Wright, London.

Kreiberg, L. and Treiman, B. R. (1962). Dentists and the practice of dentistry as viewed by the public. *Journal of American Dental Association*, **64**, 806–21

Lancet (1988). Health promotion at work. *Lancet*, **2**, 832.

Ledwith, F. (1986). Can evaluation be effective or even cost effective? *Health Education Research*, **1**, 295–8.

Levine, R. (ed.) (1989). *The scientific basis of dental health education*. Health Education Authority, London.

Likert, R. (1932). A technique for the measurement of attitudes. *Archives of Psychology*, **140**, 44–53.

Marsh, C. (1982). *The survey method: the contribution of surveys to sociological explanation*. Allen and Unwin, London.

Mausner, J. S. and Kramer, S. (1985). *Epidemiology — an introductory text*, pp. 58–9 and 348–51. W. B. Saunders Co., Philadelphia.

Nettleton, S. (1986). Understanding dental health beliefs: an introduction to ethnography. *British Dental Journal*, **161**, 145–7.

Orlandi, M. A. (1986). The diffusion and adoption of worksite health promotion innovations: an analysis of barriers. *Preventive Medicine*, **15**: 522–36.

Osgood, C. E., Suci, G. J., and Tannenbaum, P. H. (1957). *The measurement of meaning*. University of Illinois Press.

Player, D. A. and Leathar, D. S. (1981). Developing socially sensitive advertising. In *Health education and the media*, (ed. D. S. Leathar, G. B. Hastings, and J. K. Davies), pp. 187–98 Pergamon Press, London.

Rossi, P. H., Freeman, H. E., and Wright, S. (1979). *Evaluation, a systematic approach*. Sage, Beverly Hills.

Schou, L. (1987). Use of mass media and active involvement in a national dental campaign in Scotland. *Community Dentistry Oral Epidemiology*, **15**, 14–18.

Schou, L. and Blinkhorn, A. S. (1990). Combining commercial, health boards and GDPs sponsorship in an effort to improve dental attendance for young school leavers. *British Dental Journal*, **169**, 324–6.

Sorensen, G., Hunt, M. K., Morris, D. H., Donnelly, G., Freeman, L., Ratcliffe, B. J., et al. (1990). Promoting healthy eating patterns in the worksite: the Treatwell intervention model. *Health Education Research*, **5**, 505–15.

Thurstone, L. L. (1928). Attitudes can be measured. *American Journal of Sociology*, **33**, 529–54.

Todd, J. E. and Dodd, T. (1985). *Children's dental health in the United Kingdom 1983*. HMSO, London.

Tones, K., Tilford, S., and Robinson, Y. (1990). *Health education, effectiveness and efficiency*, pp. 32–4. Chapman Hall, London.

Wanless, J., Brough, D., and Alfred, M. (1990). *Helping people learn through experience.* Macmillan, Intek Ltd, Hove.

Warner, K. E., Wickizer, T. M., Wolfe, R. A., *et al.* (1988). Economic implications of work place health promotion programmes: a review of the literature. *Journal of Occupational Medicine,* **30**: 106–12.

Winkler, J. D., Kanouse, D. E., and Ware, J. E. Jr (1982). Controlling for acquiescence response set in scale development. *Journal of Applied Psychology,* **67**, 555–61.

INDEX